W0037060

DRUGS AND IMMUNE RESPONSIVENESS

BIOLOGICAL COUNCIL
The Co-ordinating Committee for Symposia
on Drug Action

DRUGS AND IMMUNE RESPONSIVENESS

Edited by

J. L. TURK

and

DARIEN PARKER

*Institute of Basic Medical Sciences,
Royal College of Surgeons of England
and University of London*

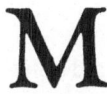

© Institute of Biology Endowment Trust Fund, 1979

Softcover reprint of the hardcover 1st edition 1979

All rights reserved. No part of this publication may be reproduced or transmitted, in any form or by any means, without permission

First published 1979 by
THE MACMILLAN PRESS LTD
London and Basingstoke
Associated companies in Delhi Dublin
Hong Kong Johannesburg Lagos Melbourne
New York Singapore and Tokyo

Typeset by
Reproduction Drawings Ltd, Sutton, Surrey

British Library Cataloguing in Publication Data

Drugs and Immune Responsiveness *(Conference), London,*
1978
 Drugs and immune responsiveness.
 1. Immunosuppressive agents–Congresses
 I. Turk, John Leslie   II. Parker, Darien
 III. Biological Council. Co-ordinating Committee
 for Symposium on Drug Action
 615'.7   RM263

 ISBN 978-1-349-04638-6   ISBN 978-1-349-04636-2 (eBook)
 DOI 10.1007/978-1-349-04636-2

This book is sold subject to the standard conditions of the Net Book Agreement

Biological Council Co-ordinating Committee for Symposia on Drug Action

Report of a symposium held on 17 and 18 April 1978 in London at The Middlesex Hospital Medical School

Sponsored by:

Biochemical Society
British Biophysical Society
British Pharmacological Society
British Society for Immunology
Chemical Society
Nutrition Society
Pharmaceutical Society of Great Britain
Physiological Society
Royal Society of Medicine
Society for Applied Bacteriology
Society for Drug Research
Society for Endocrinology
Society of Chemical Industry Fine Chemicals Group

The organisers are grateful to the following for the generous financial support which made the meeting possible:

The Wellcome Trust
Beecham Group Limited
Boehringer Ingelheim Limited
The Boots Company Limited
Ciba-Geigy (UK) Limited
Glaxo Holdings Limited
Hoechst UK Limited
Imperial Chemical Industries Limited
Janssen Pharmaceutical Limited
Lilly Research Centre Limited
Eli Lilly and Company Limited
May and Baker Limited

Merck Sharp and Dohme Limited
Ortho Pharmaceutical Limited
Organon Laboratories Limited
Pfizer Limited
Pharmacia (Great Britain) Limited
Reckitt and Colman Limited
Roche Products Limited
Sandoz Products Limited
Smith Kline and French Laboratories Limited
Smith and Nephew Research Limited
Syntex Pharmaceuticals Limited

Organised by a symposium committee consisting of:

J. L. Turk (Chairman and Hon. Secretary)
R. R. A. Coombs,
Janet M. Dewdney
D. R. Stanworth
D. W. Straughan

Symposium Contributors

Dr G. Baschang, Pharmaceuticals Division, Ciba-Geigy Ltd, Basel, Switzerland

Dr A. Brownbill, Pharmaceuticals Division, Ciba-Geigy Ltd, Basel, Switzerland

Dr J. E. T. Corrie, MRC Radioimmuno-assay Team, 2 Forrest Road, Edinburgh EH1 2QW

Dr J. De Cree, Clinical Research Unit, St Bartholomeus, 2060 Merksem, Belgium

Dr G. E. Davies, Imperial Chemical Industries Ltd, Alderley Park, Macclesfield, Chesire SK10 4TG

Dr F. M. Dietrich, Pharamaceuticals Division, Ciba-Geigy Ltd, Basel, Switzerland

Dr P. Dukor, Pharmaceuticals Division, Ciba-Geigy Ltd, Basel, Switzerland

Dr Janet M. Dewdney, Beecham Pharma-ceuticals, Brockham Park, Betchworth, Surrey RH3 4AJ

Dr G. L. Floersheim, Kanonsspital Zurich, Dermatologische Universitätsklinik, 8091 Zurich, Switzerland

Dr R. H. Gisler, Pharmaceuticals Division, Ciba-Geigy Ltd, Basel, Switzerland

Dr G. Harris, Division of Experimental Pathology, Kennedy Institute, Bute Gardens, London W6 7DW

Dr I. Hunneyball, Research Department, The Boots Co. Ltd, Nottingham NG2 3AA

Dr W. M. Hunter, MRC Radioimmunoassay Team, 2 Forrest Road, Edinburgh EH1 2QW

Professor J. Landon, Department of Chemi-cal Pathology, St. Bartholomew's Hospital, London EC1A 7BE

Professor T. Lehner, Department of Oral Immunology and Microbiology, Guy's Hospital, London SE1 9RT

Dr E. Mihich, Roswell Park Memorial Institute, 666 Elm Street, Buffalo, New York 14263, U.S.A.

Dr Darien Parker, Department of Pathology, Royal College of Surgeons of England, Lincoln's Inn Fields, London WC2A 3PN

Dr L. Polak, Department of Pharmaceutical Research, c/o Hoffmann-La Roche & Co. Ltd, CH 4002 Basel, Switzerland

Dr G. Schumann, Pharmaceuticals Division, Ciba-Geigy Ltd, Basel, Switzerland

Dr Elizabeth Shaw, Department of Bacteriology, St Bartholomew's Hospital, London EC1A 7BE

Dr F. G. Staber, Pharmaceuticals Division, Ciba-Geigy Ltd, Basel, Switzerland

Dr D. R. Stanworth, Department of Immunology, The Medical School, Birmingham B15 2TJ

Dr J. Symoens, Department of Clinical Research, Janssen Pharmaceutica, B-2340 Beerse, Belgium

Dr L. Tarcsay, Pharmaceuticals Division,
Ciba-Geigy Ltd, Basel, Switzerland

Professor J. L. Turk, Department of
Pathology, Royal College of Surgeons of
England, Lincoln's Inn Fields, London
WC2A 3PN

Professor A. L. de Weck, Inselspital Bern,
Institut für klinische Immunologie,
3010 Bern, Switzerland

Dr L. Wide, Department of Clinical
Chemistry, University Hospital, S-750
14 Uppsala 14, Sweden

Dr M. Wilton, Department of Oral
Immunology and Microbiology, Guy's
Hospital, London SE1 9RT

Foreword

It is particularly apt that the Biological Council's Co-ordinating Committee for Symposia on Drug Action should have chosen the subject of 'Drugs and Immune Responsiveness' for this year's symposium. The interphase between pharmacology and immunology has always been very close. However, in the past few years it has been recognised that a new scientific discipline—immunopharmacology—has been with us for some time. New fields are always heralded by the publication of a new journal in that particular discipline and we are about to see the publication of two new journals of 'immunopharmacology' this year. However, the British Society for Immunology already recognised the new discipline seven years ago and has held regular immunopharmacology workshops. The value of immunopharmacology has also been recognised for many years by the pharmaceutical industry, both in the United Kingdom and abroad.

Immunopharmacology is derived from two areas in the interphase between immunology and pharmacology. The first is the area of mediator production in allergic reactions. This started with the classical field of mediators of anaphylaxis and has now been extended to include the field of lymphokines and could also be considered to encompass other mediators of inflammation such as complement. However, it is with the second branch of the subject, the relationship between drugs and the immune response, that this symposium is particularly concerned.

As a result of the need for drugs that would suppress the immune response following surgery, a number of intensive research programmes have developed to search for new compounds with immunosuppressive properties. In addition much progress has been achieved in understanding the mode of action of such compounds, many of which have been found to act as anti-inflammatory agents in arthritic diseases. A further, and more recent development, has been the search for therapeutic means of increasing the immune response. Augmentation of the immune response has been achieved by a strategic use of immunoactive drugs known to interfere with immunoregulatory mechanisms. This has been supplemented by the discovery of new families of compounds with the special property of augmenting the immune response. In addition, the field of allergic reactions to drugs has always been a strong one. Research into experimental models of drug allergy is associated with the illustrious names of Karl Landsteiner, Merrill Chase and Johann Frey and current research is in the tradition of these masters. Finally, immunology has contributed highly sensitive techniques to the assay of drugs and similar compounds in biological fluids.

This book includes contributions in these fields not only from the United Kingdom but from Belgium, Sweden, Switzerland and the United States of America. It also shows a good balance of contributions from the pharmaceutical industry and academic establishments and emphasises the strong collaboration that now exists between industry and the universities.

The symposium was held on 17 and 18 April, 1978 at the Middlesex Hospital Medical School. We should like to express our gratitude to Mrs Joan Kruger and Mrs Judith Levitt for help with the organisation. The financial support of the interested societies and pharmaceutical industries is gratefully acknowledged.

J. L. Turk
Darien Parker

London, May 1978.

Contents

1

Immunosuppressive effects of miscellaneous agents

G. L. Floersheim (Department of Dermatology,
Universitätsspital, Gloriastrasse, 31, 8091 Zurich,
Switzerland)

It was tempting to call this survey 'immunosuppression by non-immunosuppressive agents'. The term immunosuppressive agent or immunosuppressant applies to a group of compounds with cytotoxic and antiproliferative properties belonging to such classes as alkylating agents, antimetabolites and antimitotics. These drugs display a general antiproliferative activity and most are used in cancer chemotherapy. They affect immune responsiveness by suppressing lymphoid tissue and its antigen-triggered proliferation. As cytotoxic drugs in cancer and as immunosuppressants in organ transplantation, autoimmune and allergic diseases, these agents have been dealt with extensively. This is also true for steroids and antilymphocyte serum, immunosuppressants that do not belong to the class of antiproliferative agents and which I shall omit from the following considerations. Traditional immunosuppressive agents such as cyclophosphamide, methotrexate, 6-mercaptopurine or azathioprine have other activities as well as immunosuppression—for example anti-inflammatory properties (Billingham *et al.*, 1967; Turk *et al.*, 1968; Stevens and Willoughby, 1969; Arinoviche and Loewi, 1970; Fitzgerald *et al.*, 1971; Steinberg *et al.*, 1972)—other compounds exert immunosuppressive side-effects.

This chapter looks at the immunosuppressive actions of substances that do not belong to the group of traditional cytotoxic–antiproliferative agents. In other words, not only immunosuppressants have immunosuppressive properties. As this field is rapidly expanding, it is impossible to give a comprehensive account within the allotted space, and I shall therefore limit myself to a discussion of immunosuppression in the following contexts:

Immunosuppressive effects of miscellaneous agents
- (1) Micro-organisms
  - (a) Bacteria
  - (b) Protozoa and other parasites
  - (c) Viruses

(2) Metabolic immunosuppression (free fatty acids; diabetes)
(3) Niridazole
(4) Diverse means and conditions
(5) Endogenous substances such as prostaglandin and serum factors
(6) Agents acting on the nervous system

IMMUNOSUPPRESSION BY MICRO-ORGANISMS

Bacteria

The seminal observation that micro-organisms may *decrease* immune responsiveness
was made in 1908 by von Pirquet. He found that the tuberculin reaction, a typical
expression of cell-mediated immunity, was depressed in patients with measles infection (von Pirquet, 1908). The same applies also to other clinical infections such as
pertussis (Caraffa, 1932), typhus (Wu and Reimann, 1931), scarlet fever (Mitchell
et al., 1935), influenza (Bloomfield and Mateer, 1919), rubella (Debré and Papp,
1926) and brucellosis (Alivisatos *et al.*, 1962; Renoux and Renoux, 1977). Subsequently, depressed tuberculin sensitivity was also seen in patients treated with
measles and other viral vaccines (Mellman and Wetton, 1963; Starr and Berkovich,
1964; Brody *et al.*, 1964).

Experimentally, the first demonstrations of decreased immune responses by
micro-organisms were probably the observations by Condie *et al.* (1955) and by
Franzl and MacMaster (1961) that bacterial lipopolysaccharides suppressed antibody formation in mice. This finding was soon extended and it became established
that with certain time intervals, dosages and routes of application, bacterial endotoxins depressed humoral immunity (Bradley and Watson, 1964; Whang and
Neter, 1967).

In 1965 we provided an experimental demonstration that *Bacillus pertussis*
inhibits cellular immunity (Floersheim, 1965a). The tuberculin reaction in guinea
pigs was markedly depressed by a single injection of pertussis vaccine. The inhibition was more profound than the one that could be achieved with maximally
tolerated doses of conventional immunosuppressants administered with similar
timing. These findings were extended when it was demonstrated that pertussis
vaccine as well as BCG may facilitate the growth of syngeneic experimental
tumours (Floersheim, 1967b; Hirano *et al.*, 1967; Piessens *et al.*, 1970; Yoo *et al.*,
1975) (table 1.1).

In the following years, immunosuppression was demonstrated with other bacterial micro-organisms (Schwab, 1975). Impressive effects were seen with group A
streptococci. A product from the cytoplasm of this very common natural pathogen
in man produced significant suppression of 19S and 7S antibody responses to
sheep erythrocytes in mice (Malakian and Schwab, 1968; Cunningham and Watson,
1978). Streptococcal, as well as products from *Salmonella typhimurium*, also suppressed adjuvant disease in rats, an immunologically mediated arthritis (Quagliata
and Taranta, 1972). Also, *Mycobacterium leprae* led to impaired immunity
(Bullock, 1968; Turk and Bryceson, 1971). Chemically, the active cytoplasmic
fraction of bacteria was identified as teichoic acid (Miller and Jackson, 1973) or as
a glycolipid (Stanislavsky *et al.*, 1977).

Potent effects were also provided by *Pseudomonas aeruginosa*. Noticing pro-

Table 1.1   Effect of *B. pertussis* on the incidence of YLI lymphoma after the transplantation of various cell doses in C57L mice

No. of tumour cells	Treatment (no. of mice)		Tumour incidence (no. of takes, less no. of regressions) at days			
		12	15	19	33	50
10^4	Controls (20)	0	0	7	4	4
	B.pertussis (20)	1	5*	12	8	8
10^5	Controls (21)	1	2	5	6	7
	B.pertussis (21)	4	12*	16*	10	10
10^6	Controls (14)	4	1	0	0	0
	B.pertussis (15)	7	5	8*	7*	8*
10^7	Controls (10)	8	6	6	5	5
	B.pertussis (9)	7	7	8	7	7

*Difference statistically significant. Within 30–60 min after the subcutaneous inoculation of the tumour cells, control mice received 0.1 ml of saline and the mice in the experimental groups were treated with an intraperitoneal dose of 2×10^9 *B. pertussis* organisms in 0.1 ml of saline (from Floersheim, 1967*b*)

longed survival of skin allografts in patients with extensive burns and pseudomonas sepsis, Stone *et al.* (1967) initiated the inquiry into the immunosuppressive capacities of this organism. Experimentally, we found that parenteral application of a lyophilisate from pseudomonas inhibited the tuberculin reaction in guinea pigs and the skin allograft reaction in mice, in doses as small as 1 µg per kg body weight corresponding to a therapeutic index of up to 1000 (Floersheim *et al.*, 1971). The pseudomonas product was also effective in inhibiting antibody formation, adjuvant-induced arthritis and experimental allergic encephalomyelitis (Floersheim *et al.*, 1972).

A therapeutic index approaching 1000 was also seen with *Salmonella typhi* and *S. paratyphi* endotoxins against the tuberculin reaction in guinea pigs (Hopff *et al.*, 1967 (table 1.2). In addition to the tuberculin reaction, these products depressed also a cutaneous graft-*versus*-host (GvH) reaction in chicken (Floersheim, 1969).

It is not clear by which mechanism bacterial agents exert immunosuppression. The same applies for the well-known adjuvant effect of these agents (Johnson *et al.*, 1956; Merrit and Johnson, 1965; Munoz, 1964; Dresser *et al.*, 1970; Neter, 1977). Among the possible explanations, thymolysis (Landy *et al.*, 1965; Rowlands *et al.*, 1965; Huldt *et al.*, 1973), inhibition of the reticuloendothelial system and of phagocytosis (Hanna and Watson, 1968), changes in lymph-node architecture (MacMaster and Franzl, 1968), alterations of lymphocyte and granulocyte kinetics and distribution (Dresser *et al.*, 1970) may be considered.

The interactions between stimulatory and suppressive effects of bacterial agents await elucidation (Howard *et al.*, 1973; Lyons and Friedman, 1978). Moreover, antigenic competition was shown to be unlikely to account for bacterial immuno-suppression (Quagliata and Taranta, 1972). On the other hand, inhibition of mito-gen-induced lymphocyte transformation by *Pseudomonas putida* (Hunt *et al.*, 1977) or streptolysin A (Andersen and Cone, 1973) might provide a clue for the

Table 1.2   Effect of bacterial endotoxins on the tuberculin reaction in guinea pigs

Group	Dosage (mg/kg)	% increase in skin thickness at 8 h	24 h	48 h
Controls		24 ± 13	66 ± 24	54 ± 22
E. coli 0128:B12	0.001	11 ± 11*	29 ± 22†	27 ± 24
S. typhi 0901	0.03	9 ± 12	14 ± 16†	12 ± 16†
S. typhi 0901	0.001	10 ± 8*	21 ± 17†	29 ± 13†
S. marcescens	0.03	0 ± 4‡	0 ± 7‡	3 ± 11‡
S. marcescens	0.001	9 ± 12*	19 ± 15†	15 ± 10†

* $P < 0.05$; † $P < 0.01$; ‡ $P < 0.001$. The bacterial lipopolysaccharides (Difco) were injected by the intraperitoneal route 30 min before and 8 h after the intracutaneous challenge with 750 IU of tuberculin (Berna). The controls received only saline intraperitoneally. The intensity of the tuberculin reaction was gauged by the increase in skin thickness at the reaction site (Floersheim, 1965*b*). Groups consisted of six guinea pigs.

Table 1.3   Modulation of lymphocyte-mediated cytotoxicity (LMC) by cyclic nucleotides

Increase of cyclic AMP	→	LMC reduced	by	↑ Adenylate cyclase
				− Prostaglandin E$_1$
				− Choleraenterotoxin
				− Isoproterenol
				↓ Phosphodiesterase
				− Theophyllin
				− Papaverin
				− Alkylating agents?
Increase of cyclic GMP	→	LMC augmented	by	↑ Guanylate cyclase
				− Cholinergic agonists
				− Insulin
				− PHA, Con A

Besides the modulating effect of cyclic AMP and cyclic GMP on lymphocyte cytotoxicity, mitogen responses, haemolytic plaque formation and IgE-mediated release of histamine from human basophils are similarly affected. PHA, Phytohaemagglutinin; Con A, concanavalin A.

mechanism of action. Moreover, it is known that *Vibrio cholerae* enterotoxin stimulates adenylate cyclase leading to increased concentrations of cyclic AMP (table 1.3). In general, the increase of cellular cyclic AMP is intepreted as being connected with inhibition of immune reactivity (Strom *et al.*, 1973; Henney *et al.*,

1973; Bourne *et al.*; 1974; Watson, 1975). It is tempting to assume that endotoxins from other Gram-negative bacteria may affect cyclic AMP as does cholera entero-toxin. It is also tempting to speculate that in analogy to the sensitisation of mice by pertussis organisms to histamine and other mediator substances (Malkiel and Hargis, 1964), other bacteria may share this effect and that some forms of chronic infective asthma or rhinitis may be due to bacteria that perhaps sensitise to endo-genous mediators. Finally, the modulatory role of cyclic AMP in immune responsiveness could provide an explanation for the relationship between im-munity and the autonomous nervous system. It will be interesting to see how the effects of *B. pertussis* on β-adrenergic function (Fishel *et al.*, 1964), cyclic AMP concentrations in lymphocytes (Parker and Morse, 1973) and immune respons-iveness may be related.

Summarising the observations on the modification of immune responsiveness by bacteria, one is struck by the fact that the same agents can affect immunity in both ways. It is not entirely clear when these agents inhibit immunity and when they stimulate it. For instance, given before antigen, endotoxin may accelerate antibody production and depress T-cells, but given after sensitisation T-cell activity is enhanced (Lagrange *et al.*, 1975; Skopinska, 1978). It seems important to learn which factors and treatment schedules will tip the balance, sometimes so pro-foundly, towards either stimulation or suppression (Hanna and Watson, 1973). For instance, *Corynebacterium*-infected mice retain skin grafts longer (Jossifides *et al.*, (1964), and remissions of rheumatoid arthritis may be seen in patients subjected to typhoid vaccine (Archer, 1951), but increase of immune reactivity is exemplified in patients with bronchial carcinoma, where an infectious pleural empyema may pro-long survival (Ruckdeschel *et al.*, 1972). It is also somewhat disturbing to consider that even with the agents used in tumour immunotherapy, *Corynebacterium parvum* and BCG. both effects can be found. *C. parvum*, besides stimulating macrophages and increasing the resistance to experimental tumours, has also been shown to inhibit T-cell functions such as GvH reactions, mixed lymphocyte reactions, PHA-responsiveness (Howard *et al.*, 1973) and to *suppress* cell-mediated immunity against tumours (Kirchner *et al.*, 1975) and parasitic infections (Ruitenberg and Sterenberg, 1973), possibly by activating suppressor cells. Such an activation of suppressor cells may also account for the prolonged survival of skin allografts in mice pretreated with donor-strain tissue extract and *B. pertussis* (Kilshaw *et al.*, 1975). On the other hand, the mitigation of GvH disease by donor pretreatment with endotoxin does not seem to be mediated by the generation of suppressor cells (Rose *et al.*, 1976). As with *C. parvum*, enhancement of tumour growth (rat mammary carcinoma) has also been seen experimentally with BCG (Piessens *et al.*, 1970). The effect of endotoxins on tumour growth is dose dependent: small doses increase animal survival, whereas larger doses increase tumour growth (Strausser and Bober, 1972). Also, both BCG (Ohrbach-Arbouys and Poupon, 1978) and *C. parvum* (Scott, 1972) have been shown to reduce the responsiveness of immunocytes. Fortunately, tumour enhancement has so far not been a major problem in human malignancies subjected to adjuvant immunotherapy. However, a report that melanoma patients receiving tumour-cell vaccine and BCG die earlier than controls (McIllmurray *et al.*, 1977) requires a cautious assessment of the otherwise pre-dominantly encouraging results involving bacterial immunotherapy in cancer patients.

Protozoa and other parasites

Mice infected with the rodent malaria parasite *Plasmodium berghei* show a diminished response to antigens such as sheep erythrocytes (Salaman *et al.*, 1969; Wedderburn, 1974), human γ-globulin (Greenwood *et al.*, 1971) or tetanus toxoid (Voller *et al.*, 1972). A defect in the macrophage function was held to be responsible. Delayed-type hypersensitivity reactions such as skin graft survival were not impaired (Greenwood *et al.*, 1971). Also, infections with *Plasmodium yoelii* depressed the antibody response to bovine serum albumin in mice, possibly by a reduction of cells contributing to the primary antibody production (McBride and Micklem, 1977). The plasmodia have also been shown to compromise T-cell function (Bomford and Wedderburn, 1973; Jayawardena *et al.*, 1975). Clinically, selective immunosuppression to some, but not all, antigens was seen in children with malaria (McGregor and Barr, 1962; Greenwood *et al.*, 1972).

Plasmodia, also trypanosomes, reduce antibody formation in experimental animals (Goodwin *et al.*, 1972; Hudson *et al.*, 1976) and impair for example the rejection of nematodes (Urquhart *et al.*, 1973). Patients with trypanosomal infection, such as sleeping sickness, showed depressed humoral and cellular immunity (Greenwood *et al.*, 1973). Immunosuppression is also seen in toxoplasmosis (Strickland *et al.*, 1972; Huldt *et al.*, 1973) and syphilis (Levene *et al.*, 1969; Wicher and Wicher, 1977). It has been suggested that free fatty acids, generated from the parasites, complement activation and polyclonal B-cell stimulation by a trypanosomal B-cell mitogen with depression of specific antibody responses, may contribute to the trypanosomal immunosuppression (Assoku *et al.*, 1977). Moreover, the generation of suppressor cells has been shown in experimental trypanosomiasis (Jayawardena and Waksman, 1977). Of course, some components of the pathogenesis of malarial and trypanosomal disease may be related to the interactions between parasites and the immune system of the hosts.

An intriguing consequence of immunodepression in multiple parasitic infections by protozoa may also be the low incidence of autoimmune disease, such as rheumatoid arthritis, in some parts of the tropics (Greenwood *et al.*, 1970). This hypothesis is supported by the suppression of autoimmune disease in NZB and (NZB × NZW)$_{F1}$ mice by *Plasmodium berghei* infection (Greenwood and Voller, 1970). Moreover, the high prevalence of Burkitts lymphoma predominantly in malaria-infected areas may have an immunological explanation (Ziegler *et al.*, 1972).

Besides the wealth of reports indicating immunosuppression by protozoa, increasing evidence suggests also immunosuppressive effects by larger parasites (Terry, 1978), such as mites (*Demodex canis*) in dogs (Corbett *et al.*, 1975) and in mice by *Trichinella spiralis*, which is likely to act by inducing suppressor cells (Barriga, 1978). The potential immune deficiency in helminthic infestations is also expressed by the profound depletion of macrophages in rabbits with cysticercosis (Hopff, 1967) and by increased tumour growth in hosts infected with the nematode *Nippostrongylus brasiliensis* (Keller *et al.*, 1971). Parasites have also been shown to release immunosuppressive factors (Capron *et al.*, 1977).

Viruses

I have already mentioned von Pirquet's (1908) observation that tuberculin-positive children become negative a few days before a measles rash appears and later revert. He also noted an activation of tuberculous disease after measles and that the symptoms of chronic nephritis disappeared during measles. Since this discovery, the propensity of certain viruses to alter the immune function of the infected host has been well recognised (Kantor, 1975). For instance, patients with acute infectious mononucleosis (Mangi *et al.*, 1975) and influenza have depressed delayed cutaneous hypersensitivity as well as an increased incidence of bacterial superinfections (Martin *et al.*, 1959). This immune defect is thought to be due to the ability of viruses to depress the chemotactic responsiveness of monocytes (Kleinermann *et al.*, 1975). Also measles virus seems to inhibit the migration of human leucocytes (Nordal *et al.*, 1975). The measles immunosuppressive effect was also attributed to an unspecific activation of T-lymphocytes, as the majority of human T-lymphocytes have binding sites for measles virus (Valdimarsson *et al.*, 1975). The reverse has been reported for Epstein–Barr virus, which binds to B- but not to T-lymphocytes (Jondal and Klein, 1973). It is suggested that cell-associated measles virus may activate human lymphocytes non-specifically.

Experimentally, the first indications that virus-infected animals had decreased humoral and cellular immune responses appeared in the early 1960s (Old *et al.*, 1960; Fahey and Humphrey, 1962; Peterson *et al.*, 1963; McCarthy, 1964; Dent *et al.*, 1965; Siegel and Morton, 1966; Odaka *et al.*, 1966). An extensive study of the non-specific immunodepressive effect of Friend and other oncogenic murine RNA viruses such as Rauscher and Moloney virus was done by Salaman (Salaman, 1969; Bennett and Steeves, 1970). It was found that Friend virus reduced predominantly the number of IgM antibody-producing cells against sheep erythrocytes when given before the antigen, probably by altering the function or the commitment of the involved splenic cells (Friedmann and Ceglowski, 1968). Antigenic competition was thought unlikely to explain this effect—rather viral leukaemogenesis (Siegel and Morton, 1966). Also cell-mediated responses were reduced in virus-infected mice (Bendinelli and Asherson, 1968), including lymphocytic choriomeningitis virus (Silberman *et al.*, 1978).

As a further explanation of the immunosuppressive viral effects, interferon production may be invoked. Indeed, several reports have demonstrated that if interferon is given before contact with antigen it prevents, perhaps by antiproliferative effects (Buffet *et al.*, 1978), both humoral antibody formation and delayed-type hypersensitivity reactions in mice (Brodeur and Merigan, 1974; Gisler *et al.*, 1974; Hirsch *et al.*, 1974; De Maeyer-Guignard *et al.*, 1975). It is noteworthy in this context that, like chemical (Stjernswärd, 1969) and physical carcinogens, oncogenic viruses depress immunity.

A new light is cast on possible viral interactions with immunity by experiments in which antibodies to endogenous C-type RNA-viruses in mice cause immunosuppression, consistent with the hypothesis that viral antigen plays a receptor-like role in lymphoid cellular interaction (Moroni and Schumann, 1977).

METABOLIC IMMUNOSUPPRESSION (FREE FATTY ACIDS; DIABETES)

Metabolic changes are known to affect immune reactivity. Two aspects of metabolic immunosuppression will be dealt with briefly, namely the effects of free fatty acids and of insulin. Immunodepression occurring in uraemia and other diseases characterised by deviations and errors of metabolism, will not be considered.

In 1964, during studies on the influence of drugs on cellular immune reactions, it was noted that the immunosuppressive effect of oestrogen preparations on skin allograft survival in mice was in part due to the vehicle in which the hormone was dissolved. This solvent, which consisted of 80 per cent arachis oil, led by itself, with a dose corresponding to 24 μl daily per mouse, to a slight but distinct prolongation of skin graft survival in the order of 20 to 30 per cent (Floersheim, 1964; Floersheim, 1965b). More convincingly, an immunoregulatory role of polyunsaturated fatty acids (PUFAs) was suggested by other authors. Mertin *et al.* (1974, 1976) reported that PUFAs, especially linoleic and arachidonic acids, would inhibit the response of lymphocytes *in vitro* to antigenic stimuli. Moreover, a significant prolongation of skin and tumour allograft survival was demonstrated in mice treated with linolenic, linoleic and arachidonic acids (Mertin, 1976) or fed on high-fat diets (Santiago-Delpin and Szepsenwol, 1977). Despite some failures to observe effects by PUFAs on manifestations of cellular immunity *in vivo* such as adjuvant-induced arthritis in rats (Delbarre, 1975) or graft survival (Brock and Field, 1975; Salaman and Millar, 1975), on the whole positive findings prevailed. Indeed, in human renal-transplant patients receiving standard immunosuppression, a diet enriched with a PUFA from oil of evening primose (*Oenothera*) and consisting of linoleic and linolenic acids led to a significantly better functional graft survival in the early post-transplant period (McHugh *et al.*, 1977). A polyunsaturated fatty acid diet also induced dramatic recoveries in cases with Guillain–Barré syndrome (Bower and Newsholme, 1978).

The mechanism by which PUFA prolongs graft survival remains the subject of debate. Effects on the lymphoid and reticuloendothelial system (Meade and Mertin, 1976), on platelet aggregation or on lymphocyte function may have a role. Steroid-induced lymphocytolysis can be mimicked with PUFAs (Turnell *et al.*, 1973). At any rate, absorbed PUFAs have easy access to recirculating lymphocytes *via* the thoracic duct as chylomicrons. It is tempting to explain the effect by the fact that PUFAs are biochemical precursors of prostaglandins. PUFA-derived prostaglandins have been shown to inhibit cell-mediated immune responses *in vitro*; this effect is accompanied by increases in lymphocytic cyclic AMP concentrations (Lichtenstein *et al.*, 1972). On the other hand, dietary deficiency of PUFAs was associated with relative immunopotentiation as indicated by accelerated rejection of skin grafts and decreased incidence and rate of development of methylcholanthrene-induced tumours in mice (Mertin and Hunt, 1976). It remains to be seen whether biguanides, such as phenformin which inhibits fatty acid oxidation, can counteract metabolic immunodepression (Dilman, 1977).

Another metabolic condition known to be accompanied by abnormal immunological activity is diabetes mellitus. It has been implicated both as an explanation for its pathogenesis as an autoimmune disease (Goldstein *et al.*, 1970; Nerup *et al.*, 1971; Nerup and Binder, 1973; Bottazzo *et al.*, 1974; Lendrum *et al.*, 1975; Huang and MacLaren, 1976), and as a reason for the increased proneness to infection suffered by diabetics (Mahmoud *et al.*, 1976).

In diabetics, several parameters of cellular function and immune reactivity such as phagocytosis (Bybee and Rogers, 1964), chemotaxis of polymorphonuclear leucocytes (Mowat and Baum, 1971) and responsiveness of lymphocytes to mitogens (MacCuish *et al.*, 1974) are depressed. Moreover, the second-set skin allograft response in streptozotocin-induced diabetic rats (Friedmann and Beyer, 1977) and other cellular reactions, including the granulomatous response to *Schistosoma mansoni* eggs in diabetic mice, is absent (Mahmoud *et al.*, 1976). Both responses can be restored by insulin. The immune defect was not correlated with hyperglycaemia, but it may be related to the observation that stimulated lymphocytes develop insulin receptors and that insulin augments lymphocyte-mediated cytotoxicity (Strom *et al.*, 1975).

With regard to our previous look at free fatty acids, it is noteworthy that diabetic subjects display an abnormally high concentration of free fatty acids in the plasma, which is due to their increased mobilisation from the peripheral fat deposits. This lipolytic activity is inhibited by insulin, which also lowers cellular cyclic AMP concentrations. Accordingly, reduced immune capacity of diabetes may be due to increased free fatty acids associated with this disease.

Moreover, the secretion of free fatty acids is stimulated by β-adrenergic agonists (Nogrady *et al.*, 1977) and in stressful situations (Cardon and Gordon, 1959), allowing one to postulate links between nervous activity with elevated levels of catecholamines and increased concentrations of free fatty acids. By this mechanism, a correlation between stress and immunosuppression could be explained. Lastly, increased free fatty acids, which are known to occur in cancer patients (Mueller and Watkin, 1961), may provide an explanation for the immunological anergy often encountered in patients with malignant disease. At any rate, free fatty acids might link nutrition, lipid metabolism, diabetes and the nervous system to immunity It would also be interesting to know whether increased PUFAs are a consequence or the cause of increased neoplastic activity.

NIRIDAZOLE

Among the miscellaneous chemical agents that display immunosuppressive effects, niridazole appears to deserve particular interest. Niridazole is a nitrothiazole derivative which has been in use for over 10 years for the clinical treatment of schistosomiasis. Besides its antischistosomal effect, niridazole also depresses the chronic granulomatous reaction of the host to eggs trapped in tissue (Mahmoud and Warren, 1974)—a manifestation of delayed hypersensitivity with an important bearing on the pathogenesis of the disease.

Following this observation, the immunosuppressive activity of niridazole was amply confirmed. I must admit that I missed this discovery when I screened niridazole in 1966 with a series of other miscellaneous agents in the mouse skin allograft reaction. Although at 80 mg/kg per day p.o. in C⁻ mice it prolonged the survival of CBA skin grafts from a control value of 9.8 days to 11.5 days, little attention was paid to this finding and no follow-up work was done as in the same series, for example, the potent mushroom toxin α-amanitin at a dose of 0.06 mg/kg per day prolonged the graft survival to 12.2 days and, more importantly, the methylhydrazine derivatives of the procarbazine type provided conspicuously superior results (Floersheim, 1967*a*).

None the less, clear-cut inhibition by niridazole of several manifestations of cellular immunity was shown some years later by Mahmoud and colleagues, including the inhibition of cutaneous hypersensitivity and skin allograft rejection in mice (Mahmoud *et al.*, 1975) as well as heterotopic cardiac allograft rejection (Salaman *et al.*, 1977) and experimental allergic encephalomyelitis (Paterson *et al.*, 1977) in rats. Interestingly, antibody titres were only marginally depressed (Pelley *et al.*, 1975).

Manifestation of cellular immunity *in vitro*, such as the mixed lymphocyte reaction and antigen-induced macrophage migration inhibition (Daniels *et al.*, 1975; Jones *et al.*, 1977), was reduced by the sera of guinea pigs or rats treated with niridazole, but not by niridazole itself, thus indicating that a metabolite of the antischistosomal compound was the active immunosuppressant. Clearly, such an immunosuppressive agent, with considerable T-cell specificity and without overt toxicity to the haemopoietic system, would have a great potential in the treatment of autoimmune disease and transplant patients. Immunosuppression in humans has been confirmed by the abrogation of cutaneous delayed hypersensitivity in schistosome-infected patients treated with niridazole (Webster *et al.*, 1975). However, clinical trials of niridazole or of a metabolite for purposes other than worm infestations deserve keen anticipation.

DIVERSE MEANS AND CONDITIONS

It is beyond the scope of this survey to cover immunosuppression by all miscellaneous drugs and means. Many of them appear highly interesting and potentially relevant.

Let me first mention the effect of diet. It can be said—perhaps a bit over-simplified—that in general malnutrition leads to a depression of humoral immunity, but cell-mediated immune responses are left intact. Effects of protein calorie restriction include increased susceptibility to infection, prolonged survival of (NZB × NZW)$_{F1}$ mice with autoimmune disease (Fernandes *et al.*, 1976*a*) and suppression of spontaneous mammary carcinoma in C3H mice (Fernandes *et al.*, 1976*b*). With regard to PUFAs, we have already mentioned that a diet high in PUFA may favour transplant survival and tumour development but inhibit autoimmune disease.

Then immunosuppression or altered macrophage function has been described with age, pregnancy (Purtilo *et al.*, 1972), uraemia (Wilson *et al.*, 1965), cancer (Frost and Lance, 1973; Glasgow *et al.*, 1974; Robinson *et al.*, 1974; Hršak and Marotti, 1975; Ting *et al.*, 1977), in particular with Hodgkin's disease and chronic lymphatic leukaemia, in burn patients (Hakim, 1977; Ninnemann *et al.*, 1978) with GvH reactions, with surgical interventions (Berenbaum *et al.*, 1973; Howard and Simmons, 1974; Vose and Mongdil, 1975) and ultraviolet radiation (Spellman and Daynes, 1977), which has been claimed to induce suppressor cells, with oestrogens (Lurie *et al.*, 1949; Kappas *et al.*, 1963; Floersheim, 1964; 1965*a*; Arnason and Richman, 1969; Waltman *et al.*, 1971; Barnes *et al.*, 1974), and human chorionic gonadotropin (Jenkins *et al.*, 1972), with noxious agents such as tobacco and lead, heroin (Brown *et al.*, 1974) and marihuana, drugs like hydantoin (Grob and Herold, 1972; Levo *et al.*, 1975), with enzymes like L-asparaginase (Hersh, 1973), with antiviral and antibacterial agents including tilorone (Wildstein *et al.*, 1976), chloramphenicol (Weisberg *et al.*, 1964) and rifampicin (Pǎunescu, 1970), with antihistamines (Boyd and Smith, 1960; Floersheim, 1964; Floersheim, 1965*a*; Jamieson, 1976), with deficiency of iron, vitamin A (Krishan *et al.*, 1974) or pyridoxal phosphate, with reticuloendothelial-system blockading agents such as colloidal carbon, thorotrast and incomplete Freunds' adjuvant (Chakrabarty and Friedman, 1971), with hyperchlorinated water (Fidler, 1977) and so on. The list of agents displaying immunosuppressive activity is growing weekly. Nevertheless, these effects should not be considered a final consequence of overt or overwhelming toxicity, because they may occur at otherwise well-tolerated doses and conversely may not be seen with other agents at near-lethal dosages. Berenbaum and Brown (1964), for instance, did not observe depression of antibody formation in mice treated with caffeine, boric acid, sodium nitrite, neomycin, polymixin and bacitracin at the approximate LD_{80}. This establishes the important point that toxicity as such does not necessarily cause immunosuppression.

If I ought to select a group of substances, I would select agents from fungal micro-organisms. Micro-organisms seem to offer an untapped source of immunosuppressive compounds. I shall only mention two fungal metabolites, which have been studied in Basel by Borel and colleagues. One agent is ovalicin (Borel *et al.*, 1974), an antibiotic isolated from *Pseudorotium ovalis*, and the other is the antilymphocytic agent cyclosporin A, a cyclic decapeptide from the fungi *Cylindrocarpum lucidum* and *Trichoderma polysporum*. Cyclosporin A is comparable with antilymphocyte serum both with regard to effectiveness and lack of myelotoxicity (Borel *et al.*, 1976; Calne *et al.*, 1978; Green and Allison, 1978). It is thought to act by interfering at an early stage in antigenic triggering of immunocompetent lymphoid cells.

ENDOGENOUS SUBSTANCES (PROSTAGLANDIN AND SERUM FACTORS)

Among the endogenous biologically and pharmacologically active agents, some deserve mention with regard to immunosuppression. One is prostaglandin (Goldyne, 1977). This unsaturated fatty acid derivative, with multiple pharmacological activities, has been reported to depress antibody formation (Zurier and Quagliata, 1971), to inhibit adjuvant-induced arthritis (Aspinall and Cammarata, 1969), to prolong survival of skin allografts and xenografts (Quagliata *et al.*, 1972; Kakita *et al.*, 1975) and to inhibit lymphocyte transformation after PHA-stimulation. The latter effect is thought to be due to increased intracellular cyclic AMP concentrations through stimulation of adenylate cyclase activity by prostaglandin E_1 (PGE_1) (Smith *et al.*, 1971). Indomethacin, an inhibitor of prostaglandin synthesis, reduced skin graft survival (Anderson *et al.*, 1977) and increased lymphocyte responses in patients with Hodgkin's disease (Goodwin *et al.*, 1977). Prostaglandin was produced by suppressor cells which were elevated in patients with Hodgkin's disease.

This finding may also explain the puzzling clinical observation that procarbazine treatment may reverse the anergic tuberculin reaction in patients with Hodgkin's disease (W. Bollag, personal communication), perhaps by affecting suppressor cells in this situation to a greater extent than normal.

Finally, the high prostaglandin content of seminal plasma may account for the suppressive effect of this material on lymphocyte activation as well as the poor immunological response in males to genital infections with *Neisseria gonorrhoeae* (Stiles and Erickson, 1975). It has also been suggested that prostaglandin secreted by cancer cells might be responsible for the non-specific immunosuppression seen in cancer patients, but no significantly elevated prostaglandin concentrations were found (Harvey *et al.*, 1977).

Normal mammalian serum seems to contain factors with immunosuppressive capabilities such as an α-globulin as described by a number of authors (Kamrin, 1959; Sims and Freeman, 1966; Jennings and Oates, 1967; Mannick and Schmid,

1967; Mowbray *et al.*, 1969; Veit and Michael, 1969; Nelken, 1973). This agent is not cytotoxic and may have a role in the homoeostasis of the immune system. It has also been associated with the immune anergy in experimental malignancy (Hršak and Marotti, 1975; Ting *et al.*, 1977) and in human cancer patients (Glasgow *et al.*, 1974). It is thought to inhibit antigen recognition by lymphocytes, to depress predominantly T-cell functions as well as phagocytosis (Nimberg *et al.*, 1975).

Whether pregnancy is accompanied by immunosuppression has been debated for some time. Hormonal changes, biogenic polyamines degraded by pregnancy factors (Gaugas and Curzen, 1978), α-foetoprotein (Zimmerman *et al.*, 1977), increased suppressor T-cell levels and suppressive properties of a pregnancy associated α-macroglobulin have been implicated and studied mostly by methods of immunological assessment *in vitro* (Stimson, 1976).

AGENTS ACTING ON THE NERVOUS SYSTEM

The modification of immune responsiveness by agents acting on the central nervous system is a newly emerging area of investigation and little information is available. The field of brain and the immune system has emerged only recently from a somewhat mystical demimonde on the fringe of respectability with a review article by Stein *et al.* (1976).

It is known, however, that psychosocial factors such as housing, fighting and stress may modify the susceptibility of animals to viral and parasitic infection as well as to neoplasia. In several instances, stress-induced immunosuppression was ascertained. For instance, lymphocytes from rats with multiple pregnancies (retired breeders) displayed reduced T-cell mitogen responses and a depressed mixed-lymphocyte reaction compared with female virgin rats of similar age that had not had to brave challenges such as encounters with males, gestation, parturition and rearing progeny (Lattime and Strausser, 1977).

Although other reports confirm that temporary stress depresses immune reactivity (Folch and Waksman, 1974), it has been shown that prolonged exposure to, for example, sound stress may also enhance it (Monjan and Collector, 1977). Anyway, immune processes may be related to hypothalamic function and mediated by neuroendocrine and autonomous nervous activity. Hypothalamic lesions have been demonstrated in several instances to be correlated with depressed humoral and cellular immune responses. Only very limited information is available that agents acting on nervous structures modify immune reactivity such as the slight prolongation by diazepam (Valium) of survival of mouse and rat skin allograft (Ballantyne and Harper, 1977) or the effect of a combination of neurotropic agents on several parameters of humoral and cellular immunity (Pierpaoli and Maestroni, 1977). Sublethal doses of reserpine suppressed antibody formation probably through starvation (Duker *et al.*, 1966).

I shall only mention in passing that adrenergic and cholinergic agonists and antagonists, interfering with intracellular levels of cyclic AMP and cyclic GMP, may affect immune responsiveness. In general, the correlation between effects afforded by these agents *in vitro* and *in vivo* has not been elaborated, and whenever the effects by one of them are termed '*modulation* of immune responsiveness' one cannot forget that modulus is only a diminutive from modus, the measure, and that modulation may reflect a change of disposition rather than a genuine modification of immunity, as documented, for example, by a significant abrogation of the allograft reaction.

As far as I know, significant effects of such agents which affect lymphocyte function and cytotoxicity *in vitro* on responses *in vivo*, on the other hand, have only been shown with endotoxins, which stimulate adenylate cyclase and thus the formation of cyclic AMP. However, caffeine, which inhibits phosphodiesterase, did not affect antibody production in mice at near-lethal doses (Berenbaum and Brown, 1964). To enter in some depth into the biochemical basis of immune regulation and to chart the many genetic provisions, feedback systems and signals, mediators, messenger molecules, surface and membrane intricacies, regulatory cascades and interactions of stimulated and suppressed populations and sub-populations would make Newton's dictum—*natura enim simplex est*—nature is by all means simple—somewhat outdated.

In passing, it might be mentioned that procarbazine belongs to a class of agents with strong inhibitory effect on brain monoaminooxydases. But to relate its potent immunosuppressive activity *in vivo* to any influence on the central nervous system is pure speculation.

OUTLOOK

I have attempted to survey immunosuppression from an unconventional angle, namely by reviewing immunosuppressive effects exerted by agents that are not included in the category of cytotoxic immunosuppressive drugs. Since immuno-suppressive effects of agents used for other purposes and of widely distributed micro-organisms and nutrients are recognised at a rapid rate, and since alteration of immune responsiveness may have pathogenetic and therapeutic implications in a spectrum of diseases, which equally seems to increase monthly and which extends from cancer and infection over metabolic and degenerative diseases such as diabetes and arthritis to conditions like alopecia areata and male infertility, it appeared worthwhile to attempt to review this topic.

Of course, the pathological significance of some alteration of lymphocyte reactivity or macrophage function is far from clear. Often alterations of immune function as suggested and recognised by methods *in vitro* fail to emerge clearly if methods are followed *in vivo*. I might cite, as an example, chalones obtained from lymphoid organs which were strongly inhibitory to mitogen stimulation of mouse spleen lymphocytes *in vitro* (Hiestand *et al.*, 1977), but which failed to provide significant or reproducible effects on manifestations of immunity *in vivo*, such as haemolytic plaque formation, skin allograft survival, GvH reactions and lymph node weight assay (Borel *et al.*, 1978). Nevertheless, the balance of immune homoeostasis may well be tipped in one or other direction by quite subtle influences with highly relevant pathological or beneficial consequences.

If the evidence for the alteration of immune responsiveness by most of the mentioned agents is satisfactory, the mechanisms by which these over-all changes in reactivity are brought forward are still by and large elusive. It is probably safe to say that the observed effects are not due to over-all toxicity. But the knowledge of changes at the cellular, anatomical or biochemical level are, at best, fragmentary. This is not surprising if we consider that even with the proper immunosuppressive agents, except for some biochemical causes of their general antiproliferative properties and for their well-characterised over-all effects, we have scanty information on which components of the immune network are affected, or on whether their main target are T or B cells, cellular or humoral immunity.

In quite a few instances, the potency of some of these miscellaneous immunosuppressants is comparable with the one afforded by the *sensu strictu* class of immunosuppressants. Bearing in mind that side-effects of the former agents are often less threatening than the bone marrow toxicity of the standard compounds, the clinical use of such unconventional immunosuppressants in autoimmune disease and in the induction of graft tolerance may rid immunosuppressive therapy of its current limitations. Combined treatments, such as the use of PUFAs (McHugh *et al.*, 1977) or niridazole (Salaman *et al.*, 1977), in analogy to the standard protocol in renal transplantation or other synergistic regimens (Storb *et al.*, 1974), need to be exploited. This second generation of diverse immunosuppressive agents is likely to come forward with no, or with less, or perhaps with specific cytotoxicity. Their introduction constitutes a challenge to immunopharmacology as the discovery of agents enhancing the immune function.

SUMMARY

(1) *Micro-organisms* including viruses, bacteria and protozoa (and their products) may depress immune reactivity. Quantitative aspects such as dose dependency and timing, as well as mode of action, relation to adjuvanticity and impact of parasitic immunosuppression on infectious, autoimmune and malignant disease need to be studied.

(2) The use of miscellaneous immunosuppressants without bone marrow toxicity, such as niridazole, *combined* with standard antiproliferative immunosuppressants should increase the efficacy of immunosuppressive protocols.

(3) *Prostaglandin* seems to have a central role in immunosuppression. It is released by T-suppressor cells, which are activated by some of the miscellaneous immunosuppressants including micro-organisms, and it is also induced by dietary and metabolic factors such as free fatty acids as well as by nervous impulses, thus linking the nervous system to immunity and, perhaps, cancer.

(4) Reports of the modulatory effects on the immune reactivity by the most diverse agents and conditions and as side effects of drugs used for other purposes accumulate at an accelerating rate. These findings establish the concept of *concomitant immunosuppression*. With regard to the pathogenetic role of immunity in a rapidly widening spectrum of diseases and inflammatory processes, concomitant immunosuppression may have an important place in the expanding discipline of immunopharmacology.

REFERENCES

Alivisatos, G. P., Marketos, N. and Vava, Z. (1962). Die Immunitätsparalyse bei Brucellosen. *Z. Immun. forschg and Experimentelle Therapie*, **122**, 291

Andersen, B. R. and Cone, R. (1974). Inhibition of human lymphocyte blast transformation by streptolysin O. *J. Lab. clin. Med.*, **84**, 241

Anderson, C. B., Jaffee, B. M. and Graff, R. J. (1977). Prolongation of murine skin allografts by prostaglandin E_1. *Transplantation*, **23**, 444

Archer, B. J. (1951). Remission in rheumatoid arthritis following fever therapy with liver damage., *N.Y. St. J. Med.*, **51**, 2657

Arinoviche, R. and Loewi, G. (1970). Comparison of the effects of two cytotoxic drugs and of antilymphocytic serum. On immune and non-immune inflammation in experimental animals. *Ann. rheum. Dis.*, **29**, 32

Arnason, B. G. and Richman, D. P. (1969). Effect of oral contraceptives on experimental demyelinating disease. *Archs Neurol.* **21**, 103

Aspinall, R. L. and Cammarata, P. S. (1969). Effect of prostaglandin E_2 on adjuvant arthritis. *Nature*, **224**, 1320

Assoku, R. K. G., Tizard, I. R. and Nielsen, K. H. (1977). Free fatty acids, complement activation, and polyclonal B-cell stimulation as factors in the immunopathogenesis of African trypanosomiasis. *Lancet*, **ii**, 956

Ballantyne, D. L. and Harper, A. D. (1977). Prolongation of survival in mouse tail skin allografts by Valium (diazepam). *Transplantation*, **23**, 163

Barnes, E. W., McCuish, A. C., Loudon, N. B., Jordan, J. and Irvine, W. J. (1974) Phytohaemagglutinin – induced lymphocyte transformation and circulating autoantibodies in women taking oral contraceptives. *Lancet*, **i**, 898

Barriga, O. O. (1978). Depression of cell-mediated immunity following inoculation of *Trichinella spiralis* extract in the mouse. *Immunology*, **34**, 167

Bendinelli, M. and Asherson, G. L. (1968). Effect of Friend virus infection on contact sensitivity. *Rep. Brit. Emp. Cancer, Campgn.*, **45**, 137

Bennett, M. and Steeves, R. A. (1970). Immunocompetent cell functions in mice infected with Friend leukemia virus. *J. Natl. Cancer Inst.*, **44**, 1107

Berenbaum, M. C. and Brown, I. N. (1964). Dose–response relationships for agents inhibiting the immune response. *Immunology*, **7**, 65

Berenbaum, M. C., Fluck, P. A. and Hurst, N. P. (1973). Depression of lymphocyte responses after surgical trauma. *Br. J. exp. Path.*, **54**, 597

Billingham, M. E. J., Robinson, B. V. and Gaugas, J. M. (1967). Two antiinflammatory components in antilymphocytic serum. *Nature*, **214**, 1138

Bloomfield, A. L. and Mateer, J. G. (1919). Changes in skin sensitiveness of tuberculin during epidemic influenza. *Am. Rev. Tuberc.*, **3**, 166

Bollag, W. (Personal communication)

Bomford, R. and Wedderburn, N. (1973). Depression of immune response to moloney leukaemia virus by malarial infection. *Nature*, **242**, 471

Borel, J. F., Lazary, S. and Stähelin, H. (1974). Immunosuppressive effects of ovalicin-semicarbozone. *Agents and Actions*, **4**, 357

Borel, J. F., Feurer, C., Gubler, H. U. and Stähelin, H. (1976). Biological effects of cyclosporin A: a new antilymphocytic agent. *Agents and Actions*, **6**, 468

Borel, J. F., Feurer, C., Hiestand, P. C. and Stähelin, H. (1978). The effects of fractions (chalones) obtained from lymphoid organs on the immune response *in vivo*. *Agents and Actions*, **8**, 523

Bottazzo, G. F., Florin-Christensen, A. and Doniach, D. (1974). Islet-cell antibodies in diabetes mellitus with autoimmune polyendocrine deficiencies. *Lancet*, **ii**, 1279

Bourne, H. R., Lichtenstein, L. M. Melmon, K. L., Henney, C. S., Weinstein, Y. and Shearer, G. M. (1974). Modulation of inflammation and immunity by cyclic AMP. *Science*, **184**, 19

Bower, B. D. and Newsholme, E. A. (1978). Treatment of idiopathic polyneuritis by a polyunsaturated fatty-acid diet. *Lancet*, **i**, 583

Boyd, J. F. and Smith, A. N. (1960). The effect of compound 48/80 on the autograft and homograft reaction. *Br. J. exp. Path.*, **41**, 259

Bradley, S. G. and Watson, D. W. (1964). Suppression by endotoxin of the immune response to actinophage in the mouse. *Proc. Soc. exp. Biol. Med.*, **117**, 570

Brock, J. and Field, E. J. (1975). Unsaturated fatty acids and transplantation. *Lancet*, **ii**, 1382

Brodeur, B. R. and Merigan, T. C. (1974). Suppressive effect of interferon on the humoral immune response to sheep red blood cells in mice. *J. Immun.*, **113**, 1319

Brody, J. A., Overfield, T. and Hammes, L. M. (1964). Depression of the tuberculin reaction by viral vaccines. *New Engl. J. Med.*, **271**, 1294

Brown, S. M., Stimmel, B., Taub, R. N., Kochwa, S. and Rosenfield, R. E. (1974). Immunologic dysfunction in heroin addicts. *Archs intern. Med.* **134**, 1001

Buffet, R. F., Caivo, A. M. and Custer, W. A. (1978). Antiproliferative activity of highly
    purified mouse interferon: Brief communication. *J. natn. Cancer Inst.*, **60**, 243
Bullock, W. E. (1968). Studies of immune mechanisms in leprosy. I. Depression of delayed
    allergic response to skin test antigens. *New Engl. J. Med.*, **278**, 298
Bybee, J. D. and Rogers, D. E. (1964). The phagocytic activity of polymorphonuclear
    leucocytes obtained from patients with diabetes mellitus. *J. Lab. clin. Med.*, **64**, 1
Calne, R. Y., White, D. J. G., Rolles, K., Smith, D. P. and Herbertson, B. M. (1978). Pro-
    longed survival of pig orthotopic heart grafts treated with cyclosporin A. *Lancet*, **i**, 1183
Capron, A., Camus, D., Dessaint, J.-P. and Le Boubennec-Fischer, F. (1977). Alteration de la
    réponse immune au cours des infections parasitaires. *Anns d'Immunologie (Institut
    Pasteur)*, **128 C**, 541
Caraffa, C. (1932). Contributo clinico allo studio dell'allergia tuberculclinica nelle diverse
    fasi della pertosse. *Clin. Pediat.*, **14**, 935
Cardon, P. V., Jr. and Gordon, R. S., Jr. (1959). Rapid increase of plasma unesterified fatty
    acids in man during fear. *J. psychosom. Res.*, **4**, 5
Chakrabarty, A. S. and Friedman, H. (1971). Immunosuppressive effects of incomplete
    Freunds' adjuvant on hemolitic antibody-forming cells in spleens of immunized mice. *J.
    Immun.*, **106**, 1389
Condie, R. M., Zak, S. J. and Good, R. A. (1955). Effect of meningococcal endotoxin on
    resistance to bacterial infection and the immune response in rabbits. *Fedn. Proc.*, **14**, 459
Corbett, R., Bauks, K., Hinrichs, D. and Bell, T. (1975). Cellular immune responsiveness in
    dogs with demodectic mange. *Transplant. Proc.*, **7**, 555
Cunningham, C. M. and Watson, D. W. (1978). Suppression of antibody response by
    group A streptococcal pyrogenic exotoxin and characterization of the cells involved.
    Infect. Immun., **19**, 470
Daniels, J. C., Warren, K. S. and David, J. R. (1975). Studies on the mechanism of suppression
    of delayed hypersensitivity by the antischistosomal compound Niridazole. *J. Immun.*,
    115, 1414
Debré, R. and Papp, K. (1926). Sur la cuti-reaction tuberculinique du cours de la rougeole
    et rubéole. *C. r. Soc. Biol.*, **95**, 29
Delbarre, F. (1975). Unsaturated fatty acid and cellular immunity. *Lancet*, **ii**, 720
De Maeyer-Guignard, J., Cachard, A. and De Maeyer, E. (1975). Delayed-type hypersenstivity
    to sheep red blood cells: inhibition of sensitization by interferon. *Science*, **190**, 574
Dent, P. B., Peterson, R. D. A. and Good, R. A. (1965). A defect in cellular immunity during
    the incubation period of passage A leukaemia in C3H mice. *Proc. Soc. exp. Biol. (N.Y.)*,
    119, 869
Dilman, V. M. (1977). Metabolic immunodepression which increases the risk of cancer.
    Lancet, **ii**, 1207
Dresser, D. W., Wortis, H. H. and Anderson, H. R. (1970). The effect of pertussis vaccine
    on the immune response of mice to sheep erythrocytes. *Clin. exp. Immun.*, **7**, 817.
Dukor, P., Salvin, S. B., Dietrich, F. M., Gelzer, J., Hess, R. and Loustalot, P. (1966). Effect
    of reserpine on immune reactions and tumor growth. *Eur. J. Cancer*, **2**, 253
Fahey, J. L. and Humphrey, J. H. (1962). Effect of transplantable plasma-cell tumours on
    antibody response in mice. *Immunology*, **5**, 110
Fernandes, G., Yunis, E. J. and Good, R. A. (1976*a*). Influence of diet on survival of mice.
    Proc. natn. Acad. Sci. U.S.A., **73**, 1279
Fernandes, G., Yunis, E. J. and Good, R. A. (1976*b*). Suppression of adenocarcinoma by the
    immunological consequences of calorie restriction. *Nature*, **263**, 504
Fidler, I. J. (1977). Depression of macrophages in mice drinking hyperchlorinated water.
    Nature, **270**, 735
Fishel, C. W., Szentivanyi, A. and Talmage, D. W. (1964). Adrenergic factors in *Bordetella
    pertussis*- induced histamine and serotonin hypersensitivity in mice. In *Bacterial endotoxins*
    (eds. Landy, M. and Braun, W.) Rutgers University Press, New Jersey, pp. 474
Fitzgerald, T. J., Williams, B. and Uyeki, E. M. (1971). Effects of antimitotic and anti-
    inflammatory agents on sodium urate-induced paw swelling in mice. *Pharmacology*, **6**,
    265.
Floersheim, G. L. (1964). Beeinflussbarkeit der Transplantationsimmunität durch Pharmaka.
    Helv. physiol. Acta, **22**, 241
Floersheim, G. L. (1965*a*). Effect of Pertussis vaccine on the tuberculin reaction. *Int. Archs
    Allergy*, **26**, 340

Floersheim, G. L. (1965*b*). Pharmakologische Beeinflussbarkeit cellulärer Immunität. *Z. naturwiss.- med. Grundlagenforsch.*, **2**, 307

Floersheim, G. L. (1967*a*). Drug-induced tolerance for skin allografts across the H-2 barrier in adult mice. *Science*, **156**, 951

Floersheim, G. L. (1967*b*) Facilitation of tumor growth by Bacillus pertussis. *Nature*, **216**, 1235

Floersheim, G. L. (1969). Suppression of cellular immunity by Gram-Negative bacteria. *Antibiotica Chemother. Basel*, **15**, 407

Floersheim, G. L., Hopff, W. H., Gasser, M. and Bucher, K. (1971). Impairment of cell-mediated immunoresponses by Pseudomonas aeruginosa. *Clin. exp. Immun.*, **9**, 241

Floersheim, G. L., Borel, J. F., Wiesinger, D. and Kis, Z. (1972). Antiarthritic and Immunosuppressive effects of *Pseudomonas aeruginosa*. *Agents and Actions*, **2**, 231

Folch, H. and Waksman, B. H. (1974). The splenic suppressor cell. I. Activity of Thymus-dependent adherent cells: changes with age and stress. *J. Immun.*, **113**, 127

Franzl, R. E. and MacMaster, P. D. (1961). Effect of bacterial lipopolysaccharides on hemolysin formation in mice. *Fedn. Proc.* 20, 26

Friedman, E. A. and Beyer, M. M. (1977). Immune competence of the streptozotocin-induced diabetic rat. I. Absent second set skin allograft response. *Transplantation*, **24**, 367

Friedman, H. and Ceglowski, W. S. (1968). Cellular basis for the immunosuppressive properties of a leukaemogenic virus. *Nature*, **218**, 1232

Frost, P. and Lance, E. M. (1973). Abrogation of lymphocyte trapping by ascitic tumors. *Nature*, **246**, 101

Gaugas, J. M. and Curzen, P. (1978). Polyamine interaction with pregnancy serum in suppression of lymphocyte transformation. *Lancet*, i, 18

Gisler, R. H., Lindhal, P. and Gresser, I. (1974). Effects of interferon on antibody synthesis *in vitro. J. Immun.*, **113**, 438

Glasgow, A. H., Nimberg, R. B. Menzoian, J. O., Saporoschetz, I., Cooperband, S. R., Schmid, K. and Mannick, J. A. (1974). Association of anergy with an immunosuppressive peptide fraction in the serum of patients with cancer. *New Engl. J. Med.*, **291**, 1263

Goldstein, D. E., Drash, A., Gibb, J. and Blizzard, R. M. (1970). Diabetes mellitus: The incidence of circulating antibodies against chyroid, gastric and adrenal tissue. *J. Pediatr.* **77**, 304

Goldyne, M. E. (1977). Prostaglandins and the modulation of immunological responses. *Int. J. Dermatol.*, **16**, 701

Goodwin, L. G., Green, D. G., Guy, M. W. and Voller, A. (1972). Immunosuppression during trypanosomiasis. *Br. J. exp. Path.*, **53**, 40

Goodwin, J. S., Messner, R. P., Bankhurst, A. D., Peake, G. D., Saiki, J. H. and Williams, R. C. (1977). Prostaglandin-producing suppressor cells in Hodgkin's disease. *New Engl. J. Med.* 247. 963

Green, C. J. and Allison, A. C. (1978). Extensive prolongation of rabbit Ridney allograft survival after short-term cyclosporin A treatment. *Lancet*, i, 1182

Greenwood, B. M. and Voller, A. (1970). Suppression of autoimmune disease in New Zealand mice associated with infection with malaria. I. (NZB × NZW) $_{F1}$ hybrid mice. *Clin. exp. Immun.*, **8**, 793

Greenwood, B. M., Herrick, E. M. and Voller, A. (1970). Can parasitic infection suppress autoimmune disease? *Proc. R. Soc. Med.*, **63**, 19

Greenwood, B. M., Playfair, J. H. L. and Torrigiani, G. (1971). Immunosuppression in murine malaria. I. General characteristics. *Clin. exp. Immun.*, **8**, 467

Greenwood, B. M., Bradley-Moore, A. M., Palit, A. and Bryceson, A. D. M. (1972). Immunosuppression in children with malaria. *Lancet*, i, 169

Greenwood, B. M., Whittle, H. C. and Molyneux, D. H. (1973). Immunosuppression in African trypanosomiasis. *Trans. R. Soc. trop. Med. Hyg.*, **67**, 846

Grob, P. J. and Harold, G. E. (1972). Immunological abnormalities and hydantoins, *Br. med. J.*, **2**, 561

Hakim, A. A. (1977). An immunosuppressive factor from serum of thermally traumatized patients. *J. Trauma*, **17**, 908

Hanna, E. E. and Watson, D. W. (1968). Host–parasite relationships among group A streptococci. IV. Suppression of Antibody response by streptococcal pyrogenic exotoxin. *J. Bact.*, **95**, 14

Hanna, E. E. and Watson, D. W. (1973). Enhanced immune response after immunosuppression by streptococcal pyrogenic exotoxin. *Infect. Immunity*, 7, 1009

Harvey, H. A., Allegra, J. C., Demers, L. M., Luderer, J. R., Brenner, D. E., Trautlein, J. J., White, D. S., Gillin, M. A. and Lipton, A. (1977). Immunosuppression and human cancer: role of prostaglandins. *Cancer*, 39, 2362

Henney, C. S., Lichtenstein, L. M., Gillespie, E. and Rolley, R. T. (1973). *In vivo* suppression of the immune response to alloantigen by cholera enterotoxin. *J. clin. Invest.* 52, 2853

Hersh, E. M. (1973). Immunosuppressive enzymes. *Transplant. Proc.*, 5, 1211

Hiestand, P. C., Borel, J. F., Bauer, W., Kis, Z. L., Magnee, C. and Stähelin, H. (1977). The effects of fractions (chalones) obtained from lymphoid organs on lymphocyte proliferation *in vitro*. *Agents and Actions*, 7, 327

Hirano, M., Sinkovics, J. G., Shullenberger, C. C. and Howe, C. D. (1967). Murine lymphoma: augmented growth in mice with pertussis vaccine-induced lymphocytosis. *Science*, 158, 1061

Hirsch, M. S., Ellis, D. A., Black, P. H., Monaco, A. P. and Wood, M. L. (1974) Immunosuppressive effects of an interferon preparation *in vivo*. *Transplantation*, 17, 234

Hopff, W. H. (1967). Makrophagenausbeute bei Kaninchen mit Cysticercen. *Helv. physiol. Acta*, 25, 397

Hopff, W. H., Floersheim, G. L. and Bucher, K. (1967). Alteration der Tuberkulinreaktion durch mikrobielle Polysaccharide. *Helv. physiol. Acta*, 25, 1

Howard, J. G., Scott, M. T. and Christie, G. H. (1973). Cellular mechanisms underlying the adjuvant activity of *Corynebacterium parvum* interactions of activated macrophages with T and B lymphocytes. In *Immunopotentiation*. Ciba Foundation Symposium 18, ASP (Elsevier Excerpta Medica, North-Holland) Amsterdam, p. 101

Howard, R. J. and Simmons, R. L. (1974). Acquired immunologic deficiencies after trauma and surgical procedures. *Surg. Gynecol. Obstet.*, 139, 771

Hršak, I. and Marotti, T. (1975). Mechanism of the immunosuppressive effect of Ehrlich ascitic tumor. *Eur. J. Cancer*, 11, 181

Huang, S. W. and MacLaren, N. K. (1976). Insulin-dependent diabetes: a disease of autoaggression. *Science*, 192, 64

Hudson, K. M., Byner, C., Freeman, J. and Terry, R. J. (1976). Immunodepression, high IgM levels and evasion of the immune response in murine trypanosomiasis. *Nature*, 264, 256

Huldt, G., Gard, S. and Olovson, S. G. (1973). Effect of *Toxoplasma gondii* on the thymus. *Nature*, 244, 301

Hunt, C. V., Khan, W., Friedman, G. and Honck, J. C. (1977). *In vitro* inhibition of human peripheral blood lymphocyte transformation by an extract of *Pseudomonas putida*. *Immunology*, 33, 209

Jamieson, S. W. (1976). Promethazine (Phenergan) in the treatment of rat cardiac allografts. *Transplantation*, 21, 69

Jayawardena, A. N. and Waksman, B. H. (1977). Suppressor cells in experimental trypanosomiasis. *Nature*. 265, 539

Jayawardena, A. N., Targett, G. A. T., Lenchars, E., Carter, R. L., Doenhoff, M. J. and Davies, A. J. S. (1975). T-cell activation in murine malaria. *Nature*, 258, 149

Jenkins, D. M., Acres, M. G., Peters, J. and Riley, J. (1972). Human chorionic gonadotropin and the fetal allograft. *Am. J. Obstet. Gynec.*, 114, 13

Jennings, J. F. and Oates, C. M. (1967). Studies on the non-specific depression of the immune response. *J. exp. Med.*, 126, 557

Johnson, A. G., Gaines, S. and Landy, M. (1956). Studies on the O-Antigen of *Salmonella typhosa*. V. Enhancement of antibody response to protein antigens by the purified lipopolysaccharide. *J. exp. Med.*, 103, 225

Jondal, M. and Klein, G. (1973). Surface markers on human B and T lymphocytes. II. Presence of Epstein-Barr virus receptors on B lymphocytes. *J. exp. Med.*, 138, 1365

Jones, B. M., Bird, M., Howells, M., Massey, P. R., Millar, D., Miller, J. J., Reeves, S. and Salaman, J. R. (1977). Inhibition of human mixed lymphocyte reactions by sera and urine dialysates from niridazole-treated rats. *Transplantation*, 24, 134

Jossifides, I. A., Gutzait, L., Brand, M. and Tocantins, L. M. (1964). Enhanced survival of skin homografts in mice with a bacterial infection. *Ann. N. Y. Acad. Sci.*, 114, 487

Kakita, A., Blanchard, J. and Fortner, J. G. (1975). Effectiveness of prostaglandin E_1 and procarbazine hydrochloride in prolonging the survival of vascularized cardiac hamster-to-rat xenograft. *Transplantation*, 20, 439

Kamrin, B. B. (1959). Successful skin homografts in mature non-littermate rats treated with fractions containing alpha-globulins. *Proc. Soc. exp. Biol. Med.*, 100, 58

Kantor, F. S. (1975). Infection, anergy and cell-mediated immunity. *N. Engl. J. Med.*, 292, 629

Kappas, A., Jones, H. E. H. and Roitt, I. M. (1963). Effects of steroid sex hormones on immunological phenomena. *Nature*, 198, 902

Keller, R., Ogilvie, R. M. and Simpson, E. (1971). Tumour growth in nematode-infected animals. *Lancet*, i, 678

Kilshaw, P. J., Brent, L. and Pinto, M. (1975). Suppressor T cells in mice made unresponsive to skin allografts. *Nature*, 255, 489

Kirchner, H., Glaser, M. and Herberman, R. B. (1975). Suppression of cell-mediated tumour immunity by *Corynebacterium parvum*. *Nature*, 257, 396

Kleinerman, E. S., Snyderman, R. and Daniels, C. A. (1975). Depressed monocyte chemotaxis during acute influenza infection. *Lancet*, ii, 1063

Krishan, S., Bhuyan, U. N., Talwar, G. P. and Ramalingaswami, V. (1974). Effect of vitamin A and protein-calorie undernutrition on immune responses. *Immunology*, 27, 383

Lagrange, P. H., Mackaness, G. B., Miller, T. E. and Pardon, P. (1975). Expression of bacterial lipopolysaccharide on the induction and expression of cell-mediated immunity. I. Depression of the afferent arc. II. Stimulation of the afferent arc. *J. Immunol.*, 114, 442

Landy, M., Sanderson, R. P., Bernstein, M. T. and Lerner, E. M. (1965). II Involvement of thymus in immune response of rabbits to somatic polysaccharides of Gram-negative bacteria. *Science*, 147, 1591

Lattime, E. C. and Strausser, H. R. (1977). Arteriosclerosis. Is stress-induced immune suppression a risk factor? *Science*, 198, 302

Lendrum, R., Walker, G. and Gamble, D. R. (1975). Islet-cell antibodies in juvenile diabetes mellitus of recent onset. *Lancet*, i, 880

Levene, G. M., Turk, J. L., Wright, D. J. M. and Grimble, A. G. S. (1969). Reduced lymphocyte transformation due to plasma factor in patients with active syphilis. *Lancet*, ii, 246

Levo, Y., Markovitz and Trainin, N. (1975). Hydantoin immunosuppression and carcinogenesis. *Clin. exp. Immun.*, 19, 521

Lichtenstein, L. M., Gillespie, E. and Bone, H. R. (1972). The effects of a series of prostaglandins on *in vitro* models of the allergic response and cellular immunity. *Prostaglandins*, 2, 519

Lyons, S. F. and Friedman, H. (1978). Cellular mechanism of cholera toxin − mediated modulation of *in vitro* hemolysin formation by mouse immunocytes. *J. Immun.*, 120, 452

Lurie, M. B., Harris, T. N., Abramson, S. and Allison, J. M. (1949). Constitutional factors in resistance to infection. II. The effect of estrogen on tuberculin skin sensitivity and on the allergy of the internal tissues. *Am. Rev. Tuber.*, 59, 186

MacCuish, A. C., Urbaniak, S. J., Campbell, C. J., Duncan, L. J. P. and Irvine, W. J. (1974). Phytohemagglutinin transformation and circulating lymphocyte subpopulations in insulin-dependent diabetic patients. *Diabetes*, 23, 708

MacMaster, P. D. and Franzl, R. E. (1968). The primary immune response in mice. II. Cellular responses of lymphoid tissue accompanying the enhancement or complete suppression of antibody formation by a bacterial endotoxin. *J. exp. Med.*, 127, 1109

Mahmoud, A. A. F. and Warren, K. S. (1974). Anti-inflammatory effects of tartaric emetic and niridazole: suppression of schistosome egg granuloma. *J. Immun.*, 112, 222

Mahmoud, A. A. F., Mandel, M. A., Warren, K. S. and Webster, L. T., Jr. (1975). Niridazole. II. A potent long acting suppressant of cellular hypersensitivity. *J. Immun.*, 114, 279

Mahmoud, A. A. F., Rodman, H. M., Mandel, M. and Warren, K. S. (1976). Induced and spontaneous diabetes mellitus and suppression of cell-mediated immunologic responses. Granuloma formation, delayed dermal reactivity and allograft rejection. *J. Clin. Invest.* **57**, 362

Malakian, A. and Schwab, J. J. (1968). Immunosuppressant from group A streptococci. *Science,* **159**, 880

Malkiel, S. and Hargis, B. J. (1964). Anaphylactic reactions in mice induced by *Bordetella pertussis* lipopolysaccharide. *J. Allergy,* **35**, 306

Mangi, R. J., Niederman, J. C. and Kelleher, J. E., Jr. (1975). Depression of cell-mediated immunity during acute infectious mononucleosis. *N. Engl. J. Med.,* **291**, 1149

Mannick, J. A. and Schmid, K. (1967). Prolongation of allograft survival by an alpha-globulin isolated from normal blood. *Transplantation,* **5**, 1231

Martin, C. M., Kunin, C. M., Gottlieb, L. S. and Finland, M. (1959). Asian Influenza A in Boston, 1957–1958. II. Severe staphylococcal pneumonia complicating influenza. *Archs intern Med.,* **103**, 532

McBride, J. S. and Micklem, H. S. (1977). Immunosuppression in murine malaria. II. The primary response to bovine serum albumin. *Immunology,* **33**, 253

McCarthy, R. E. (1964). Modification of the immune response of mice to skin homografts and heterografts by Ehrlich ascites carcinoma. *Cancer Res.,* **24**, 915

McGregor, I. A. and Barr, M. (1962). Antibody response to tetanus toxoid inoculation in malarious and non-malarious Gambian children. *Trans. R. Soc. trop. Med. Hyg.,* **36**, 364

McHugh, M. I., Wilkinson, R., Elliott, R. W., Field E. J., Dewar, P., Hall, R. R., Taylor, R. M. R., and Uldall, P. R. (1977). Immunosuppression with polyunsaturated fatty acids in renal transplantation. *Transplantation,* **24**, 263

McIllmurray, M. B., Embleton, M. J., Greeves, W. G., Langman, M. J. S. and Deane, M. (1977). Controlled trial of active immunotherapy in management of stage II B malignant melanoma. *Br. med. J.,* **1**, 540

Meade, C. and Mertin, J. (1976). The mechanism of immunoinhibition by arachidonic and linoleic acid: effects on the lymphoid and reticuloendothelial systems. *Int. Archs. allergy appl. Immun.,* **51**, 2

Mellman, W. J. and Wetton, R. (1963). Depression of the tuberculin reaction by attenuated measles virus vaccine. *J. Lab. clin. Med.,* **61**, 453

Merrit, K. and Johnson, A. G. (1965). Studies on the adjuvant action of bacterial endotoxins on antibody formation. *J. Immun.,* **94**, 416

Mertin, J. (1976). Effect of polyunsaturated fatty acids on skin allograft survival and primary and secondary cytotoxic response in mice. *Transplantation,* **21**, 1

Mertin, J. and Hunt, R. (1976). Influence of polyunsaturated fatty acids on survival of skin allografts and tumor incidence in mice. *Proc. natn. Acad. Sci. U.S.A.,* **73**, 928

Mertin, J., Hughes, D., Shenton, B. K. and Dickinson, J. P. (1974). *In vitro* inhibition by unsaturated fatty acids of the PPD- and PHA-induced lymphocyte response. *Klin. Wschr.* **52**, 248

Mertin, J., Shenton, B. K. and Field, E. J. (1976). Unsaturated fatty acids in multiple sclerosis. *Br. med. J.,* **2**, 777

Miller, G. A. and Jackson, R. W. (1973). The effect of a *Streptococcus pyrogenes* teichoic acid on the immune response of mice. *J. Immun.,* **110**, 148

Mitchell, A. G., Nelson, W. E. and Le Blanc, T. J. (1935). Studies in immunity. V. Effect of acute diseases on reaction of skin to tuberculin. *Am. J. Dis. Child.,* **49**, 695

Monjan, A. A. and Collector, M. I. (1977). Stress-induced modulation of the immune response. *Science,* **196**, 307

Moroni, C. and Schumann, G. (1977). Are endogenous C-type viruses involved in the immune system? *Nature,* **269**, 600

Mowat, A. G. and Baum, J. (1971). Chemotaxis of polymorphonuclear leucocytes from patients with diabetes mellitus. *N. Engl. J. Med.,* **284**, 621

Mowbray, J. F., Boylston, A. W., Milton, J. D. and Weksler, M. (1969). Studies on the mode of action of immunosuppressive ribonucleases. *Antibiotica Chemother.,* **15**, 384

Mueller, P. S. and Watkin, D. M. (1961). Plasma unesterified fatty acid concentrations in neoplastic disease. *J. Lab. clin. Med.,* **57**, 95

Munoz, J. (1964). Effect of bacteria and bacterial products on anti-body response. *Adv Immunol.,* **4**, 397

Nelken, D. (1973). Normal immunosuppressive protein (NIP). *J. Immun.*, 110, 1161

Nerup, J. and Binder, C. (1973). Thyroid, gastric and adrenal autoimmunity in diabetes mellitus. *Acta Endocr. (Kbh)*, 72, 279

Nerup, J., Andersen, O. O., Bendixen, G., Egeberg, J. and Poulsen, J. E. (1971). Antipancreatic cellular hypersensitivity in diabetes mellitus. *Diabetes*, 20, 424

Neter, E. (1977). Endotoxins and the immune response. *Curr. topics Microbiol.*, 47, 82

Nimberg, R. B., Glasgow, A. H., Menzoian, J. O., Constantin, M. B., Cooperband, S. R., Mannick, J. A. and Schmid, K. (1974). Isolation of an immunosuppressive peptide fraction from the serum of cancer patients. *Cancer Res.*, 35, 1489

Ninnemann, J. L., Fisher, J. C. and Frank, H. A. (1978). Prolonged survival of human skin allografts following thermal injury. *Transplantation*, 25, 69

Nogrady, S. G., Hartley, J. P. R. and Seaton, A. (1977). Metabolic effects of intravenous salbutamol in the course of acute severe asthma. *Thorax*, 32, 559

Nordal, H. J., Frøland, S. S., Vandvik, B. and Norby E. (1975). Measles-virus-induced migration inhibition of human leucocytes: an immunologically unspecific phenomenon? *Lancet*, ii, 1266

Odaka, T., Ishii, H., Yamanuva, K. and Yamamoto, T. (1966). Inhibitory effect of Friend leukaemia virus infection on the antibody formation to sheep erythrocytes in mice. *Jap. J. exp. Med.*, 36, 277

Old, L. J., Clarke, D. A., Benacer, B. and Goldsmith, M. (1960). The reticuloendothelial system and the neoplastic process. *Ann. N. Y. Acad. Sci.*, 88, 264

Orbach-Arbouys, S. and Poupon, M. F. (1978). Active suppression of *in vitro* reactivity of spleen cells after BCG treatment. *Immunology*, 34, 431

Page, A. R., Condie, R. R. and Good, R. A. (1962). Effect of 6-mercaptopurine on inflammation. *J. exp. Med.*, 40, 519

Parker, C. W. and Morse, S. I. (1973). The effect of *Bordetella pertussis* on lymphocyte cyclic AMP and metabolism. *J. exp. Med.*, 137, 1078

Paterson, P. Y., Harvey, J. M. and Webster, L. T. (1977). Niridazole suppression of experimental allergic encephalomyelitis in Lewis rats. *J. Immun.*, 118, 2151

Păunescu, E. (1970). *In vivo* and *in vitro* suppression of humoral and cellular immunological response by rifampicin. *Nature*, 228, 1118

Pelley, R. P., Pelley, R. J., Stavitsky, A. B., Mahmoud, A. A. F. and Warren, K. S. (1975). Niridazole, a potent long-acting suppressant of cellular hypersensitivity. II. Minimal suppression of antibody responses. *J. Immun.*, 115, 1477

Peterson, R. D. A., Hendrickson, R. and Good, R. A. (1963). Reduced antibody forming capacity during the incubation period of passage A leukaemia in C3H mice. *Proc. Soc. exp. Biol. (N.Y.)*, 114, 517

Pierpaoli, W. and Maestroni, G. J. M. (1977). Pharmacological control of the immune response by blockade of the early hormonal changes following antigen injection. *Cell. Immun.*. 31, 355

Piessens, W. F., Lachapelle, F. L., Legros, N. and Hennson, J. C. (1970). Facilitation of rat mammary tumor growth by BCG. *Nature*, 228, 1210

von Pirquet, C. E. (1908). Das Verhalten der kutanen Tuberkulinreaktion während der Masern *Dtsch. med. Wschr.*, 34, 1297

Purtilo, D. T., Hallgrew, H. M. and Yunis, E. J. (1972). Depressed maternal lymphocyte response to phytohaemogglutinin in human pregnancy. *Lancet*, i, 769

Quagliata, F. and Taranta, A. (1972). Suppression of adjuvant disease by bacterial extracellular products. *Ann. rheum. Dis.*, 31, 500

Quagliata, F., Lawrence, V. J. W. and Phillips-Quagliata, J. M. (1972). Prostaglandin E_1 as a regulator of lymphocyte function. Selective action on B lymphocytes and synergy with procarbazine in depression of immune responses. *Cell. Immun.*, 3, 198

Renoux, M. and Renoux, G. (1977). Brucellosis, immunosuppression and levamisole. *Lancet*, i, 372

Robinson, E., Sher, S. and Mekori, T. (1974). Lymphocyte Stimulation by phytohemagglutinin and tumor cells of malignant effusions. *Cancer Res.*, 34, 1548

Rose, W. C., Rodey, G. E., Rimm, A. A., Truitt, R. L. and Bortin, M. M. (1976). Mitigation of graft-versus-host disease in mice by treatment of donors with bacterial endotoxin. *Expl. Hemat.*, 4, 90

Rowlands, D. T., Claman, H. N. and Kind, Phyllis D. (1965). The effect of endotoxin on the thymus of young mice. *Am. J. Path.* **46**, 165

Ruckdeschel, J. C., Codish, S. D., Stranahan, A. and McKneally, M. F. (1972). Postoperative empyema improves survival in lung cancer. *New Engl. J. Med.,* **287**, 1013

Ruitenberg, E. J. and Steerenberg, P. A. (1973). Possible immunosuppressive effect of *Corynebacterium parvum* on infection with *Trichinella spiralis. Nature New Biol.,* **242**, 149

Salaman, J. R. and Millar, D. (1975). Linoleic acid as an immunosuppressive agent. *Lancet,* i, 857

Salaman M. H. (1969). Immunodepression by viruses. *Antibiotica Chemother.,* **15**, 393

Salaman, M. H., Wedderburn, N. and Bruce-Chwatt, L. J. (1969). The immunodepressive effect of a murine plasmodium and its interaction with murine oncogenic viruses. *J. gen. Microbiol.* **59**, 383

Salaman, J. R., Bird, M., Godfrey, A. M., Jones, B., Millar, D. and Miller, J. (1977). Prolonged allograft survival with niridazole, azathioprine and prednisolone. *Transplantation,* **23**, 29

Santiago-Delpin, E. A. and Szepsenwol, J. (1977). Prolonged survival of skin and tumour allografts in mice on high-fat diets: Brief communication. *J. Nat. Cancer Inst.,* **59**, 571

Schwab, J. J. (1975). Suppression of the immune response by micro-organisms. *Bact. Rev.,* **39**, 121

Scott, M. T. (1972). Biological effects of the adjuvant *Corynebacterium parvum.* Inhibition of PHA, mixed lymphocyte and G-v-H reactivity. *Cell. Immun.,* **5**, 251

Siegel, B. V. and Morton, J. L. (1966). Depressed antibody response in the mouse infected with Rauscher leukaemia virus. *Immunology,* **10**, 559

Silberman, S. L., Jacobs, R. P. and Cole, G. A. (1978). Mechanisms of hemopoietic and immunological dysfunction induced by lymphocytic choriomeningitis virus. *Infect. Immun.,* **19**, 533

Sims, F. H. and Freeman, J. W. (1966). The depression of the immune response by serum protein fractions. *Immunology,* **11**, 175

Skopinska, E. (1978). The effect of lipopolysaccharide (LPS) on the development of cell-mediated immunity to transplantation antigens. *Transplantation* (in the press)

Smith, J. W., Steiner, A. L. and Parker, C. W. (1971). Human lymphocyte metabolism. Effects of cyclic and non-cyclic nucleotides on stimulation by phytohemagglutinin. *J. clin. Invest.,* **50**, 442

Spellman, C. W. and Daynes, R. A. (1977). Modification of immunological potential by ultraviolet radiation. II. Generation of suppressor cells in short-term UV-irradiated mice. *Transplantation,* **24**, 120

Stanislavsky, E. S., Bogdanova, V. V., Kirpatovsky, I. D. and Zhvanetskaya, M. I. (1977). Isolation and immunochemical characteristics of the immunosuppressive substance from *Escherichia coli. J. Hyg. Epidemiol. Microbiol. Immun.,* **21**, 84

Starr, S. and Berkovich, S. (1967). Effect of measles gamma-globulin-modified measles and vaccine measles on the tuberculin test. *New Engl. J. Med.,* **270**, 386

Stein, M., Schiavi, R. C. and Camerino, M. (1976). Influence of brain and behaviour on the immune system. *Science,* **191**, 435

Steinberg, A. D., Plotz, P. H., Wolff, S. M., Wong, V. G., Agus, S. G. and Decker, J. L. (1972). Cytotoxic drugs in treatment of non-malignant diseases. *Ann. intern. Med.,* **76**, 619

Stevens, J. E. and Willoughby, D. A. (1969). The antiinflammatory effect of some immuno-suppressive agents. *J. Path. Bact.,* **97**, 367

Stiles, D. P. and Erickson, R. P. (1975). Suppressive effect of seminal plasma on lymphocyte activation. *Nature,* **253**, 727

Stimson, W. H. (1976). Studies on the immunosuppressive properties of a pregnancy-associated α-macroglobulin. *Clin. exp. Immun.,* **25**, 149

Stjernswärd, J. (1969). Immunosuppression by carcinogens. *Antibiotica Chemother. (Basel),* **15**, 213

Stone, H. H., Given, K. S. and Martin, J. D. (1967). Delayed rejection of skin homografts in *Pseudomonas sepsis. Surg. Gynec. Obstet.,* **124**, 1067

Storb, R., Floersheim, G. L., Weiden, P. L., Graham, T. L., Kolb, H. J., Lerner, K. G., Schroeder, M. L. and Thomas, E. D. (1974). Effect of prior blood transfusions on marrow grafts abrogation of sensitization by procarbazine and antithymocyte serum. *J. Immun.,* **112**, 1508

Strausser, H. R. and Bober, L. A. (1972). Inhibition of tumour growth and survival of aged mice inoculated with Moloney tumour transplants and treated with endotoxin. *Cancer Res.*, 32, 2156

Strickland, G. T., Voller, A., Pettit, L. E. and Fleck, G. D. (1972). Immunodepression associated with concomitant toxoplasma and malarial infection in mice. *J. infect. Dis.* 126, 54

Strom, T. B., Bear, R. A. and Carpenter, C. B. (1975). Insulin-induced augmentation of lymphocyte-mediated cytotoxicity. *Science*, 187, 1206

Strom, T. B., Carpenter, C. B., Garovoy, M. R., Austen, K. F., Merrill, J. P. and Kalinen, M. (1973). The modulating influence of cyclic nucleotides upon lymphocyte-mediated cytotoxicity. *J. exp. Med.*, 138, 381

Terry, R. J. (1978). Immunodepression in parasite infections. In *Immunity in parasitic diseases.* Inserm. Paris p. 161

Ting, C. C., Tsai, S. C. and Rogers, M. J. (1977). Host control of tumor growth. *Science*, 197, 571

Turk, J. L. and Bryceson, A. D. M. (1971). Immunological phenomena in leprosy and related diseases. *Adv. Immun.*, 13, 209.

Turk, J. L., Willoughby, D. A. and Stevens, J. E. (1968). An analysis of the effects of some types of antilymphocyte sera on contact hypersensitivity and certain models of inflammation. *Immunology*, 14, 683

Turnell, R. W., Clarke, L. H. and Burtor, A. F. (1973). Studies on the mechanism of corticosteroid-induced lymphocytolysis. *Cancer Res.*, 33, 203.

Urquhart, G. M., Murray, M., Murray, P. K., Jennings, F. W. and Bate, E. (1973). Immunosuppression in *Trypanosome brucei* infections in rats and mice. *Trans. R. Soc. trop. Hyg.* 67, 528

Valdimarsson, H., Agnarsdottir, G. and Lachmann, P. J. (1975). Measles virus receptor on human T-lymphocytes. *Nature*, 255, 554

Veit, B. C. and Michael, J. G. (1969). Immune response suppression by an inhibitor in normal and immune mouse serum. *Nature New Biol.*, 235, 238

Voller, A., Gall, D. and Manawadu, B. R. (1972). Depression of the antibody response to tetanus toxoid in mice infected with malaria parasites. *Z. Tropenmed. Parasit.*, 23, 152

Vose, B. M. and Mondgil, G. C. (1975). Effect of surgery on tumour-directed lymphocyte responses. *Br. med. J.*, 2, 56

Waltman, S. R., Burde, R. M. and Berrios, J. (1971). Prevention of corneal homograft rejection by oestrogens. *Transplantation*, 11, 194

Watson, J. D. (1975). The influence of intracellular levels of cyclic nucleotides on cell proliferation and the induction of antibody synthesis. *J. exp. Med.*, 141, 97

Webster, L. T., Butterworth, A. E., Mahmoud, A. A. F., Mngola, E. N. and Warren, K. S. (1975). Suppression of delayed hypersensitivity in schistosome-infected patients by niridazole. *New Engl. J. Med.*, 292, 1144

Wedderburn, N. (1974). Immunodepression produced by malarial infection in mice. In *Parasites in the immunized host: mechanisms of survival.* Ciba Foundation Symposium 25 (New Series) Elsevier. Excerpta Medica. North-Holland, Amsterdam, London and New York p. 123

Weisberg, A. S., Dancel, T. M. and Hoffman, A. (1964). Suppression of antibody synthésis and prolongation of homograft survival by chloramphenicol. *J. exp. Med.*, 120, 183

Whang, H. Y. and Neter, E. (1967). Immunosuppression by endotoxin and its lipoid A component. *Proc. Soc. exp. Biol. N.Y.*, 124, 919

Wicher, V. and Wicher, K. (1977). *In vitro* cell response to *Treponema pallidum* infected rabbits. II. Inhibition of lymphocyte response to phytohaemagglutinin by serum of *T. pallidum*-infected rabbits. *Clin. exp. Immun.*, 29, 501

Wildstein, A., Stevens, L. E. and Hashim, G. (1976). Skin and heart allografted prolongation in tilorone-treated rats. *Transplantation*, 21, 129

Wilson, W. E. C., Kirkpatrick, C. H. and Talmage, D. W. (1965). Suppression of immunologic responsiveness in Uremia. *Ann. intern. Med.*, 62, 1

Wu, C. J. and Reimann, H. A. (1931). Effect of typhus fever on intracutaneous tuberculin reaction. *Nat. Med. J. China*, 17, 210

Yoo, T. J., Kuo, C. Y. and Stagner, J. I. (1975). Effect of *Bordetella pertussis* vaccine on growth of hepatoma. *Lancet*, i, 402

Ziegler, J. L., Bluming, A. Z., Morrow, R. H. Jr., Cohen, M. H., Fife, E. H. Jr., Finerty, J. F.

and Woods, R. (1972). Burkitt's lymphoma and malaria. *Trans. R. Soc. Trop. Hyg.,* **66,** 285
Zimmermann, E. F., Voorting-Howking, M. and Micheal, J. G. (1977). Immunosuppression by mouse sialylated α-foetoprotein. *Nature,* **265,** 354
Zurier, R. B. and Quagliata, F. (1971). Effect of prostaglandin E_1 on adjuvant arthritis. *Nature,* **234,** 304

2
Drug selectivity in the suppression of the immune response

E. Mihich (Department of Experimental Therapeutics and Grace Cancer Drug
Center, Roswell Park Memorial Institute, New York State Department of Health,
Buffalo, New York, U.S.A.)

Chemotherapy is a relatively effective treatment for certain types of neoplastic
diseases. In fact, by using drugs alone or in combination, good quality life can be
prolonged and, in some cases, complete remission can be obtained with no evidence
of the disease being found five years or more after diagnosis. These therapeutic
results are obtained in patients with certain types of choriocarcinoma, Wilm's
tumour, Burkitt's lymphoma, acute lymphocytic leukaemia and certain tumours
of the skin. In the near future, chemotherapeutic treatments in conjunction with
surgery may provide additional examples of therapeutic efficacy, as in the case of
osteogenic sarcoma of the limb and of pre-menopausal breast tumours.

Notwithstanding the demonstrated value of cancer chemotherapy, substantial
improvements need to be achieved before drugs can be used broadly and effectively
in the treatment of malignancy. The anticancer agents available are not sufficiently
selective in their action on tumours, and therefore toxicity to normal tissues limits
treatment that would otherwise be required to eliminate the last tumour cell.
Because of this basic limitation, it may not be possible to overcome moderate
degrees of natural or acquired resistance if unacceptable toxicity is to be avoided.
As discussed elsewhere (Mihich, 1976, 1978a, b; Mihich et al., 1976; Mihich and
Grindey, 1977), current approaches in cancer chemotherapy are aimed at removing
these limitations and focus on (a) the development of new drugs with increased
selectivity of action, (b) the clarification of the mechanisms of selective toxicity of
known drugs, hopefully resulting in improvement in their use, (c) the development
of new combination treatments taking advantage of therapeutic synergism among
drugs used concurrently or sequentially, (d) the utilisation of additional treatment
modalities in conjunction with chemotherapy and (e) the identification and inte-
grated measurement of the critical determinants of drug action in patients, hope-

*The results from this laboratory outlined in this presentation were obtained in part with the
support of Grant CA-15142 from the National Cancer Institute, USPHS.

fully as a means of establishing individually 'tailored' treatment. Among the studies directed towards the clarification of the mechanisms of selective toxicity of anti-cancer drugs, of potential importance are those on the interactions of these drugs with the defenses of the host against tumour.

The demonstration that cells from autochthonous tumours in animals have anti-genic characteristics not present in cells from normal tissues of the adult host (Klein, 1966; Prehn, 1968; Weiss, 1969) has led to the hope that responses of the host to tumour-associated antigens might be exploited in the treatment of neo-plastic disease. As reviewed elsewhere (Mihich, 1978*b*), this expectation is suppor-ted by mostly indirect evidence suggesting that human tumours may also have tumour-associated antigens capable of stimulating host responses. Despite the fact that no firm conclusion may be reached on the effectiveness of these responses in patients or on their regulation, it seems reasonable to consider the possibility that the reduction of tumour burden by drug treatment may be followed by the elimination of residual tumour cells by existing or augmented host defenses direc-ted against the tumour.

Substantial limitations may have to be overcome to exploit tumour immunity therapeutically. Difficulties may be related to the fact that most anticancer drugs are potentially capable of suppressing host mechanisms of defense and that in many cases this is a consequence of the very antiproliferative action that is at the basis of the antitumour effect (Mihich, 1971, 1975*a*). Moreover, increased tumour growth may result from modifications of immunological regulation possibly caused by tumour, drug or immunomanipulations. Indeed the interactions between chemo-therapeutic treatment and natural or augmented host defenses are crucial in any attempt to exploit these defenses in conjunction with chemotherapy (Mihich, 1978*b*).

Immunosuppression by anticancer drugs has been repeatedly demonstrated in animals and in humans (see, Mihich, 1971, 1975*a*; Hersh, 1973, 1974). It is now considered that this action may be relatively selective because it depends on a variety of factors (a) the pharmacological characteristics of the drug, (b) the characteristics of the immunological response affected and (c) temporal factors relating drug action to the development and function of the immunological response. Consequently, the selectivity of drug action under certain conditions in a given system may not be demonstrable under different conditions or in other systems in which a certain host function is measured (Schwartz and Mihich, 1973). A few reported examples may serve to support this generalisation. Under certain condi-tions cyclophosphamide was found to inhibit preferentially B cell responses (Turk, 1973). In rabbits, 6-mercaptopurine was found to have different effects on the antibody responses to bovine gamma-globulin ranging from inhibition, or the induction of state of unresponsiveness, to stimulation, depending on the dose and schedule of drug administration and also on the amount of antigen (Chanmougan and Schwartz, 1966). Depending on dose and regimen, arabinosylcytosine was found to exert selective depression of humoral or cellular immunity (Heppner and Calabresi, 1972; Griswold *et al.*, 1972). Under certain conditions daunorubicin and adriamycin appeared to spare selectively cells of the macrophage-monocytic type within the spleen of allogeneic tumour-bearing mice (Mantovani *et al.*, 1976) or of normal mice (Orsini *et al.*, 1977). Certain treatments may cause directly or in-directly a stimulation of the defenses of the host against the tumour. So-called rebound increases of immunological responses after drug-induced suppression have been observed in animals and in humans (Swanson and Schwartz, 1967). A direct effect may be the basis of the immune augmentation reportedly induced by levamisole under certain conditions (Avery, 1976). Immuno-augmenting effects of this and other agents are discussed in detail by others (see chapters 7 and 8).

The selective immunosuppressive and immunoaugmenting effects of anticancer drugs may also be the expression of actions exerted on the mechanisms of control of the immune responses. The regulation of certain immune responses appears to depend on a variety of cell interactions. Selectivity of drug action on a cell within a multicellular target system is likely to be determined by a multiplicity of biochemical and pharmacological factors affecting the drug and its metabolic environment within that cell (Rustum *et al.*, 1976). On the basis of this notion, which is bound to have general implications in a variety of biological systems, it is possible that a drug may alter the regulation of the immune response through selective effects on specific cell subsets within the immune system. Immunomodulation by drugs through alteration of immunological control mechanisms is discussed elsewhere (see chapter 8).

The fact that anticancer drugs may exert selective effects on specific components and functions of the immune response in mice is illustrated by four examples from this laboratory. (a) The unusual time restriction found in the reversal by leucovorin of the suppression of the responses to sheep erythrocytes (SRBCs) caused by methotrexate, (b) the selective effects of methylglyoxal bis (guanyl-hydrazone) on the development of anti-SRBC antibody-forming cells and its reversal by spermidine, (c) the selective effects of a series of anticancer drugs on the function of pre-formed non-T-cell effectors involved in the responses to SRBCs and (d) the selective effects of procarbazine on the development of T-cell effectors against allogeneic tumour cells.

REVERSAL OF METHOTREXATE (MTX)-INDUCED IMMUNOSUPPRESSION BY LEUCOVORIN (CF)

The cellular basis for the action of MTX is thought to be relatively better understood than that of most of the other anticancer drugs used clinically. It is well known that the drug inhibits dihydrofolate reductase (Zakrzewski and Nichol, 1958; Werkheiser, 1961) and thus prevents the reductive formation of tetrahydrofolate cofactors in the target cells. Because MTX binds tightly to dihydrofolate reductase, only a very small amount of reduced folates may be formed in the cell until new enzyme is synthesised. Because 5, 10-methylene tetrahydrofolate is used in the synthesis of thymidylate and is concurrently oxidised to dihydrofolate, and because the pools of reduced folates in cells are interchangeable, in the presence of intracellular concentrations of MTX sufficient to inhibit pre-existing and newly formed dihydrofolate reductase, the pools of reduced folate will decrease essentially as a function of the rate of thymidylate synthetase activity (Moran *et al.*, 1975). After a time, the pools of reduced folate will be inadequate for the synthesis of thymidylate, or purine, or both. Consequently, whether and when a proliferating cell will die after inhibition of dihydrofolate reductase will depend on many interacting factors, including the size of the pools of reduced folate, the size of the pools of thymidyla e and purine, the activity of thymidylate synthetase, the kinetics of free intracellular MTX, the rate of synthesis of dihydrofolate reductase, and the metabolic needs of the cell with time (Mihich and Grindey, 1977). It should be noted, however, that although the information available is consistent with the above outline, the precise proximal cause of cell death after MTX treatment has not yet been conclusively elucidated (Bertino, 1975; Mihich *et al.*, 1976).

Antitumour treatments with high-dose MTX followed by CF rescue from limiting toxicities have been studied in animals (Goldin and Mantel, 1957) and more recently in humans (Levitt *et al.*, 1973; Frei *et al.*, 1975). These treatments are essentially based on the notion that CF is taken up by cells, enters the pools of reduced folate, and reverses MTX toxicity in animals if given within a certain time after MTX (Goldin and Mantel, 1957). In view of the arguments developed in the introduction, it is possible that host defenses play a cooperative role in the thera-peutic effects of MTX; it is therefore important to study the kinetics of CF rescue of MTX-induced immunosuppression. The biochemical pharmacological informa-tion briefly discussed above is indeed consistent with the possibility that variations in the multifactorial parameter of MTX action among different cells and cell types may result in different degrees of restriction in the rescue from different MTX tissue toxicities, by CF.

The initial evidence that MTX exerts immunosuppressive effects in a variety of animal systems has been reported in the early 1960s (Friedman *et al.*, 1962; Lochte *et al.*, 1962; Glynn *et al.*, 1963; Uy *et al.*, 1966) and has been repeatedly reviewed (Makinodan *et al.*, 1970; Mihich, 1971; Gerebtzoff *et al.*, 1972; Hersh, 1974). The reversal by CF of the suppressive effects of the drug was first demonstrated in mice immunised with typhoid–paratyphoid A and B vaccine (Berenbaum and Brown, 1965) or bearing skin allografts (Berenbaum, 1964). In these studies it was noted that the effects of MTX could be reversed only if CF was given 1 h before to 1–2 h after the drug, in contrast with the longer time-range permissible in the case of effects on body weight, and with the greater latitude found previously (Goldin and Mantel, 1957) with reference to other limiting MTX toxicities. The strict time restrictions in the reversal by CF of the MTX-induced immunosuppression found in this laboratory (Medzihradsky *et al.*, 1977) agree with the results that Berenbaum obtained in different systems.

In the studies from this laboratory, particular care was taken to use chromato-graphically purified MTX. The single intraperitoneal (i.p.) dose of 100 mg/kg MTX used corresponded to less than one-half of the LD_{50}; CF was also given i.p., at the dose of 200 mg/kg. Immunisation was by a single i.p. administration of 5×10^8 SRBCs. Spleen cells were obtained at various times after immunisation and cell suspensions were prepared by standard procedures (Cohen *et al.*, 1975). The com-plement-dependent (CDCC) and complement-independent (CICC) cellular cytoxi-city assays used in this laboratory (Mawas *et al.*, 1973) are based on ^{51}Cr release from prelabelled target cells. The CDCC was measured after incubation of effector spleen cells with target SRBCs at different ET ratios, in RPMI 1640 medium plus 5 per cent foetal calf serum, for 45 min at 37 °C in 10 per cent CO_2, followed by an additional 45 min incubation in the presence of guinea pig complement. The incuba-tion was terminated by the addition of 2 ml of cold RPMI 1640 medium. The CICC assay was carried out in the same way, except that complement was not added and the incubation was continued for 20 h. After centrifugation for 5 min at 800*g* in the cold, the radioactive label in the supernatant and pellet was measured in a gamma radiation counter and the percentage release was calculated as follows:

$$\% \text{ release} = \frac{\text{c.p.m. in supernatant}}{\text{c.p.m. in supernatant} + \text{c.p.m. in pellet}} \times 100$$

The specific release is the percentage release with sensitised spleen cells minus the percentage release with non-sensitised spleen cells.

The kinetics of the CDCC response, which reaches a peak on days 4 or 5, is similar to the kinetics of the direct anti-SRBC plaque-forming assay (Jerne and Nordin, 1963).

The CICC response reaches a peak on days 10 to 12, and the assay is dependent on the presence of IgG secreted by sensitised antibody-forming cells (AFC) in the spleen of the immunised mice. The killer cells bear receptor for the Fc portion of the antibody and thus bind to the target cells only when their antigenic determinants are complexed with the IgG secreted by the AFC. The evidence supporting the necessary involvement of both AFC and killer cells in the CICC, the characteristics of the humoral and cellular interactions occurring in the assay, and the fact that the required IgG is actually secreted during the 20 h incubation, have been reviewed (Ehrke *et al.*, 1978). Therefore the CICC against SRBCs is similar to the antibody-dependent cellular cytotoxicity (ADCC) assay, except that in the CICC the IgG is secreted by AFC in the sensitised spleen cell populations, whereas in the ADCC the IgG is present in the antisera added along with the non-sensitised spleen cell populations in the assay mixture.

In mice treated with MTX on day 2, the inhibition of both CDCC and CICC was complete on day 4 regardless of the E/T ratio used in the assay (Medzihradsky *et al.*, 1977); comparable patterns of recovery of both responses were seen on later days, with complete recovery by day 14. When CF was also given on day 2, at times ranging from 5 h before to 5 h after the administration of MTX, and the response was measured on day 4, 50 per cent reversal of the inhibition could be achieved only when CF was given at least at the same time as MTX for CDCC or at least 2–3 h before MTX for CICC. When the responses were measured on day 7, namely at the time spontaneous recovery from inhibition started to occur, CF was found to accelerate this recovery when given on day 2 as late as 6 h after MTX. When the responses were measured on day 5, the results were intermediate between those obtained on days 4 and 7.

The spontaneous recovery of the responses may be due to proliferation of cells not affected by MTX on day 2. The patterns of inhibition of CDCC and CICC were essentially similar, as were those of spontaneous recovery and CF reversal. That the effects of MTX were primarily on the proliferation of AFC precursors was suggested by the fact that the drug had no effect when given on day 0 or on day 4, namely when the responses require cell interactions during initial sensitisation or are already developed as a result of the differentiation of AFCs. It was also apparent that the majority of the cells proliferating on day 2 would have to be protected by CF in order for a complete reversal of the effects of MTX to be seen on day 4. Because it was necessary to pre-load these cells with CF to allow for only a partial response to develop by day 4, it appears that the AFC precursors have a great dependence on newly formed folate cofactors, probably because of a high ratio between proliferation requirements and available cofactor and/or preformed purines and thymidine pools. The delayed administration of CF on day 2 was, however, capable of protecting a sufficient number of cells to provide a full response on day 7, probably in concert with the cells responsible for the partial recovery seen on that day without CF rescue.

It is apparent that the spleen cells proliferating in response to sensitisation by SRBCs are inhibited by MTX by virtue of their stringent metabolic requirements. Moreover, they represent a cell subset whose full functional expression is entirely dependent on the integrity of its complete proliferating capability. Therefore this system may be a sensitive tool in studies of the selective effects of certain drugs on metabolically restricted cells and of the relevance of specific target determinants of drug action.

SELECTIVE EFFECTS OF METHYLGLYOXAL BIS(GUANYLHYDRAZONE) (MGBG)

This compound has definite activity in acute myelocytic leukaemia and malignant lymphomas, but its clinical usefulness is greatly limited by severe toxicity (Mihich, 1965, 1975*b*). In animals, as well as in humans, MGBG causes marked antiproliferative effects, namely dramatic gastrointestinal toxicity, atrophy of lymphoid tissues, bone marrow depression and immunosuppression. In addition, the drug causes hepatotoxicity, cardiotoxicity and nephrotoxicity.

Spermidine (Spd), a physiological polyamine, selectively prevented the antiproliferative effects of the drug (Mihich, 1963, 1975*b*). This observation led to the finding that MGBG specifically inhibits the activity of the putrescine-activated *S*-adenosylmethionine decarboxylase (SAMDC) (Williams-Ashman and Schenone, 1972), a key enzyme in the biosynthesis of Spd. Paradoxically, substantial increases in SAMDC activity were found in tissues from animals treated with the drug (Pegg *et al.*, 1973), presumably due to, at least in part, the enzyme stabilisation occurring as a result of the tight binding of MGBG *in vivo*, with prolongation of the apparent half-life of the enzyme. Because the biosynthesis of Spd is inhibited in animals treated with MGBG (Pegg, 1973; Corti *et al.*, 1974), this stabilised SAMDC is apparently not functional *in vivo*. In addition, the carrier-mediated transport of MGBG in leukaemic cells was competitively inhibited by Spd (Mihich *et al.*, 1974), which indicates a second site of interaction between drug and polyamine.

Because the immunosuppressive effects of the drug may cause limiting toxicity in patients (Levin *et al.*, 1965), and because the possibility exists that selective reversal of this toxicity might be achieved with Spd, the characteristics of the immunosuppressive action and the possible relationships of this action to polyamine metabolism were investigated.

The immune responses of C57BL/6Ja mice to SRBCs constituted the basic model used in this study (Bennett *et al.*, 1977). The CDCC and CICC responses were measured essentially as described in the preceding section on MTX. Three additional sets of functions were measured. (a) Those involved in the ADCC where the anti-SRBC antibody (day 11) used to pre-coat the target cells was from mice not treated with drug and killer cells were from spleen of drug-treated mice, (b) phagocytosis of target SRBCs coated by 'endogenous' antibody, namely antibody secreted by AFC from spleen of immunised mice during the 20 h of CICC incubation (CICC-Phg) and (c)phagocytosis of target SRBCs coated by 'exogenous' antibody, namely antibody added to target cells before the addition of spleen cells from non-sensitised mice (ADCC-Phg). In some tests, 'exogenous' antibody was also added with spleen cells from immunised mice to clarify the specificity of drug action on CICC and CICC-Phg (see below). The ADCC was measured by published procedures (Perlmann and Perlmann 1970; Cohen *et al.*, 1975; MacLennan, 1973). The phagocytic functions were measured by reported procedures (Hersey, 1973) as modified in this laboratory (Cohen *et al.*, 1975): for CICC-Phg and ADCC-Phg assays the incubation was the same as for CICC and ADCC respectively, except that it was stopped by the addition of 1 ml of cold water followed after 15 s by 1 ml of cold double-concentrated medium. In these two assays the basic principle is that SRBCs engulfed by phagocytic cells are protected from hypo-osmotic lysis; consequently, in this case a reduction in ^{51}Cr release from prelabelled SRBCs is the measure of phagocytosis. The animals were treated with MGBG, 85 mg/kg i.p. for five consecutive days, starting 3 h after antigen and skipping day 4; the assays were carried out on day 7, 2 days after the last injection of drug.

Table 2.1   Effects of MGBG on immune functions
of mouse spleen cells

% inhibition of response				
CDCC	CICC	ADCC	CICC-Phg	ADCC-Phg
71	85	None	40	None

Results are modified from Bennett *et al.* (1977). C57BL/6Ja mice were immunised with 5×10^8 SRBCs on day 0 and the spleen cells were tested on day 7. MGBGttreatment and assays were as described in the text. Each assay was carried out at an effector cell/target cell ratio of 50:1 for 20 h, except for the CDCC which was at a ratio of 10:1 for a total of 1.5 h. The percentage inhibition was calculated on the basis of per cent of ^{51}Cr release for lytic assays and reciprocal of per cent of ^{51}Cr release for phagocytic assays (see text).

As summarised in Table 2.1, MGBG caused a marked inhibition of the development of the CDCC and CICC responses, and a substantial inhibition of the CICC-Phg. In contrast, the drug had no effect on ADCC or ADCC-Phg. The inhibition of the CICC-Phg assay was reversed when 'exogenous' antibody was added to the incubation mixture (results not shown), this indicates that the inhibition of the CICC-Phg was not due to the effects of drugs on phagocytic cells, interference with target SRBC coating by antibody, or inhibition of the phagocytosis of antibody-coated target cells. This conclusion is consistent with the results of the lytic assays: the inhibition of the CICC, when contrasted with the lack of inhibition of the ADCC, indicates that the effect on CICC is not due to effects of drugs on killer cells, on SRBC coating by antibody or on binding of killer cells to antibody-coated SRBCs. The data as a whole are consistent with the conclusion that MGBG inhibits the development of AFCs in the spleen of immunised mice.

The pattern of drug effects shown in table 2.1 could be reproduced when spleen cells adherent to columns of nylon wool were used as effectors. In contrast, except for ADCC and ADCC-Phg, no response was seen with non-adherent effector cells, which further indicates the non-T nature of the effectors involved in CDCC, CICC and CICC-Phg assays, all of which require the presence of AFCs in sensitised spleen. MGBG had no effect on the two responses involving 'exogenous' antibody, regardless of whether adherent or non-adherent effector cells were used, in confirmation of the results summarised in table 2.1.

The activity of SAMDC was increased by about 40–50-fold in spleen cells from mice treated with MGBG, and this increase was not affected by immunisation. It is of interest that a 60-fold increase in SAMDC activity was found when nylon-adherent cells from drug-treated mice were assayed, whereas only a 6–16-fold increase was seen in non-adherent cells. To exclude artifacts possibly caused by nylon wool column separation, the same assays were carried out with spleen cell populations separated through adherence to monolayers of antibody-coated SRBCs, and the results obtained were similar to those found with nylon wool-separated cells.

In additional studies, the uptake of ^{14}C-labelled MGBG in non-separated and nylon wool-separated cells was measured after incubation with 10 μM of the labelled compound *in vitro* for 15 min by published procedures (Dave and Mihich, 1972). Immunisation and pretreatment with MGBG *in vivo* did not affect uptake *in vitro*. Consistent with the greater effects of MGBG on immunological functions and SAMDC activity of adherent cells, the uptake of the drug was about 40 per cent higher in the adherent than in the non-adherent cells.

The lack of effect on phagocytic cells and their function, on binding of antibody to target cells, on killer cells and their function and on the actual secretion of antibody from sensitised cells in the CICC and CICC-Phg assays, was confirmed in experiments in which 100 μM MGBG was present in the incubation mixture of the various assays.

The most likely explanation of the results outlined above is that the drug inhibits the proliferation of AFC precursors. The possibility that the drug affects T-helper cells cannot be excluded on the basis of the immunological data, but it seems unlikely in view of the much greater increase in SAMDC activity, and the greater drug uptake observed in non-T-cell-enriched fractions compared with T-cell-enriched fractions. That the effect of MGBG is on a proliferation compartment of the immune response to SRBCs is further suggested by the fact that Spd completely reversed the immunosuppressive effects and greatly decreased the increase in SAMDC activity caused by the drug (Bennett *et al.*, 1978). Indeed this polyamine is known to reverse selectively the antiproliferative effects of MGBG without affecting those on non-proliferating tissues (Mihich, 1975*b*).

The studies on MGBG summarised herein provide evidence for selectivity of cellular effects of an antiproliferative agent, and attest to the well-accepted notion that B-cell proliferation plays a key role in the responses to SRBCs, whether the AFCs function is assessed directly by measurements of CDCC or indirectly by measurements of CICC and CICC-Phg. The usefulness of biochemical measurements of target determinants of drug action and of pharmacological measurements of the kinetics of intracellular drug concentrations as tools in the further verification of specificity of drug action within a multicellular system is also indicated by these results.

SELECTIVITY OF INHIBITION BY DRUGS OF EFFECTOR FUNCTIONS INVOLVED IN RESPONSES TO SRBCs IN SPLEEN CELLS

The action of anticancer drugs on the immune system has been most frequently studied in terms of effects on the development of the immune responses. Notwithstanding the unquestionable value of the information thus obtained, it is also important to measure drug effects on the function of the actual effector cells involved in these responses. The identification of the selectivity of drug action on immune effectors may be important in cancer therapeutics because in humans it is likely that the initial responses to tumour-associated antigens have probably already occurred at the time diagnosis is initially made and chemotherapy instituted (Mihich, 1971).

The selective effects of 24 agents on the effector functions involved in the responses to SRBCs of spleen cells from C3Hf/He mice have been investigated in this laboratory (Ehrke *et al.*, 1978). Most of the agents studied also have antitumour activity. The assay systems used were those described in the preceding section. CDCC, CICC, ADCC, CICC-Phg and ADCC-Phg (see table 2.2 for conditions). The effectors were developed in immunised mice not treated with drugs, and the drugs were added to the assay incubation mixtures in at least three concentrations. Control values for the conditions of assay utilised are presented in table 2.2. The agents studied and the results obtained are summarised in table 2.3. As shown in this table, the 24 agents can be divided into seven groups on the basis of their action on the effector functions studied. During the 4 h of incubation, the drugs could affect four sets of phenomena. (a) Synthesis, secretion and/or release of antibodies (CDCC and CICC), (b) binding of antibody to target cells (CDCC and

Table 2.2 Maximal control values obtained in the five tests using
^{51} Cr-labelled SRBCs as targets.
The C3Hf/He effector cells for the CDCC and CICC tests were
sensitised to SRBCs *in vivo*. In the CDCC test the effector and target
cells were incubated for 45 min, then guinea pig complement was added
and the incubation was continued for another 45 min. In both CICC
tests the incubations were for 4 h. In the ADCC tests non-sensitised
C3Hf/He spleen cells were used as effector cells and the target cells
were precoated with specific antisera before combining effector and
target cells. The incubation time for the ADCC tests was also 4 h.
Results are reprinted from Ehrke *et al.* (1978) by permission of
Cancer Research, Inc.

Test	Maximum effector/ target ratio used	Maximum specific effect (% ± s.e.)
CDCC	20:1	87 ± 4*
CICC lysis	50:1	44 ± 6*
ADCC lysis	30:1	48 ± 5*
CICC phagocytosis	50:1	32 ± 5†
ADCC phagocytosis	30:1	26 ± 5†

*per cent specific release ± s.e.
†per cent specific protection ± s.e.

Table 2.3 Selectivity of inhibition of normal and immune C3H spleen effector functions by various agents *in vitro*

Group number	Drugs*	CICC† Phagocytosis	CICC† Lysis	ADCC† Phagocytosis	ADCC† Lysis	CDCC†
1	5-FUdr, DTIC, Ara C, hydroxyurea, procarbazine, streptozotocin	−‡	−	−	−	−
2	Maytensine, MTX	±‡	−	−	−	−
3	Bleomycin	±	±	±	−	−
	2-Deoxyglucose	+‡	±	±	−	−
	Actinomycin D	+	±	+	−	−
	AD, DR, N^6-benzyladenosine	+	±	+	−	−
4	Cycloheximide, puromycin	+	+	+	−	−
5	CB, colchicine, VCR	+	+	+	+	−
	Levamisole	+	+	±	+	−
6	Prednisolone, BCNU, acridine derivative	+	+	+	+	±
7	IPAR	S‡, ±	+	S‡, ±	±	−

Values are reprinted from Ehrke *et al*. (1978) by permission of Cancer Research, Inc. (The acridine derivative listed is 4′-(9-acridinyl-amino)methane sulphon-*m*-anisidide methanesulphonate salt.)

*Range of molarity tested: 2-deoxyglucose 5×10^{-3}–10^{-5}; Prednisolone 5×10^{-3}–10^{-6}; Levamisole and N^6-benzyladenosine 10^{-3}–10^{-5}; MTX, Bleomycin and IPAR 10^{-3}–5×10^{-6}; Colchicine 10^{-3}–10^{-6}; FUdR, DTIC, Ara C, Hydroxyurea, Procarbazine and Streptozotocin 5×10^{-4}–5×10^{-6}; BCNU 5×10^{-4}–10^{-6}; AD, Actinomycin D and acridine derivative 10^{-4}–10^{-6}; Puromycin and Vincristine 10^{-4}–5×10^{-7}; Cycloheximide 10^{-4}–10^{-8}; DR 5×10^{-5}–$5 \times$ CB 5×10^{-5}–10^{-7}; Maytensine 10^{-6}–10^{-11}.

†Assay conditions are as given for table 2.2.
‡−Indicates no effect; ± indicates significant inhibition but the highest drug concentration tested did not reduce the value obtained to lower than 50 per cent of control; + indicates inhibition to values lower than 50 per cent of controls; and S indicates stimulation of response.

CICC), (c) killer cells-dependent phenomena (ADCC and CICC) and (d) phago-cytosis (ADCC-Phg and CICC-Phg). The effects of the seven groups of drugs need to be interpreted in the light of these four basic sets of functions.

The six anticancer agents in group 1 exert some type of immunosuppressive action *in vivo* (Gerebtzoff *et al.*, 1972; Hersh, 1974) and inhibit DNA synthesis albeit at different metabolic levels. DNA synthesis is not expected to be an essential factor in the implementation of the preformed effector functions studied and therefore it may not be too surprising that these agents had no effect.

Maytensine and MTX inhibited CICC-Phg only. This effect did not seem to affect phagocytic function *per se* because when the target cells were precoated with antibody (ADCC-Phg), no inhibition was seen. Antibody production, excretions or binding to target cells may represent the site of action even though the CICC was not affected. It is also possible that macrophage functions in non-sensitised spleen (as tested with ADCC-Phg) and in sensitised spleen (as tested with CICC-Phg) are different, and that this accounts for the differences in sensitivity to these two drugs.

The six agents in group 3 inhibited ADCC-Phg and CICC-Phg and, to a much lesser degree, CICC. They did not affect ADCC. The addition of heat-inactivated, day 11 anti-SRBC antiserum to the CICC prevented the effects on CICC (results not shown). This prevention, and the lack of effect on ADCC, suggest that the inhibition of the CICC by these agents is based on effects on antibody production or secretion from AFC and not on antibody binding to target cells. The effects on phagocytic functions, however, must also involve a direct action on phagocytic cells because the ADCC-Phg was inhibited and this inhibition was slightly less than that of the CICC-Phg.

The two protein inhibitors in group 4 inhibited markedly the three tests affected by the agents in group 3. The reason for separating these two agents is that they strongly inhibited the CICC. Although antibody synthesis represents an obvious site of action, the inhibition of ADCC-Phg also in this case implies a direct action on the phagocytic cell. The lack of inhibition of the CDCC further supports the conclusion that in this test antibody is preformed at the time the effector cell is incubated with the target cell (Mawas *et al.*, 1973).

The four agents in group 5 inhibited all the tests, except in CDCC. Three of these agents are known to interact with microtubules or microfilaments and these interactions probably lead to impairment in cell motility and changes in cyto-logical appearance (Creasey, 1975). The other drug, levamisole, has also been reported to affect cell motility and it has been postulated that microtubule assembly may be the site involved (Anderson *et al.*, 1976). Therefore a basic common pattern of cellular action seems to tie these agents within a group and may be related to the effects on immune effector functions observed.

The three agents in group 6 inhibited all the tests, possibly through non-specific toxicity. It should be stressed, however, that no non-specific lysis of the target cells was observed. Also, because it has been suggested that preformed antibody is released in the CDCC assay, it might be argued that only antibody present on the surface of AFCs could be released even if the secreting cells were damaged by an agent. Indeed the CDCC was not inhibited to less than 50 per cent of control values by these drugs.

N^6-Isopentenyladenosine was the only agent that caused an augmenting effect, namely the augmentation in the phagocytosis tests. This compound has been shown to accumulate at the plasma membrane and to affect the transport of uridine and cytosine (Hakala *et al.*, 1975). This accumulation of the drug in the membrane may be related to the effects seen.

The results outlined above clearly indicate that several agents may exert a selective action on certain preformed effector functions, and not on others, within the heterogeneous spleen cell population involved in the responses to SRBCs. Moreover, no correlation is readily apparent between reputedly known proximal site of biochemical action and selectivity of drug effect, nor between antiproliferative action and selective effects on effector cells. The selectivity of action on effector cell functions, demonstrated *in vitro*, provides a set of examples that may have a counterpart in the sensitivity of effector functions *in vivo*.

EFFECTS OF PROCARBAZINE ON THE DEVELOPMENT OF T-CELL EFFECTORS AGAINST ALLOGENEIC TUMOUR CELLS

C57BL/6J mice inoculated i.p. with 3×10^7 washed P815 cells develop humoral and cellular immune responses, which are measured by using spleen cells as effectors. The CDCC assay developed in this laboratory (Mawas *et al.*, 1973) measures the humoral response, whereas the CICC assay measures the cell-bound response. It should be stressed that against allogeneic tumour cells the CICC measures a T-cell effector response, in contrast with the CICC against SRBCs discussed in the preceding sections.

In this system the CDCC reaches a peak on days 5 or 6 and terminates around day 10; the CICC reaches a peak around day 12 and decreases by day 14. The effects of procarbazine were examined in these two systems (Hoffmann *et al.*, 1978) and the CDCC and CICC were measured on days 5 and 10 respectively. The drug was given at doses ranging from 100 to 400 mg/kg as a single i.p. or i.v. (intravenous) injection given on days 0, 1, 2, 4, 6 or 8 after immunisation. When the drug was given on days 0 or 1, there was little or no inhibition of the CICC response at non-toxic doses, and the inhibition was maximal when the drug was given on days 4 or 6. When the drug was given on day 8, the CICC was not inhibited as much with respect to day 10 controls, but it was indeed blocked at a level similar to that reached in the controls on day 8. The inhibitory effects were dose-dependent. In contrast with the unusual time-dependence for maximal inhibition of the CICC by procarbazine, cyclophosphamide at doses of 75 and 150 mg/kg i.p. inhibited this response maximally regardless of day of administration. This inhibition was possibly related to general lymphotoxicity as shown by reduction in spleen size and cell numbers. Daunorubicin inhibited the CICC maximally when given on day 2, at a number of doses ranging from slightly active to slightly toxic. Thus, in contrast with the two agents chosen for comparison and with the majority of drugs tested by others in similar systems, procarbazine appears to have little effect during the early stages of sensitisation of the CICC response. It seems reasonable to assume on the basis of the time of maximal inhibition that at non-toxic doses procarbazine inhibits primarily the proliferation of precursor T-effector cells. The lack of measurable effects of procarbazine on the CICC when the drug is given on days 0 or 1 should be contrasted with its inhibitory effects on the CDCC at the same time.

The example provided by procarbazine indicates the possibility that certain anti-cancer agents may inhibit selectively T-effector cell-dependent responses at sites beyond the stage of early sensitisation, which is notoriously sensitive to the majority of the immunosuppressive drugs studied. This also implies the possibility that drugs affect ongoing responses against established tumours.

CONCLUDING REMARKS

As mentioned initially, the study of the selectivity of action of anticancer agents represents one of the major approaches followed in attempts to improve the design of optimal treatments with available drugs used alone or in combination. Should it prove possible to reduce the toxicity of an effective anticancer agent to normal tissues without altering its antitumour potency, major therapeutic advantages might be achieved. Among the normal tissues frequently affected by anticancer agents are those involved in the development and functions of host defense. Indeed immunosuppression represents a major untoward effect in cancer chemotherapy and in some cases may drastically limit the usefulness of a treatment and may lead to such secondary effects as the development of severe opportunistic infections. If host mechanisms of defense do operate against human tumours and if they are instrumental in determining the outcome of certain chemotherapeutic treatments, the therapy-limiting effects of drug-induced immunosuppression will be only too apparent.

Anticancer and antiproliferative agents may exert specific selective effects on the development and functions of the various components of the immune response. This would be expected on theoretical grounds because data obtained primarily in tumour and other non-immune systems indicate that multiple biochemical and pharmacological determinants of drug action are different in different cell types and in the same cell type at different functional stages. Therefore it should not be too surprising that in recent years several examples of selectivity of drug action within the immune system have been obtained in a variety of experimental systems. Some of the observations recently made in this laboratory have been discussed.

As suggested by the example provided by MTX plus CF rescue, the early stages of certain immune responses may be under stringent restrictions in terms of the metabolic requirements, which are probably derived from the need to synthesise DNA in the face of a relatively rapid utilisation of small intracellular pools of essential cofactors and metabolites. In contrast, DNA synthesis is probably irrelevant to the function of preformed effectors, where the unique selectivity of drug action may nevertheless be found to be based on different biochemical and pharmacological mechanisms. The example provided by MGBG indicates that good correlations may exist between the selectivity of drug action on the develop-ment of certain immune effectors and the specificity of cellular effects in terms of drug uptake or inhibition of a target enzyme. The initial study of the effects of procarbazine suggests that this agent, unlike many anticancer drugs, is substantially more effective on proliferating T-cell effectors and precursors than on the cells involved in the early stages of this response.

Whereas examples of selectivity of drug action in the immune system may be expected to be found in greater numbers in the foreseeable future, it becomes increasingly important to identify the specific cellular and biochemical basis for these effects and to relate them to the mechanisms of regulation and control of the immune responses. It is indeed likely that a drug may have different effects on a strictly regulated and dynamic multicellular system such as the immune response, depending not only on its pharmacological characteristics and the parameters of dose, regimen and time of treatment, but also on the functional status of the often opposing mechanisms of regulation operating in the target system. This functional status may depend on specific relationships among cells and on specific biochemical phenomena in these cells, which in turn may be determinants of drug action. The clarification of the mechanisms of controls within the immune system and their definition in metabolic terms may in time provide opportunities for a pharmacological intervention aimed at causing therapeutically favourable modulations of the immune responses.

REFERENCES

Anderson, R., Glover, A., Koornhof, H. J. and Rabson, A. R. (1976). *J. Immun.*, 117, 428
Avery, W. K. (1976). *Ann. N. Y. Acad. Sci.*, 277, 260
Bennett, J., Ehrke, J., Dave, C. and Mihich, E. (1977). *Biochem. Pharmac.*, 26, 723
Bennett, J., Ehrke, J., Fadale, P., Dave, C. and Mihich, E. (1978). *Biochem. Pharmac.*, (in press)
Berenbaum, M. C. (1964). *Lancet*, ii, 1363
Berenbaum, M. C. and Brown, I. N. (1965). *Immunology*, 8, 251
Bertino, J. R. (1975). In *Antineoplastic and Immunosuppressive Agents II*, (eds. A. C. Sartorelli and D. G. Johns), Springer-Verlag, New York
Chanmougan, D. and Schwartz, R. S. (1966). *J. exp. Med.*, 124, 363
Cohen, S. A., Ehrke, M. J. and Mihich, E. (1975). *J. Immun.*, 115, 1007
Corti, A., Dave, C., Williams-Ashman, H. G., Mihich, E. and Schenone, A. (1974). *Biochem. J.*, 139, 351
Creasey, W. A. (1975). In *Antineoplastic and Immunosuppressive Agents II*, (eds. A. C. Sartorelli and D. G. Johns), Springer-Verlag, New York
Dave, C. and Mihich, E. (1972). *Biochem. Pharmac.*, 21, 2681
Ehrke, M. J., Cohen, S. A. and Mihich, E. (1978). *Cancer Res.*, 38, 521
Frei, E. III, Jaffe, N., Tattersall, M. H. N., Pitman, S. and Parker, L. (1975). *New Engl. J. Med.*, 292, 846
Friedman, R. M., Baron, S. and Buckler, C. (1962). *Blood*, 20, 115
Gerebtzoff, A., Lambert, P. H. and Miescher, P. A. (1972). *A. Rev. Pharmac.*, 12, 287
Glynn, J. P., Bianco, A. R. and Goldin, A. (1963). *Nature*, 198, 1003
Goldin, A. and Mantel, N. (1957). *Cancer Res.*, 17, 635
Griswold, D. E., Heppner, G. H. and Calabresi, P. (1972). *Cancer Res.*, 32, 298
Hakala, M. T., Slocum, H. K. and Gryko, G. J. (1975). *J. cell. Physiol.*, 86, 281
Heppner, G. H. and Calabresi, P. (1972). *J. natn. Cancer Inst.*, 48, 1161
Hersey, P. (1973). *Transplantation*, 15, 282
Hersh, E. M. (1973). In *Cancer Medicine*, (eds. J. F. Holland and E. Frei III), Lea and Febiger, Philadelphia
Hersh, E. M. (1974). In *Antineoplastic and Immunosuppressive Agents* I, (eds. A. C. Sartorelli and D. G. Johns), Springer-Verlag, New York
Hoffmann, C. C., Ehrke, M. J. and Mihich, E. (1978). *Proc. Am. Ass. Cancer Res.*, 19, 221
Jerne, N. K. and Nordin, A. A. (1963). *Science*, 140, 405
Klein, G. (1966). *A. Rev. Microbiol.*, 20, 223
Levin, R. H., Henderson, E., Koryn, M. and Freireich, E. J. (1965). *Clin. Pharmac. Ther.*, 6, 31
Levitt, M., Mosher, M. B., DeConti, R. C., Farber, L. R., Skeel, R. T., Marsh, J. C., Mitchell, M. S., Papac, R. J., Thomas, E. D. and Bertino, J. R. (1973). *Cancer Res.*, 33, 1729
Lochte, H. L. Jr., Levy, A. S., Guenther, D. M., Thomas, E. D. and Ferrebee, J. W. (1962). *Nature*, 196, 1110

MacLennan, I. C. M. (1973). *Contemp. Top. Immunobiol.*, **2**, 175
Makinodan, T., Santos, G. W. and Quinn, R. P. (1970). *A. Pharmac. Rev.*, **22**, 189
Mantovani, A., Tagliabue, A., Vecchi, A. and Spreafico, F. (1976). *Eur. J. Cancer*, **12**, 381
Mawas, C., Carey, T. and Mihich, E. (1973). *Cell. Immun.*, **6**, 243
Medzihradsky, J., Ehrke, J. and Mihich, E. (1977). *Biochem. Pharmac.*, **26**, 203
Mihich, E. (1963). *Cancer Res.*, **23**, 1375
Mihich, E. (1965). *Archivio Italiano di Patologia e Clinica Dei Tumori*, **8**, 153
Mihich, E. (1971). In *Prediction of Response in Cancer Chemotherapy and Immunity*,
   (ed. T. C. Hall), NCI Monograph 34, U.S. Government Printing Office
Mihich, E. (1975*a*). *Transplant. Proc.*, **7**, 275
Mihich, E. (1975*b*) In *Antineoplastic and Immunosuppressive Agents*, (eds. A. Sartorelli and
   D. Johns), Springer-Verlag, New York
Mihich, E. (1976). In *Chemotherapy*, (eds. K. Hellmann and T. A. Connors) Vol. 7, Plenum
   Publishing Corp. New York
Mihich, E. (1978*a*). *Monograph of First National Course of Chemotherapy of Solid Tumor*,
   Bologna, Italy, (ed. F. Pannuti), Editrice Universitaria Bolognese, pp. 143–180
Mihich, E. (1978*b*). *Proc. of 7th International Symposium on the Biological Characterization
   of Human Tumours*, Budapest, Hungary, Excerpta Medica, Amsterdam, (in press)
Mihich, E. and Grindey, G. (1977). *Cancer*, **40**, 534
Mihich, E., Dave, C. and Williams-Ashman, H. G. (1974). In *Proceeding 8th International
   Congress of Chemotherapy*, (ed. G. K. Daikos) Vol. 3, 845
Mihich, E., Laurence, D. J. R., Laurence, D. M. and Eckhardt, S. (1976). *UICC Technical
   Rept.*, Vol. 21, Geneva
Moran, R. G., Domin, B. A. and Zakrzewski, S. F. (1975). *Proc. Am. Ass. Cancer Res.*, **16**, 49
Orsini, F., Pavelic, Z. and Mihich, E. (1977). *Cancer Res.*, **37**, 1719
Pegg, A. E. (1973). *Biochem. J.*, **132**, 537
Pegg, A. E., Corti, A. and Williams-Ashman, H. G. (1973). *Biochem. Biophys. Res. Commun.*,
   52, 696
Perlmann, P. and Perlmann, H. (1970). *Cell. Immun.*, **1**, 300
Prehn, R. T. (1968). *Cancer Res.*, **28**, 1326
Rustum, Y. M., Grindey, G. B., Hakala, M. T. and Mihich, E. (1976). In *Advances in Enzyme
   Regulation*, (ed. G. Weber) **14**, Pergamon Press, New York and Oxford
Schwartz, H. S. and Mihich, E. (1973). In *Drug Resistance and Selectivity: Biochemical and
   Cellular Basis*, (ed. E. Mihich), Academic Press, New York
Swanson, M. A. and Schwartz, R. S. (1967). *New Engl. J. Med.*, **277**, 163
Turk, J. L. (1973). *Proc. R. Soc. Med.*, **66**, 805
Uy, Q. L., Srinivasan, T., Santos, G. W. and Owens, A. H., Jr. (1966). *Expl Hemat.*, **10**, 4
Weiss, D. W. (1969). *Cancer Res.*, **29**, 2368
Werkheiser, W. C. (1961). *J. biol. Chem.*, **236**, 888
Williams-Ashman, H. G. and Schenone, A. (1972). *Biochim. Biophys. Res. Commun.*, **46**, 288
Zakrzewski, S. F. and Nichol, C. A. (1958). *Biochim. Biophys. Acta*, **27**, 425

3

The effects of penicillamine and
other thiols on lymphoid cells

G. Harris and D. Hutchins (Division of Experimental Pathology,
Kennedy Institute of Rheumatology, Bute Gardens, London W6 7DW, U.K.)

INTRODUCTION

D-Penicillamine (D-PAm, β,β-dimethyl-D-cysteine) is now widely used to treat
rheumatoid arthritis (Hill, 1977). Although its efficacy in inducing remissions is not
in doubt, its mode of action is still unknown. The ability of D-PAm to chelate
copper and other heavy metals is the basis for its use in Wilson's disease and in lead
poisoning, but there is no evidence that this has any relevance to its therapeutic
effect in rheumatoid arthritis.

The present studies were on the effects of D-PAm and other thiols on lymphoid
cells and tissues in different cultural conditions. Since lymphoid-tissue function and
its disorder play a central though ill-defined role in the pathogenesis of inflammatory conditions such as rheumatoid arthritis, the important action of D-PAm may
be on lymphoid cells. The results obtained indicate that PAm, like other thiols,
can modulate lymphoid cell functions *in vitro* in a manner that may be related to
effects *in vivo*. Support for this was sought by studies of the action of D-PAm in
intact mice of various strains.

EXPERIMENTAL

Source of lymphocytes for culture

The spleens of CBA mice, 2–3 months old of either sex, reared at the Kennedy
Institute, were used to prepare single-cell suspensions, which were cultured as
described previously (Harris and Olsen, 1976).

Organ cultures were prepared from the spleens of New Zealand White rabbits
obtained commercially, and immunised with sheep erythrocytes (SRBCs) at
least 2 months before being killed (Harris, 1973).

Media

RPMI 1640 medium, supplemented with 5 per cent foetal calf serum (FCS; Flow
Laboratories, Irvine, Scotland), was used for culture, in duplicate, of mouse spleen
cell suspensions, either in 1 ml, 2×10^6 cells (flat-bottomed plastic vials;

Sterilin Ltd., London), or in 5 ml, 1×10^6 cells/ml (25 ml, glass universals). Eagle's minimum essential medium (MEM) was used in experiments on amino acid deprivation of the cultures. Cells were harvested in ice-cold phosphate-buffered saline (PBS), containing 2 per cent FCS. This was particularly important for cultures in serum-free medium, to ensure minimal cell losses during removal of cells from culture vessels and their centrifugation.

Table 3.1   Amino acids present in explant culture medium

Amino acids	
Non-essential	Essential
Glycine*	Threonine
Alanine	Valine
Serine*	Leucine
Aspartic acid	Isoleucine
Glutamic acid	Methionine → cysteine, cystine
Proline	Phenylalanine → tyrosine
Hydroxyproline	Histidine
Asparagine	Tryptophan
	Lysine
	Arginine

*Absent from the original Eagle's MEM

Eagle's MEM, supplemented with folic acid (10 μg/ml), hydrocortisone (5 μg/ml), glutamine (2mM), amino acids (as in table 3.1), and 10 per cent FCS was used for the culture of rabbit spleen explants (Harris, 1973). This involved culturing 5×1mm fragments of rabbit spleen in 30 mm plastic dishes (Sterilin) in 1 ml of medium containing 2×10^5 thrice-washed SRBCs. During incubation, active migration of cells from the tissue into the medium occurred, and these cells always contained the majority of cells producing antibody to SRBCs. For optimal responses, the medium required changing daily, SRBCs being continuously present. The migrating population (outgrowth) was collected daily for measurement of the immune response to SRBCs by the specific haemolytic plaque assay (Jerne and Nordin, 1963). All results given are the means of duplicate or triplicate cultures.

Concanavalin A (Con A; Sigma, London) was used to stimulate mouse spleen cells in culture. It was stored at $-20\ ^\circ$C and added to cultures at final concentrations of 3–4 μg/ml.

D-PAm was obtained as the free base or hydrochloride salt (D-PAm HCl) from various sources, including Beecham Pharmaceuticals, Sigma and Aldrich chemical companies. It was stored desiccated at 4 $^\circ$C. A stock solution (67 mM, equivalent to 10 mg of the free base/ml) in PBS, pH 7.0, was freshly prepared for each experiment, and diluted with PBS to enable the requisite amount to be added to the appropriate cultures in 50 μl portions. Other thiols, including 2-mercaptoethanol (2-ME), were handled in the same manner. For injection of mice, D-PAm HCl was first neutralised with sodium bicarbonate and diluted as required in saline immediately before i.p. (intraperitoneal) administration.

L-Cystine (BDH) solutions were prepared by dissolving the free base initially in 1M hydrochloric acid, followed by dilution as appropriate, such that the final acid concentration was 35–50mM. Cystine and cysteine refer to the L-forms of these two amino acids in these studies.

Animals
CBA, NZB × NZW F_1 hybrids (BW) and AKR mice were all reared at the Kennedy Institute.

Radioactively labelled precursors
Methyl-T [^{3}H] thymidine (15–21 Ci/mmol), [^{3}H] 5,6-uridine (46 Ci/mmol) and [^{3}H] 4,5-leucine (40 Ci/mmol) were obtained from The Radiochemical Centre, Amersham. The amounts used are given in the text, unlabelled precursors being added to the radioactively labelled ones as required. The estimation of uptake of these precursors into cells has been described in full (Harris, 1973). The results are presented as trichloroacetic acid (TCA)-precipitable counts per minute per 10^6 cells or per culture, and are the means of duplicate or triplicate cultures. All counts of cell numbers were done microscopically in a haemocytometer.

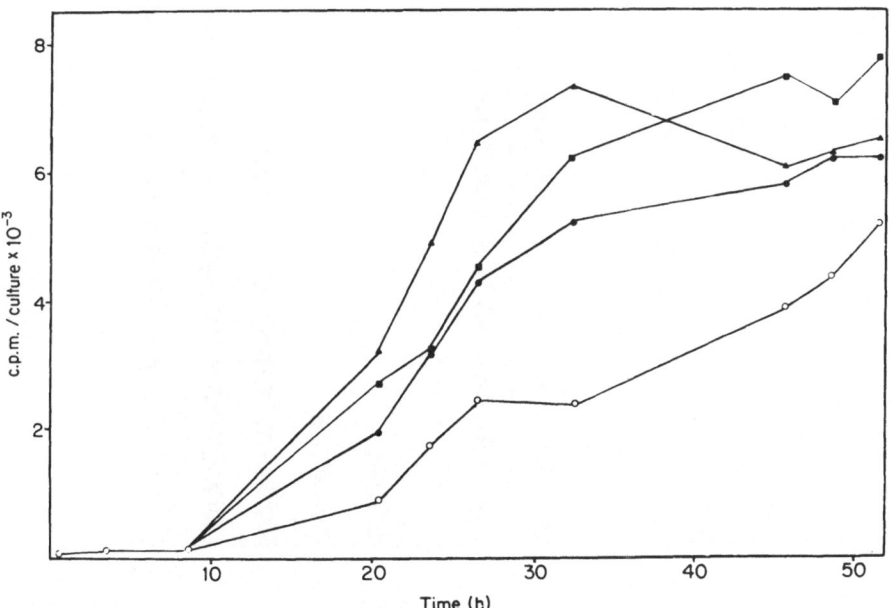

Figure 3.1   Con A-stimulated mouse spleen lymphocytes: effect of 2-mercaptoethanol on [^{3}H] thymidine incorporation in 1 ml cultures. Mouse spleen cells (2 × 10^6) were cultured in 1 ml of RPMI 1640 medium in the presence of Con A (4 µg/ml) and 2-ME was added initially at the concentrations indicated. The rate of incorporation of [^{3}H] thymidine (2 µCi/ml, 10 µM) was measured during 1 h periods at the times of culture shown as cpm/ culture. 2-ME concentrations: o—o, none; ●—●, 5 µM; ▲—▲, 50 µM; ■—■, 500 µM.

MOUSE SPLEEN CULTURES

The effects of D-PAm on the rate of incorporation of [³H] thymidine into DNA-synthesising mouse spleen lymphocytes stimulated by Con A in culture has been described in some detail (Kendall and Hutchins, 1976, 1978). This thiol compound had an immediate enhancing effect followed by profound inhibition of DNA synthesis by the stimulated cells. It was concluded that, in these cultures, D-PAm had altered the cultural environment particularly with regard to the availability of cystine in the medium, the inhibitory action resulting from the withdrawal of this amino acid from the cells by the formation of a mixed disulphide of D-PAm with cysteine.

In view of these reported effects of D-PAm, another thiol, 2-ME, was studied in 1 ml cultures of mouse spleen cells, as shown in figure 3.1. The rate of incorporation of [³H] thymidine was enhanced by 2-ME above the level of cells

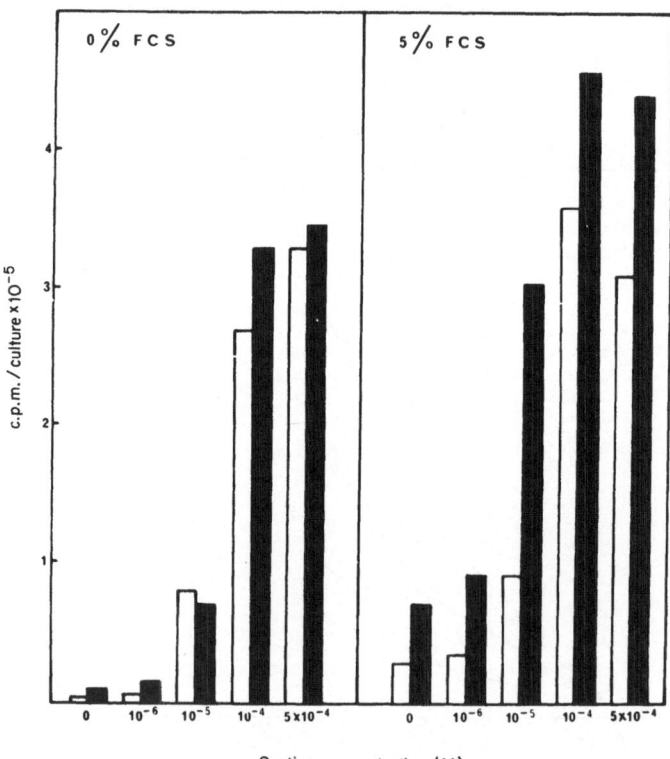

Cystine concentration (M)

Figure 3.2 Con A-stimulated mouse spleen lymphocytes: cysteine requirements in the presence and absence of FCS. Con A-stimulated mouse spleen cells were cultured for 40 h as in figure 3.1. After washing, 1×10^6 cells/ml were re-cultured in the presence or absence of 5 per cent FCS, using Eagle's MEM containing various amounts of cystine. The uptake of [³H] thymidine (2 μCi/ml, 0.1 μM) was measured as c.p.m./culture during 66–70 h of culture. □, Without 2-ME; ■, 50 μM 2-ME.

cultured with Con A alone, at all times studied and in a dose-dependent manner.

The importance of cystine for these cultures was studied, in the presence or absence of FCS, as shown in figure 3.2. Without FCS, 2-ME did not significantly influence this response to Con A, which was clearly dependent on the presence of adequate amounts of cystine ($> 10 \mu M$). When FCS was present in the medium, 2-ME corrected the deleterious effect of cystine deficiency on the uptake of [^{3}H] thymidine by the cultures, particularly when more than 1 μM cystine was present. In contrast to D-PAm, 2-ME did not produce cystine deficiency, but actually corrected its effects.

The effects of three different reducing agents on cystine-free cultures of mouse spleen cells stimulated with Con A in the presence of various amounts of FCS are shown in figure 3.3. Here [^{3}H] thymidine incorporation was measured at 60 h of culture. Both 2-ME and sodium sulphite (Na_2SO_3) enhanced the response to Con A significantly when FCS, but no added cystine, was present in the culture medium. The thiol reagent, dithiothreitol (DTT) was unexpectedly ineffective in this respect.

Harris and Olsen (1976) showed that cell division was suppressed in 1 ml cultures

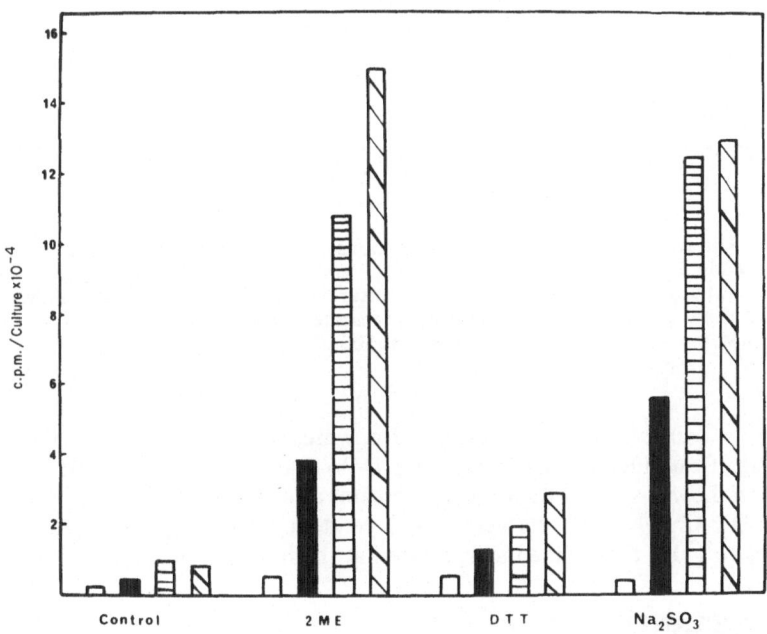

Figure 3.3 The influence of FCS on the response of mouse lymphocytes to Con A. Mouse spleen cells were cultured as in figure 3.2. After washing, the cells were continued in culture, using Eagle's MEM without cystine but with various amounts of FCS. The three reducing agents used were added at 50 μM to the washed cultures and the uptake of [^{3}H] thymidine (2 $\mu Ci/ml$, 0.1 μM) was measured as cpm/culture during 60–64 h of culture. FCS: $\square$, 0%; $\blacksquare$, 5%; $\boxminus$, 10%; $\boxtimes$, 15%.

of mouse spleen cells stimulated with Con A. In contrast, active cell growth occurred when the culture volume was increased to 5 ml. The effect of 2-ME on cells numbers in such cultures is shown in figure 3.4, 50 μM being optimal. The results showed that the most striking effects of 2-ME on lymphocyte growth

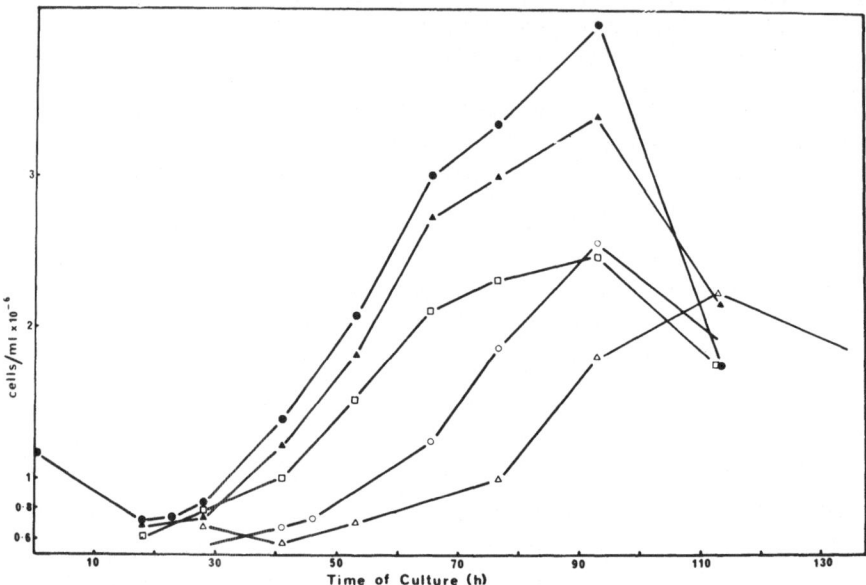

Figure 3.4   The effect of 2-mercaptoethanol on mouse spleen cultures. Mouse spleen cells were cultured in 5 ml volumes at 1×10^6/ml in the presence of Con A (4 μg/ml) and 2-ME, both added initially. The number of cells/ml of culture were counted at the times shown and are the means of triplicate cultures counted separately. 2-ME concentrations: △—△, none; ○—○, 0.5 μM; □—□, 5 μM; ▲—▲, 50 μM; ●—●, 500 μM.

occurred between 24 and 80 h of culture, after which cultures without 2-ME also showed significant increase of cell numbers. D-PAm and 2-ME were compared (figure 3.5), which showed that 2-ME produced a greater rate of DNA synthesis and cell division than D-PAm. These effects were dose-dependent, both compounds being inhibitory to [³H] thymidine incorporation at the higher concentrations used.

ORGAN EXPLANTS

In view of these findings, which suggested that cystine, probably in its reduced form cysteine, played an intrinisic role in the action of various thiols on the mouse spleen cell cultures, the effect of these agents on the immune response of organ cultures of rabbit spleen was studied. The amino acids present in the medium used to culture the explants are shown in table 3.1. The requirements of these cultures for essential and non-essential amino acids are indicated in table 3.2. Serum is source of free

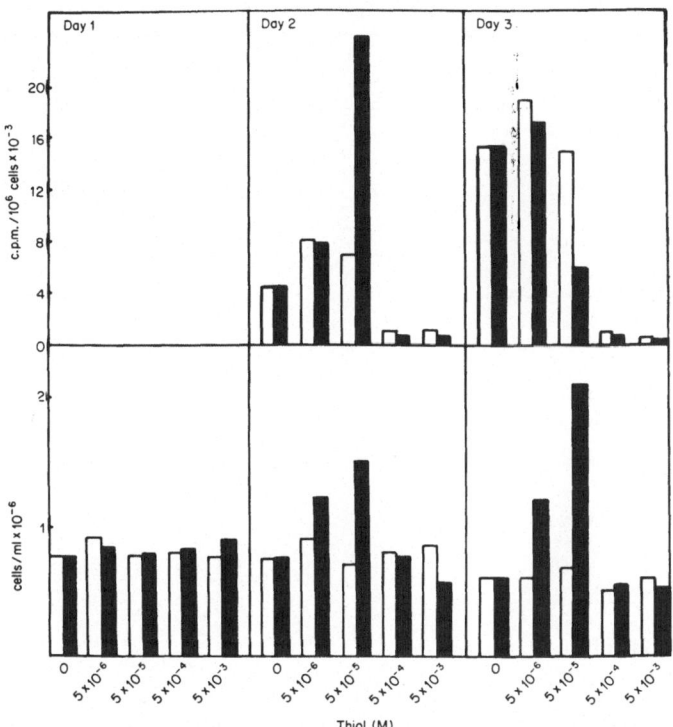

Figure 3.5 The effect of thiols on proliferation and DNA synthesis in mouse spleen culture. 2-ME and D-PAm were added initially as shown to 5 ml cultures of Con A-stimulated mouse spleen cells. The uptake of [^{3}H] thymidine (1 μCi/ml, 10 μM) was measured during 1 h periods on the days of culture indicated and are given as c.p.m./10^6 cells harvested. The cell numbers were estimated as cells/ml of culture on the days indicated. □, D-PAm; ▪, 2-ME.

amino acids (Piez *et al.*, 1960) and this could have been responsible for the partial retention of the response to SRBCs shown here in amino acid-deficient medium, 10 per cent serum supplying 10μM leucine to the cultures. The absence of cystine caused the greatest depression of this response to SRBCs.

As shown in table 3.3, 0.1 mM cystine was required for an optimal response of the explants to SRBCs, measured on days 2 and 3 of culture. The effects of cystine deficiency were significantly corrected by the presence of 2-ME. A more detailed analysis of the effects of absence of different amino acids from the medium from 24 to 72 h of culture, in the presence or absence of 2-ME, is shown in figure 3.6. These results confirmed that both cystine and glutamine were the most essential for the response of the cultures to SRBCs and that their deficiency was corrected by 2-ME. The response of explants to SRBCs, cultured in full medium, was also enhanced by the presence of 2-ME in this experiment.

The influence of various reducing and anti-oxidant agents on the response of explants to SRBCs is shown in figure 3.7. The different agents used, including

Table 3.2   Amino acid requirements of rabbit spleen explants

	Day 3 responses (% of control values)
Essential	4
Leucine	52
Methionine	32
Phenylalanine	26
Cystine	5
All essential amino acids, except for cystine	37
Non-essential	30
Non-essential and cystine	5
All amino acids	17
All amino acids, except for cystine	42

Rabbit spleen explants were cultured in Eagle's MEM with or without amino acids as shown. The responses measured were the PFCs (plaque-forming cells)/10^6 cells migrating from the explants into the medium between 48 and 72 h of culture, calculated as per cent of controls, which were explants cultured in full medium.

Table 3.3   The cystine requirements of rabbit organ explants

	PFCs/10^6 cells			
	Day 1–2		Day 2–3	
Cystine (μM)	+2-ME	−2-ME	+2-ME	−2-ME
0	5 549	2 078	30 126	4 370
5	6 115	2 203	44 488	4 755
50	10 000	2 094	98 947	13 209
100	8 434	7 843	100 666	75 102

Rabbit spleen explants were cultured in the presence of various concentrations of cystine with or without 50 μM 2-ME, as shown. The numbers of PFCs/10^6 cells migrating from the tissues into the medium were estimated at the times of culture shown.

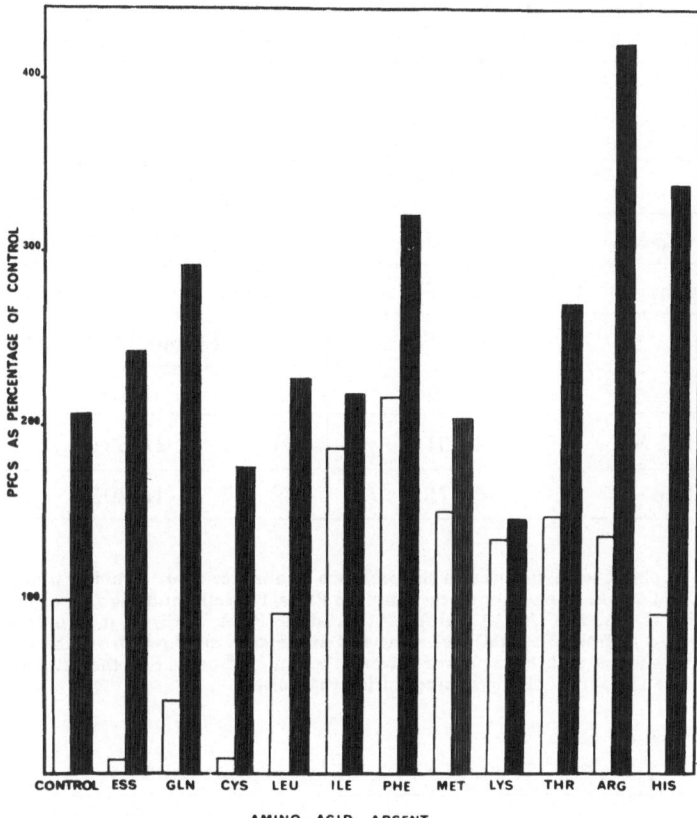

Figure 3.6 Effect of amino acid deprivation on PFC response at 72 h. Rabbit spleen explants were cultured in the presence (▫) or absence (▫) of 50 μM 2-ME in the medium defined as to the presence or absence of amino acids as shown. The numbers of PFCs/10^6 cells in the cells migrating from the explants between 48 and 72 h of culture were estimated. The results are given as per cent of the control values of explants cultured in complete medium in the absence of 2-ME.

D-PAm, enhanced the responses of the cultures to varying degrees, but these effects were influenced by the presence of cystine in the culture medium. 2-ME and glutathione alone prevented the inhibition of these tissues, owing to the absence of cystine in the culture medium. Glutathione was only effective at 0.5 mM, possibly acting as a source of cystine (cysteine).

The influence of 2-ME on the effects of cystine deprivation on the outgrowths of rabbit spleen explants was further studied as shown in table 3.4. In the absence of cystine there was a reduction of the development of antibody-producing cells, most profound on day 3 of culture. To a lesser degree than the development of antibody forming cells, the synthesis of DNA, RNA and proteins was also reduced in the absence of cystine. The addition of 2-ME to these cystine-deprived cultures restored the activities of the migrating cells of the cultures to normal levels.

Table 3.4   Effects of cystine deprivation and 2-ME on
macromolecular synthesis by spleen explants

Treatment	Antibody response (PFCs/10^6 cells)	24–48 h pulse (c.p.m./10^6 cells)		
		DNA	RNA	Protein
No cystine	616	27 900	21 291	9 699
No cystine + 2-ME	1 287	46 766	26 314	10 462
0.1 mM Cystine	1 965	41 030	24 482	14 068
		48–72 h pulse (c.p.m./10^6 cells)		
No cystine	4 660	17 324	8 181	7 440
No cystine + 2-ME	114 901	41 962	16 621	22 745
0.1 mM cystine	66 875	40 392	16 705	18 437

Rabbit spleen explants were cultured in the presence or absence of 0.10 mM cystine, with or without 50 μM 2-ME. The antibody response, as PFCs/10^6 cells, and the rate of uptake of [^{3}H] thymidine (DNA, 2 μCi/ml, 0.1 μM), [^{3}H] uridine (RNA, 2μCi/ml, 0.05 μM), and [^{3}H] leucine (protein, 5 μCi/ml, 0.12 μM) was measured in the cells migrating from the explants during the times shown, and the results are given as c.p.m./10^6 cells. For the estimation of [^{3}H] leucine uptake, leucine-free MEM was used during the pulse.

Table 3.5   The effect of 2-ME on explant cultures

Cystine (μM)	PFCs/10^6 cells at 72 h			
	FCS (%)			
	0		1	
	2-ME (μM)		2-ME (μM)	
	0	50	0	50
0	421	400	812	15 294
0.1	920	923	823	22 790
1	1 310	3 600	975	37 777
10	1 760	9 454	6 941	44 186
100	8 000	6 163	8 000	43 818

Rabbit spleen explants were cultured in the presence of various concentrations of cystine and in the presence or absence of 1 per cent FCS with or without 50 μM 2-ME. The antibody response to SRBCs was measured at 72 h as the PFCs/10^6 cells migrating from the explants into the medium between 48 and 72 h of culture.

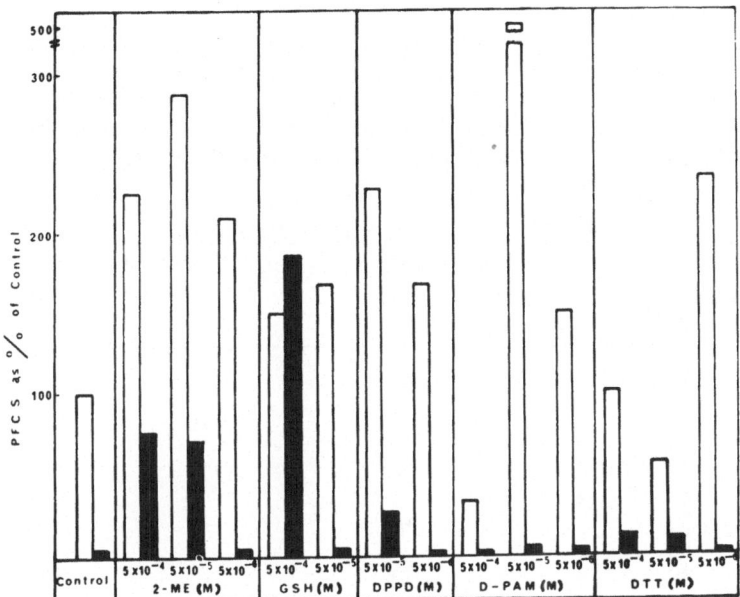

Figure 3.7 Effect of reducing agents and antioxidants on the PFC response at 72 h in rabbit spleen explant cultures. Rabbit spleen explants were cultured in the presence of 2-ME, glutathione (GTH), diphenyl-*p*-phenylenediamine (DPPD), D-PAm, or dithiothreitol (DTT) at the concentrations shown, with or without cystine. The numbers of antibody-producing cells to SRBCs (PFCs) were estimated per 10^6 cells migrating from the tissues between 48 and 72 h of culture. The results are given as per cent of the control values of explants cultured in complete medium in the absence of 2-ME. □, 100 μM cystine, ■, no cystine;

The effects of 2-ME on cystine deprivation in the presence or absence of FCS was studied as shown in table 3.5. In the absence of FCS from the medium, 2-ME did not enhance the response to SRBCs at 72 h of culture until 1 mM cystine was present and when optimal amounts of this amino acid were added, no significant differences from the controls were seen. In contrast, in the presence of only 1 per cent FCS, 2-ME overcame the effect of cystine deprivation and produced enhanced responses above control values when cystine was added to the cultures.

EFFECTS OF D-PAM *IN VIVO*

CBA mice

Mice of this strain were given D-PAm by the i.p. route in doses of 40–400 mg/kg body weight, five times weekly, for periods up to 6 months. The starting age was from before birth, i.e. pregnant mice were given the thiol after conception, and from 3 weeks to 3 months after birth. No embryotoxicity was seen when pregnant mice were given D-PAm, and all treated animals developed normally. No haematological or histological changes have been found in these mice, and their response to SRBCs was unaffected.

Drugs and Immune Responsiveness

NZB × NZW F$_1$ hybrids (BW)

Female mice of this strain have a much shorter life-span than males, owing to the earlier onset and more rapid progression of glomerulonephritis, which results in renal failure. The animals were therefore grouped according to both sex and age for the study of the effects of D-PAm. Table 3.6 shows that D-PAm improved the survival of female BW mice, particularly when treatment was begun at 24 weeks of

Table 3.6   Survival of female BW mice

Survival time (weeks)	Age of commencement of D-PAm* (weeks)			
	Nil †	4	12	24
21	9/10	10/10	9/10	9/9
28	6/10	7/8	7/10	7/9
29	3/10	5/9	5/7	7/8
33	0/10	4/6	–	7/9
40	–	2/6	4/7	7/9
60	–	–	2/5	2/9

*400mg of D-PAm HCL/kg body wt., five times weekly.
†Phosphate-buffered saline, five times weekly from 4 weeks old.

Female BW mice were treated with D-PAm at the ages shown and their survival is given in weeks from birth.

age. The disease process of treated mice was not significantly altered with respect to renal damage and to serum levels of antibodies to DNA and RNA (results not shown). Histological examination of the tissues of BW mice given D-PAm (figure 3.8) showed perivascular lymphoid cell infiltration of their organs, particularly the kidneys, lungs, liver, and to a lesser extent, the heart. Untreated mice showed similar but smaller infiltrates, confined to the kidneys, and occasionally in the lungs, at about 5–6 months in females and at 1 year in males. These perivascular infiltrates were evident in female mice after about 3 weeks treatment even when D-PAm was begun in very young animals. In male mice given D-PAm, the development of these lymphoid infiltrates was slower than in females, but was well marked after about 3 months of treatment, at ages when not found in untreated animals of the same sex.

The most unexpected finding was the occurrence of leukaemia in both male and female BW mice treated with D-PAm. This explains the failure of female mice given D-PAm, beginning at 3 weeks of age, to survive beyond 40 weeks. As shown in table 3.7 both male and female animals developed leukaemia after at least 20 weeks of treatment, whatever the starting age. Leukaemic changes in the blood (figure 3.9) are a relatively late event and the diagnosis was based on histological study of

Table 3.7 The incidence of leukaemia in BW mice given D-PAm

Age D-PAm began (weeks)	Treatment time (weeks)	Leukaemia incidence*			Total cases	
		Age (weeks)	Male	Female	Male	Female
4	20	24	—	1	4/10	5/10
	26	30	2	1		
	29	33	—	1		
	30	34	1	1		
	40	44	1	1		
12	23	35	—	1	2/10	2/10
	41	53	1	—		
	48	60	1	1		
26	31	57	2	—	4/10	2/9
	34	60	1	—		
	38	64	1	1		

*Diagnosis of leukaemia was based on histological changes in spleen, other lymphoid tissues, bone marrow, and on the presence of massive infiltration of liver, lungs and kidneys.

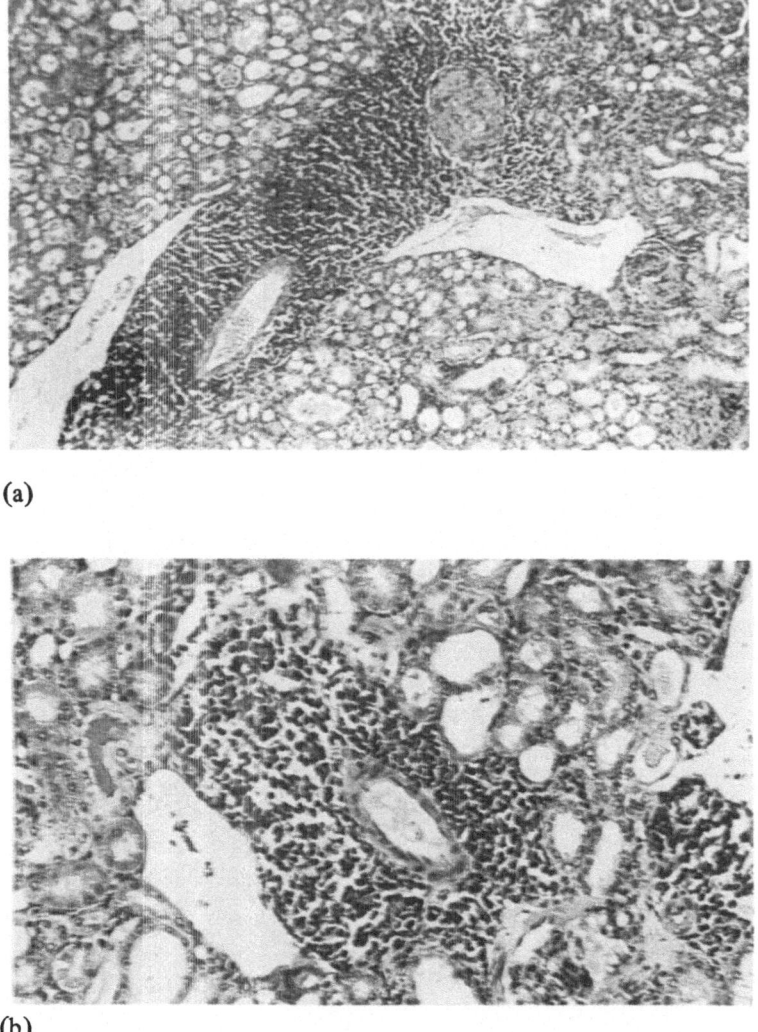

(a)

(b)

Figure 3.8   Section of kidney of a female BW mouse, age 32 weeks, treated with D-PAm for 20 weeks, showing perivascular accumulation of cells. Magnification × 25 (*a*), × 150 (*b*).

the spleen, lymph nodes, thymus and other organs (figure 3.9). When cells from the bone marrow of leukaemic donors were given to nude mice, 30 per cent of the recipients developed the same leukaemic picture as the donor animal after about 6 weeks. Further analysis is needed to clarify the relationship between the cellular infiltration of the organs of non-leukaemic mice and the development of leukaemia.

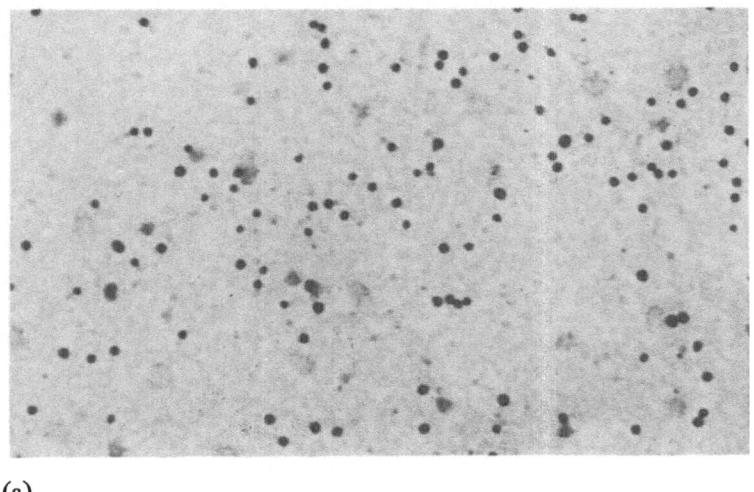

(a)

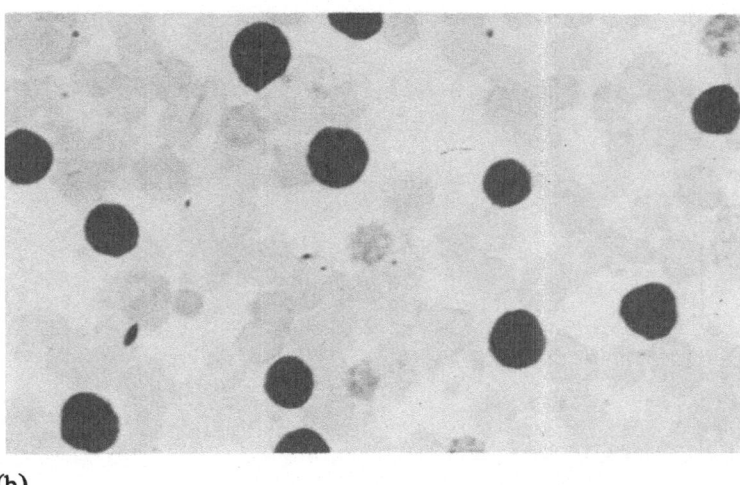

(b)

Figure 3.9 Widespread involvement of the tissues of a female BW mouse, age 26 weeks, with leukaemia after treatment with D-PAm for 22 weeks. Magnifications: (a) peripheral blood ×25 (b) peripheral blood ×250; (c) liver ×25; (d) lung ×25; (e) sternum ×25; (f) kidney ×150.

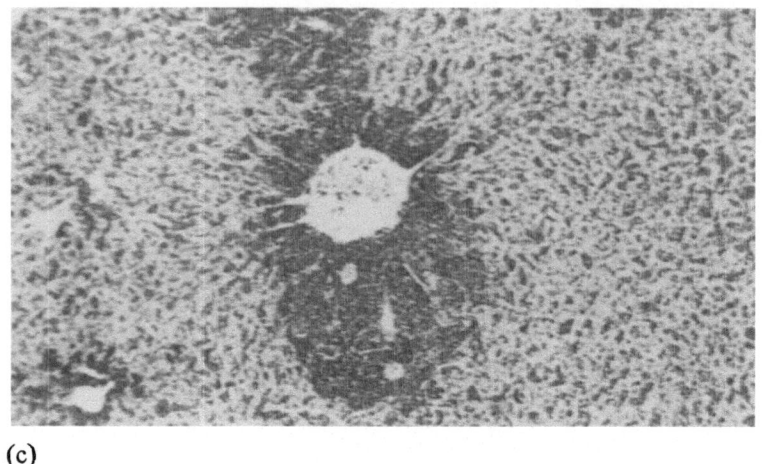

(c)

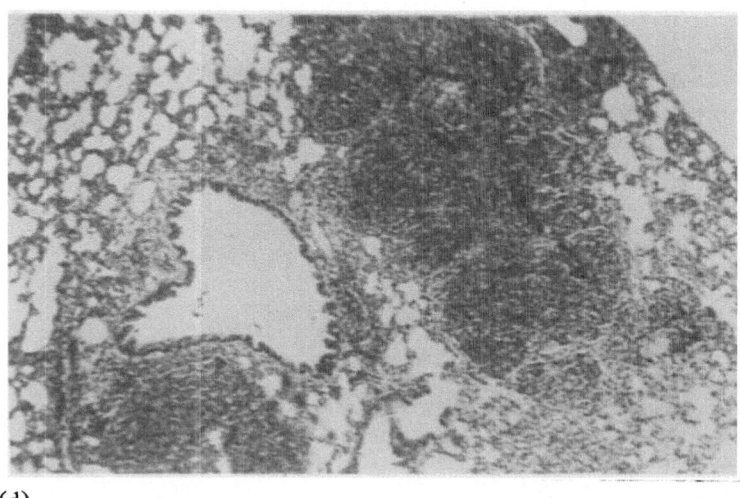

(d)

Figure 3.9 *(cont.)*

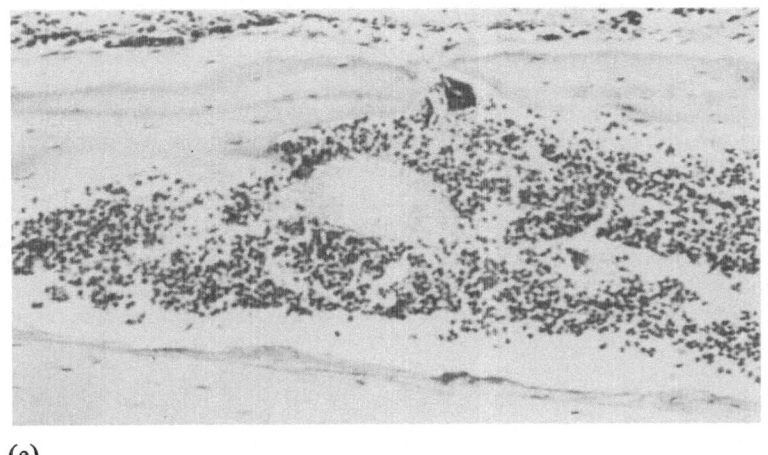

(e)

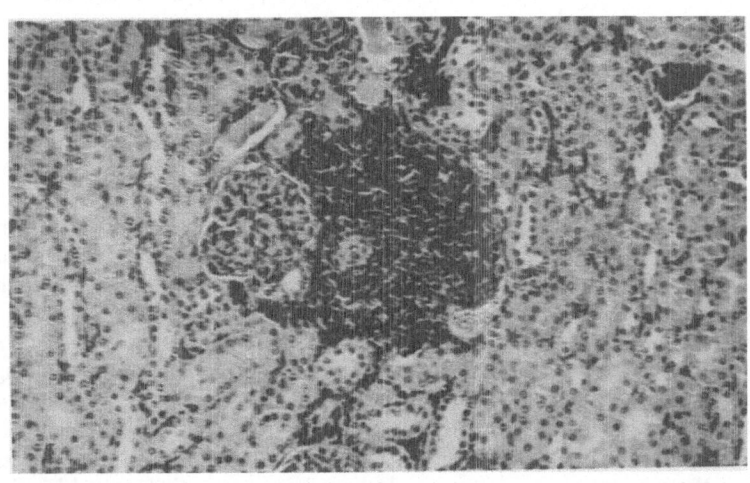

(f)

Figure 3.9 *(cont.)*

AKR mice

At about 6 months of age mice of this strain spontaneously develop lymphoblastic leukaemia, which morphologically resembles that found in the BW mice treated with D-PAm. In the AKR mouse strain the leukaemia is due to a type-C virus (Gillespie *et al.*, 1975) and the tumour is manifest at about 6 months of age in both sexes. When these animals were given D-PAm in the same dosage as the BW and CBA mice, starting at 4 weeks of age, no significant alteration in the development of this leukaemia occurred, with respect to time or nature, indicating that this thiol compound had not apparently influenced the host–virus relationship in this respect.

DISCUSSION

The present results show that thiol compounds can influence the behaviour of lymphoid cells in culture in different ways. In contrast to D-PAm, 2-ME markedly stimulated the growth of mouse lymphocytes responding to Con A. Previous studies of the action of D-PAm on such cells (Kendall and Hutchins, 1978) showed that this thiol could stimulate or inhibit the incorporation of [^{3}H] thymidine depending on its concentration, time of addition to the cultures, and time after addition that the rate of DNA synthesis was estimated.

D-PAm forms mixed disulphides with cysteine and it was suggested (Kendall and Hutchins, 1978) that this interaction resulted in an effective deprivation of the cells of cystine. It was therefore not unexpected to find that D-PAm did not counteract the effects of cystine deprivation of the cultures used here. In contrast, 2-ME could compensate for deficiency of cystine in the media both of mouse spleen suspensions and rabbit spleen explant cultures, provided FCS was present. Cystine, although not necessary for nitrogen balance in man, is essential for many cell lines in culture (Eagle *et al.*, 1958). Serum proteins bind significant amounts of half-cystine residues which can be released in the presence of inorganic reducing agents, containing sulphur, and organic thiol compounds (Eagle *et al.*, 1960). This release of protein-bound half-cystine residues was the explanation given by these authors for the growth-promoting effects of such compounds in cultures using cystine-free medium, supplemented with serum.

Freshly drawn serum contains 40–45 μM free cystine, which becomes protein-bound over a period of days (Eagle *et al.*, 1961). Therefore FCS in the concentrations used in the present experiments would have been potentially capable of contributing a minimum of 2 to 4.5 μM cystine to the culture medium by release of half-cystine residues. The lymphoid cells and tissues cultured here required 0.1 mM cystine for optimal responses to Con A or SRBCs respectively. It was therefore very unlikely that thiols such as 2-ME produced their effects to overcome deficiency of cystine by simply releasing half-cystine residues from the serum proteins present in the culture medium. The restorative effect of 2-ME on glutamine-deficient explant cultures also suggested that other mechanisms might be involved. More detailed studies of the amino acid requirements of these cultures in more fully defined medium are needed to explore this further.

Pulse and chase studies of these explant cultures, using radioactively labelled amino acids, indicate that salvage pathways, involving re-utilisation of amino acids from cellular proteins, could explain their relative independence of exogenous amino acids. The exact mechanism is not clear but involves the turnover of amino acids in an intracellular pool which is not freely exchangeable with the extracellular one of the medium. It is therefore possible that the action of thiols in these cultures could result in improvement of these salvage mechanisms, thus promoting cellular function in deficient conditions of culture.

FCS was necessary for the restorative effect of 2-ME on these cystine-deficient cultures. A direct action of 2-ME on mouse serum proteins resulting in activation of a serum factor necessary for the primary response of mouse spleen cells to SRBCs has been proposed (Opitz *et al.*, 1977). A concentration of 1mM 2-ME was used to treat the serum for these studies. At this concentration 2-ME was toxic when added directly to lymphoid cells in culture in the present studies, the most effective concentrations of 2-ME used being 5–50μM. However, the present results do show that FCS was essential for the enhancement of the cultures by thiol compounds and this could well have resulted from interaction of thiols with serum factors promoting cell functions as well as by release of half-cystine residues bound to serum proteins.

The most striking differences between 2-ME and D-PAm were the lack of effect of the latter thiol compound on the growth of Con A-stimulated mouse spleen cells and its inability, unlike 2-ME, to overcome the effects of the cystine deficiency of the medium of rabbit spleen explants responding to SRBCs. D-PAm had a significant stimulatory effect on the response of these explants to SRBCs when normal concentrations of cystine were present, but did not stimulate the growth of Con A-stimulated cells even in fully supplemented medium. These results suggested that interactions with cystine were of prime importance in determining the ultimate effects of thiol compounds on lymphoid cells in culture.

The potential for growth promotion *in vitro* by specific thiols and disulphides is found with neoplastic lymphoid cells as well as with normal lymphoid cells (Broome and Jeng, 1973). Most results of stimulation of lymphocyte activities by 2-ME and other thiols in culture have been interpreted as being due to their reducing action (see Click *et al.*, 1972). This may not be the complete explanation for these effects, since the disulphides may also be effective (Broome and Jeng, 1973). The situation is, however, complicated by the potential of living cells to reduce disulphides (Cleland, 1964). This might explain the difference of effect of D-PAm on lymphocyte cultures compared with explant cultures, on the basis of the ability of the cells to reduce the appropriate disulphides. Dithiothreitol (DTT) is a thiol that can reduce disulphides completely and should therefore, theoretically, function like 2-ME, for example by releasing half-cystine residues from serum proteins and reducing S–S compounds generally. It does not itself form stable mixed disulphides and would therefore have been expected to correct for cystine deficiency like 2-ME. That this was not the case was perhaps related to a toxic action of DTT, which might occur with sub-optimal concentrations of cystine in the culture medium.

Although the situation in intact animals and man is very different from that of cultures of lymphoid cells and tissues, thiols could have similar effects in both situations. CBA mice, which do not develop overt autoimmune disease like the BW mouse, showed no apparent effects from prolonged treatment with D-PAm, even at high doses. In contrast, treatment with D-PAm, at high doses, prolonged the lifespan of female BW mice. This treatment was associated with marked acceleration and increase of the perivascular accumulation of cells in their kidneys and other tissues in both male and female animals. The exact nature of these cells has not been fully determined but they have the appearance of lymphoid cells and mononuclear phagocytes.

Although it is popularly accepted that lymphocytic infiltration plays a role in the inflammatory process, this may not necessarily be injurious. Lymphocytes may have an important role in the protection of damaged tissues and in their healing, as has been argued elsewhere (Harris, 1978). The stimulation by D-PAm of lymphoid cells from female BW mice could perhaps be directly related to their improved viability as the result of this treatment. Although D-PAm did not significantly affect normal lymphoid tissues of CBA mice, it was possible that the cells infiltrating the organs of the BW animals were in a deleterious environment and were thus amenable to the effects of thiol compounds, as was seen in the deficient cultures using 2-ME.

Rheumatoid arthritis in man is also characterised by lymphocytic accumulations in the affected tissues, such as joint synovium. The ameliorative effects of D-PAm on this condition might therefore be produced by a direct action on the cells present in the diseased tissues, remission of the disease resulting in return of the synovium to normal. Chronic experimental arthritis in rabbits was reduced by treatment with D-PAm (Hunneyball *et al.*, 1977), but in contrast, adjuvant arthritis in rats was unaffected (Liyanage and Currey, 1972). Since these differences might be related to the different ways arthritis was induced in these two studies, care must be exercised in selecting models to study the mode of action of D-PAm and other thiols *in vivo*.

The development of leukaemia in BW mice treated with D-PAm may be evidence of the same stimulatory processes by thiol compounds reported *in vitro* (Broome and Jeng, 1973). Leukaemia as reported here does not spontaneously occur in the BW mouse. Neonatal infection of this mouse strain with a moloney-like oncornavirus failed to result in virus production or the development of thymic lymphoma as occurred in other strains (Dixon *et al.*, 1976). The lack of effect of D-PAm to change the onset and characteristics of the leukaemia of the AKR mouse, which is of known viral aetiology, may be relevant in that it suggests that host–viral relationships were unaltered by the thiol compound. The mode of action of D-PAm in precipitating leukaemia in the BW mouse therefore remains obscure. These results, however, may be related to the involvement of virus infections, including those caused by oncornavirus, in the autoimmune disease of various mouse strains.

ACKNOWLEDEMENTS

Beecham Pharmaceuticals are thanked for financial supported of this study.

REFERENCES

Broome, J. D. and Jeng, M. W. (1973). Promotion of replication in lymphoid cells by specific thiols and disulphides *in vitro*. Effects on mouse lymphoma cells in comparison with splenic lymphocytes. *J. Exp. Med.*, **138**, 574.

Cleland, W. W. (1964). Dithiothreitol, a new protective agent for-SH groups. *Biochemistry*, **3**, 480

Click, R. E., Benck, L. and Alter, B. J. (1972). Enhancement of antibody synthesis *in vitro* by mercaptoethanol. *Cell. Immunol.*, **3**, 155

Dixon, F. J., Jensen, F. C., McConahey, P. J. and Croker, B. P. (1976). Oncornaviruses and immunologic disease. In *Immunopathology*, VII Int. Symp., (ed. Miescher, P. A.), Schwafe and Co., Basel/Stuttgart, pp. 131-137

Eagle, H., Freeman, A. E. and Levy, M. (1958). The amino acid requirements of monkey kidney cells in first culture passage. *J. Exp. Med.*, **107**, 643

Eagle, H., Oyama, V. I. and Piez, K. A. (1960). The reversible binding of half-cystine residues to serum protein, and its bearing on the cystine requirements of cultured mammalian cells. *J. Biol. Chem.*, **235**, 1719

Eagle, H., Piez, K. A. and Levy, M. (1961). The intracellular amino acid concentrations required for protein synthesis in cultured human cells. *J. Biol. Chem.*, **236**, 2039.

Gillespie, D., Saxinger, W. C. and Gallo, R. C. (1975). Information transfer in cells infected by RNA tumour viruses and extension to human neoplasia. *Progr. Nucl. Acid Res. Mol. Biol.*, **15**, 1

Harris, G. (1973). The immune response of spleen explants from primed rabbits to sheep red cells (SRC). *Immunology*, **24**, 343

Harris, G. (1978). Lymphoid cells and transport of macromolecules. In *Carriers in Biology and Medicine*, (ed. G. Gregoriadis), (in press)

Harris, G. and Olsen, I. (1976). Cell division and deoxyribonucleic acid (DNA) synthesis in culture of stimulated lymphocytes. *Immunology*, **31**, 195

Hill, H. F. H. (1977). Treatment of rheumatoid arthritis with penicillamine. *Semin. Arthr. Rheum.*, **6**, 361

Hunneyball, I. M., Stewart, G. A. and Stanworth, D. R. (1977). Effect of (D) –pencillamine on chronic experimental arthritis in rabbits. *Ann. rheum. Dis.*, **36**, 378

Jerne, N. K. and Nordin, A. A. (1963). Plaque formation in agar by single antibody-producing cells. *Science*, **140**, 465

Kendall, P. A. and Hutchins, D. (1976). The effect of D-penicillamine on lymphocyte transformation *in vitro*. In *Penicillamine Research in Rheumatoid Disease*, (ed. E. Munthe), Fabritius and Sφnner, Oslo, p. 198

Kendall, P. and Hutchins, D. (1978). The effect of thiol compounds on lymphocytes stimulated in culture. *Immunology*, **35**, 189

Liyanage, S. P. and Currey, H. L. F. (1972). Failure of oral D-penicillamine to modify adjuvant arthritis or immune response in the rat. *Ann. rheum. Dis.*, **31**, 521

Opitz, H. G., Opitz, U., Lemke, H., Flad, H-D., Hewlett, G. and Schlumberger, H. D. (1977). Humoral primary immune response *in vitro* in a homologous mouse system: replacement of foetal calf serum by a 2-mercaptoethanol or macrophage activated fraction of mouse serum. *J. Immunol.*, **119**, 2089

Piez, K. A., Oyama, V. I., Levintow, L. and Eagle, H. (1960). Proteolysis in stored serum and its possible significance in cell culture. *Nature*, **188**, 59

4

The effect of D-penicillamine on humoral and cellular immune responses in animals

I. M. Hunneyball* and D. R. Stanworth (Department of Experimental Pathology, University of Birmingham, Birmingham B15 2TJ, U.K.)

INTRODUCTION

D-Penicillamine is now a well-established antirheumatic drug (Multicentre Trial Group, 1973) and has been shown to inhibit the progression of rheumatoid arthritis (Gibson *et al.*, 1976), yet its mode of action is unclear; especially as it fails to affect the traditional models of acute inflammation. Studies with the experimental antigen-induced arthritis model of Dumonde and Glynn (1962) in rabbits have shown that D-penicillamine can reduce the severity of the inflammation (Puschel *et al.*, 1976; Hunneyball *et al.*, 1977). In contrast, in the rat adjuvant arthritis model, D-penicillamine not only fails to control the swelling of the primary lesion (Liyanage and Currey, 1972), but also causes enhancement of the secondary lesions (Arrigoni-Martelli and Bramm, 1975).

Previous studies on the effect of penicillamine on the immune responses of rabbits (Tobin and Altman, 1964; Altman and Tobin, 1965) and mice (Hübner and Gengozian, 1965) were performed with the mixed (D-L) isomer and are thus difficult to interpret. More recent investigations with the pure D isomer at a dose of 200 mg/kg in rats failed to affect either the cellular or humoral response (Liyanage and Currey, 1972). In contrast, Schumacher *et al.* (1975) have reported a depression of rosette-forming cells but not plaque-forming cells in the spleens of mice in response to immunisation with sheep erythrocytes after short-term treatment with D-penicillamine at doses of 80–200 mg/kg commencing 10 days before immunisation. Dieppe *et al.* (1976) and Arrigoni-Martelli *et al.* (1976) found that in pertussis vaccine-induced pleurisy and paw oedema models in rats D-penicillamine at doses of 25–100 mg/kg could inhibit the delayed hypersensitivity reaction when administration commenced before sensitisation and continued throughout the experiment, but

*Present address: Research Department, The Boots Company Ltd., Pennyfoot Street, Nottingham NG2 3AA, U.K.

enhanced the severity of the reaction when administered around the time of challenge. These authors concluded that short-term dosing with the drug gave rise to immunostimulation, whereas long-term dosing led to immunosuppression.

All the studies described above employed relatively short-term dosing regimens compared with those used clinically in the treatment of rheumatoid arthritis. The experiments described in detail below were aimed at investigating the effects of long-term treatment (up to 400 days), with low doses of D-penicillamine, on the immune responses of normal and experimentally arthritic rabbits under a variety of dosing regimens. Both the humoral and cellular responses were monitored during the course of D-penicillamine treatment, which was designed to resemble that used clinically and resulted in a reduction in the severity of the experimentally induced monoarticular arthritis in the majority of animals treated with the drug.

EXPERIMENTAL STUDIES IN RABBITS

Adult New Zealand White × Californian rabbits were used. Ovalbumin (Sigma) emulsified in Freund's complete adjuvant (Difco) was used as antigen throughout. Animals received two to four immunisations, each containing 5 mg of ovalbumin. Monoarticular arthritis was induced experimentally by a method similar to that described by Dumonde and Glynn (1962) by intra-articular injection of a solution containing 10 mg of ovalbumin into one knee joint of animals that had been previously immunised with the antigen. Animals were skin tested before intra-articular injection to confirm the existence of a delayed hypersensitivity response.

Animals were given dry D-penicillamine powder (Distamine) daily, orally in gelatin capsules at a dose of 15–30 mg/kg body weight per day. The rabbits were divided into groups of four or five. Four dosing schedules were employed, commencing either 12 weeks before immunisation, 2 weeks before immunisation, on the day of immunisation or 16 weeks after the induction of the arthritis (i.e. during the chronic phase). Each D-penicillamine-treated group of animals was compared directly with a control group that had been treated in an identical manner, except for the administration of the drug.

Serum antibody concentrations were measured by both haemagglutination analysis, using sheep erythrocytes coated with ovalbumin via glutaraldehyde, and the reverse single radial immunodiffusion technique employing 1.5% Noble agar containing ovalbumin as described previously (Hunneyball *et al.*, 1978*a*). Concentrations of circulating immunoglobulins (IgG, IgA, IgM) were measured by single radial immunodiffusion using specific sheep antisera. Delayed hypersensitivity to ovalbumin and tuberculin PPD, measured by the peripheral blood leucocyte migration-inhibition technique of Bendixen and Søberg (1969) and skin testing, and the index of phagocytic activity, measured by the clearance of carbon from the circulation, have been described previously (Hunneyball *et al.*, 1978*b*). The stimulation of peripheral blood lymphocytes by pokeweed mitogen (PWM) and phytohaemagglutinin (PHA) (Burroughs Wellcome) was measured in 72 hour cultures by [^{3}H] thymidine uptake.

Animals were sensitised to dinitrochlorobenzene (DNCB) by two applications of 5 μl of 50 per cent DNCB in acetone 7 days apart and challenged 14 days later with 0.5 per cent DNCB in olive oil. Delayed hypersensitivity reactions were graded according to Turk (1967).

TREATMENT DURING IMMUNISATION

Initially, treatment of rabbits with D-penicillamine was started at various times before immunisation and continued daily throughout the whole immunisation phase. Treatment of normal rabbits with D-penicillamine commencing 14 days before immunisation resulted in a significant decrease in circulating levels of specific anti-ovalbumin antibody, as measured by both haemagglutination and immunoprecipitation techniques (figure 4.1). Pretreatment of the rabbits with D-penicillamine for 12 weeks before immunisation resulted in the same degree of inhibition of antibody production as treatment commencing on the day of immunisation. The effect of drug treatment on cell-mediated responses was measured by inhibition of leucocyte migration (figure 4.2). D-Penicillamine treatment markedly reduced the inhibition of migration observed in response to

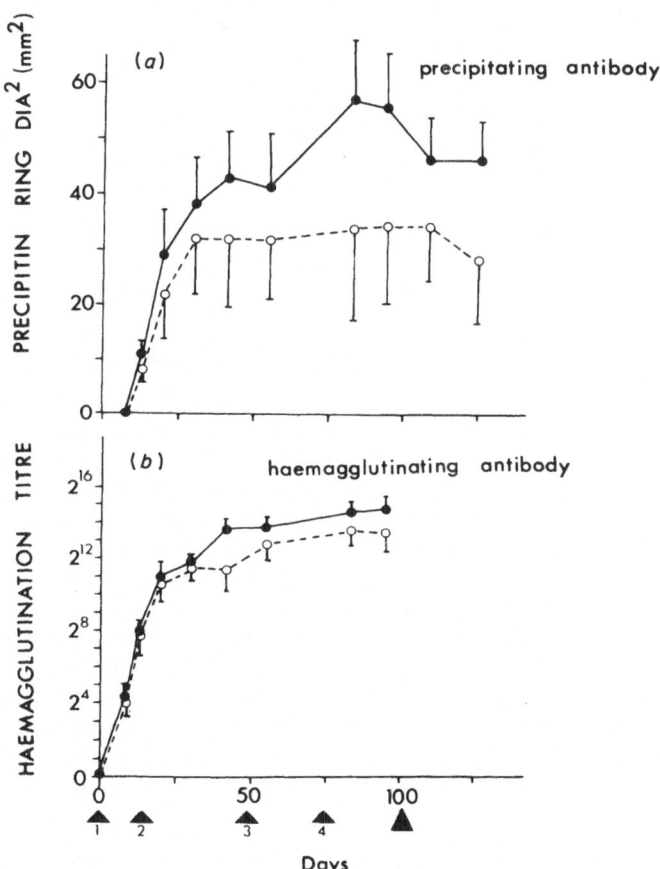

Figure 4.1 Concentration of specific precipitating antibody (*a*) and haemagglutinating antibody (*b*) directed against ovalbumin in control animals (●———●) and animals treated daily with D-penicillamine at a dose of 15 mg/kg (○– – –○) commencing 14 days before immunisation. Antigen was injected on days 0, 14, 50 and 75. Each point represents the mean of four or five animals. For clarity 1 s.d. only is shown on one side of each point.

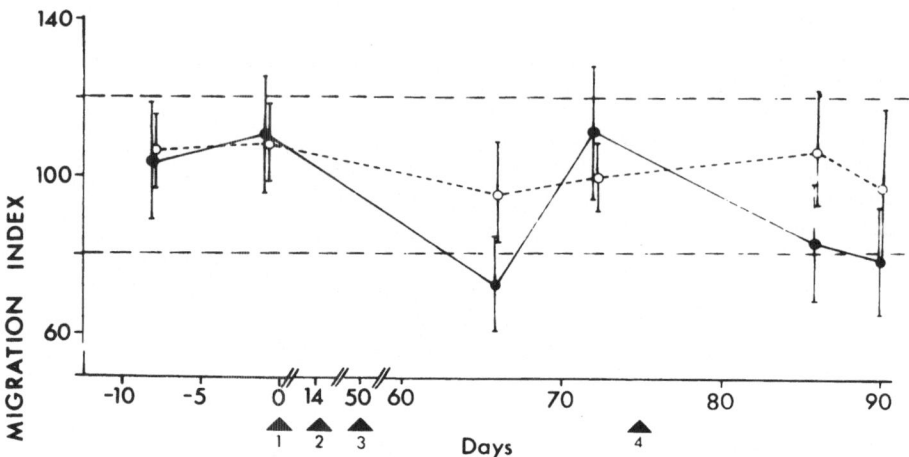

Figure 4.2   Migration inhibition by ovalbumin (100 μg/ml) of peripheral blood leucocytes
from control animals (●——●) and animals treated with D-penicillamine at a dose of 15 mg/kg
from day − 14 (○−−−○). Animals were immunised with ovalbumin on days 0, 14, 50 and 75.
Each point represents the mean ± s.d. of four animals.

immunisation with ovalbumin in untreated animals. However, at this time (after
70 days of treatment), the capacity of D-penicillamine-treated animals to produce
a cutaneous hypersensitivity reaction to ovalbumin was unaffected.

TREATMENT DURING THE COURSE OF THE EXPERIMENTAL ARTHRITIS

Antigen was injected intra-articularly into one knee joint of each of the immunised
animals described above and daily treatment with D-penicillamine continued.
Cutaneous hypersensitivity to both ovalbumin and tuberculin PPD was monitored
at regular (50 day) intervals. Intradermally (i.d.) injected ovalbumin (10–50 μg)
elicited.a strong Arthus (type 3) reaction which persisted and modulated the subsequent delayed (type 4) hypersensitivity reaction. Hence the measured lesion
must be regarded as a combined type 3–type 4 hypersensitivity reaction. I.d. injected tuberculin PPD (10–50 μg) elicited only a classical delayed reaction. Treatment
with D-penicillamine for 230 days caused a significant reduction in the diameter
of the cutaneous hypersensitivity reaction to ovalbumin, becoming more pronounced
after 410 days of treatment (figure 4.3). Comparable reductions in the height of
these cutaneous lesions could also be observed. Similarly, a time-dependent reduction in the delayed hypersensitivity reactions to tuberculin PPD could be observed,
resulting in complete abrogation of response after 410 days' treatment (figure 4.4).

TREATMENT COMMENCING DURING THE CHRONIC PHASE OF EXPERI-
MENTAL ARTHRITIS

Treatment with D-penicillamine commencing 16 weeks after the induction of the
arthritis had no effect on antibody production (figure 4.5). This contrasts with the
inhibition of antibody production observed when treatment commenced before
immunisation, which is most likely due to an effect on T cells as opposed to B cells
or plasma cells.

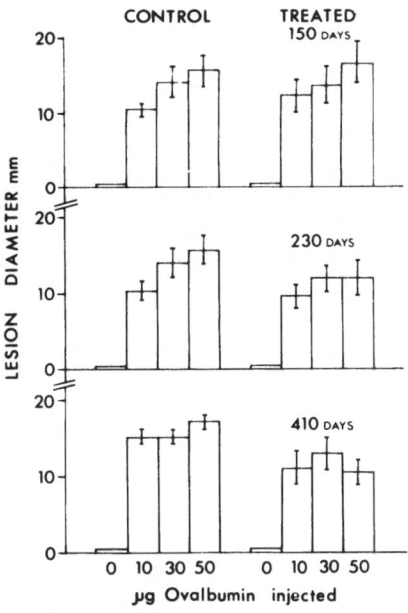

Figure 4.3 Effect of treatment with D-penicillamine (15 mg/kg) for various lengths of time, commencing 14 days before immunisation, on the diameter of the 48 h combined type 3–type 4 cutaneous hypersensitivity reactions to ovalbumin in arthritic animals. Each bar represents the mean ± s.d. of four animals.

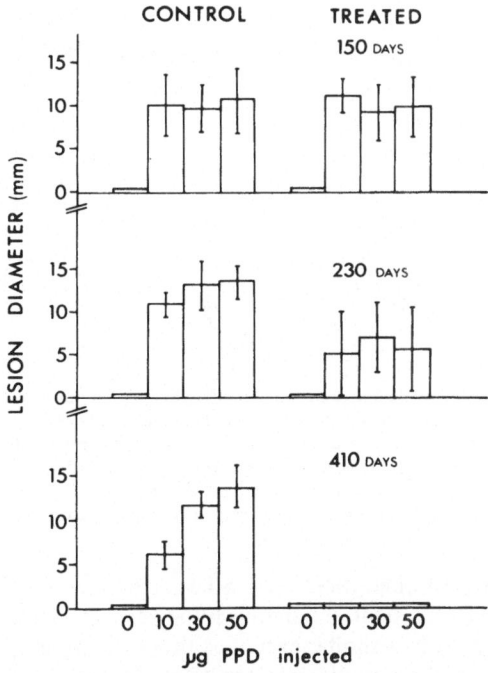

Figure 4.4 48 h-delayed cutaneous hypersensitivity reactions to i.d. injections of 10, 30 and 50 μg doses of tuberculin PPD in arthritic animals treated for 150, 230 and 410 days with D-penicillamine (15 mg/kg) commencing 12 weeks before immunisation and corresponding control animals. Each bar represents the mean ± s.d. of four animals.

Drugs and Immune Responsiveness

A marked effect on circulating concentrations of IgA was observed as a result of D-pencillamine treatment (figure 4.6). In untreated animals, serum IgA levels rose abruptly during the induction of the arthritis (intra-articular injection of antigen), but subsequently fell below the lower limit of the normal range during the chronic phase of the arthritis. Treatment with D-pencillamine reversed this fall and restored the circulating IgA to normal concentrations. It is felt that IgA, as well as reflecting the state of chronic inflammation in the joint, may also be involved in the patho-

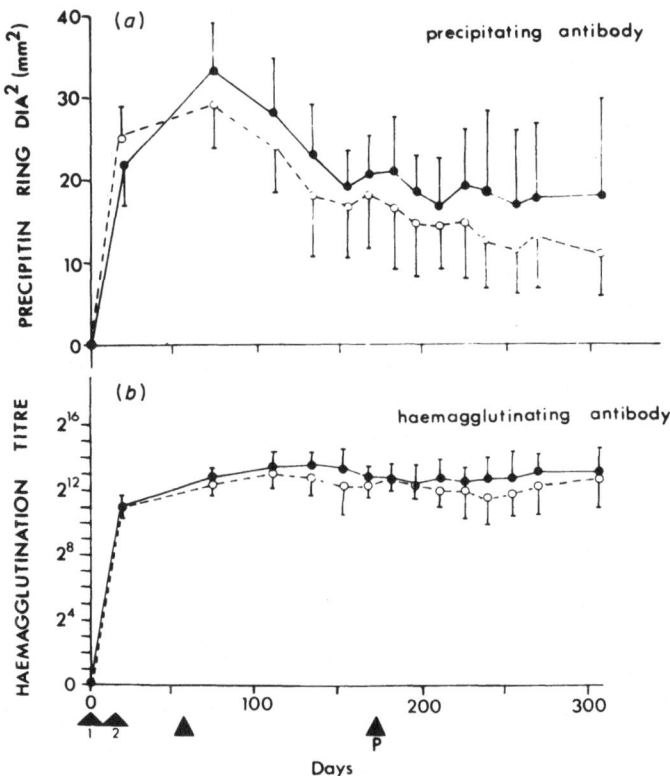

Figure 4.5 Concentration of specific precipitating antibody (*a*) and haemagglutinating antibody (*b*) directed against ovalbumin in control arthritic animals (●——●) and animals treated daily with D-penicillamine at a dose of 15 mg/kg (○---○) after immunisation and the onset of chronic arthritis. Immunising injections were given on days 0 and 14. Arthritis was induced on day 56 and D-penicillamine treatment commenced on day 171. Each point represents the mean of four animals. For clarity 1 s.d. only is shown on one side of each mean.

genesis of the lesion; although there is no other evidence for this as yet.

After 250 days of treatment, cutaneous hypersensitivity reactions in this group of rabbits were reduced to a similar extent as those described previously and lymphocyte-transformation studies performed at this time showed a reduced responsiveness to both PHA and PWM in D-penicillamine-treated animals (figure 4.7). However, sensitisation of these animals with DNCB was attempted and it was found that treatment with the drug had no effect on the production of a contact hyper-

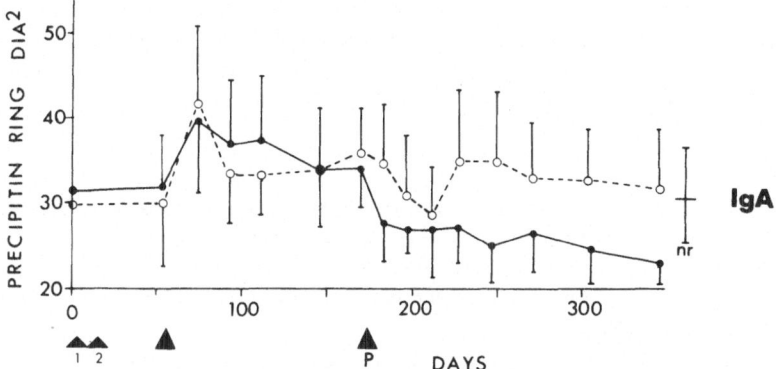

Figure 4.6 Concentrations of IgA in the serum of control arthritic animals (●——●) and animals treated daily with D-penicillamine at a dose of 15 mg/kg (○----○) after immunisation and the onset of chronic arthritis. Immunising injections were given on days 0 and 14. Arthritis was induced on day 56 and D-penicillamine treatment commenced on day 171. Each point represents the mean of four animals. For clarity 1 s.d. only is shown on one side of each point.

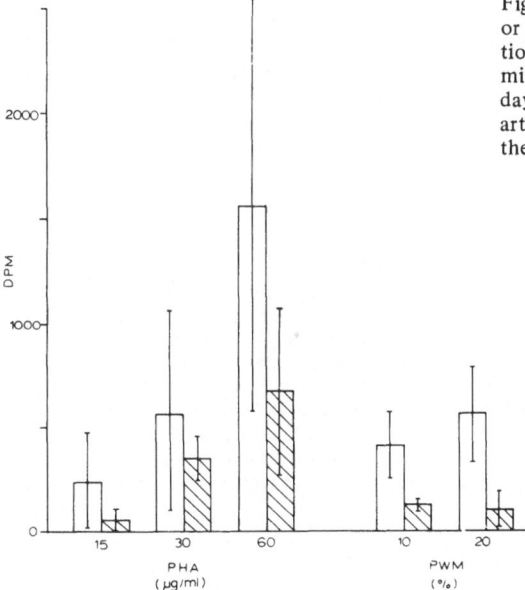

Figure 4.7 Inhibition of PHA-induced or PWM-induced lymphocyte transformation in animals treated with D-penicillamine at a dose of 15–30 mg/kg for 250 days commencing after the onset of arthritis (hatched). Each bar represents the mean ± s.d. of four animals.

sensitivity response to the subsequent challenge. These findings indicate that D-penicillamine treatment has no effect on sensitisation of the animals' lymphocytes to an antigen, but long-term treatment can reduce and abrogate the response, presumably by inhibiting the maintenance of a long-lived population of T lymphocytes such as the sensitised memory cells.

EFFECT ON MACROPHAGES

The effect of D-penicillamine treatment on macrophage function in normal rabbits was investigated. Having determined the normal phagocytic index of each animal

by carbon clearance, half the animals were treated with D-penicillamine for 50 days;
the remainder received no treatment. On remeasuring the phagocytic index it was
found that treatment with the drug had caused an increase in phagocytic index
(figure 4.8) indicating a stimulation of macrophage function.

DISCUSSION

The results show that long-term low dose D-penicillamine treatment consistently
produced a decrease in cell-mediated immune responses (presumably those mediated
by memory cells) yet appeared to have no effect on initial sensitisation of the
animals' lymphocytes. In addition, it can cause a stimulation of phagocyte, presumably macrophage, function.

It is possible that the stimulation of macrophage function observed here after
short-term treatment may account for the stimulation of delayed hypersensitivity
reactions to pertussis vaccine in rats observed by Dieppe *et al.* (1976) and Arrigoni-
Martelli *et al.* (1976). In fact Arrigoni-Martelli (1977) has shown that stimulation
of DNA synthesis in lymph-node cells by D-penicillamine *in vitro* requires the presence of macrophages. In addition, the depression of delayed hypersensitivity reaction observed here with longer treatment may correspond to the suppression
observed in the pertussis models under the long-dosage regime.

The delayed appearance of the reduction in cell-mediated responses by
D-penicillamine is consistent with the delayed action of the drug observed in both
the monoarticular experimental arthritis and rheumatoid arthritis. It is tempting

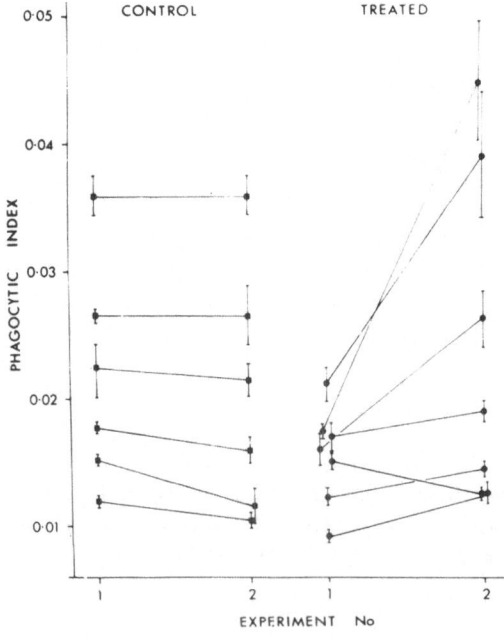

Figure 4.8 Effect of treatment
with D-penicillamine (15 mg/kg)
for 50 days on the phagocytic
index as measured by carbon
clearance. Each point represents
the mean ± s.d. for each animal.
Each animal was tested before
(expt. 1) and after (expt. 2) D-
penicillamine treatment. Control
animals received no D-penicillamine.

to speculate that D-penicillamine may therefore be reducing the number of sensitised lymphocytes entering the inflamed joints. This would correlate with the reduced mononuclear cell infiltration that we have observed in synovia from experimental monoarticular arthritic rabbits treated with D-penicillamine (Hunneyball *et al.*, 1977).

The possibility of activation of macrophage by D-penicillamine has been suggested by Willoughby (1976) and the resulting increase in phagocytic efficiency would be beneficial in rheumatoid arthritis by sequestering or removing endogenous antigens from the inflamed joints, hopefully in the absence of lysosomal enzyme release.

The inhibition of antibody production by D-penicillamine treatment commencing before immunisation, but not when treatment commenced after the onset of arthritis, is unrelated to the effect of the drug on the monoarticular arthritis, as a reduction in the severity of the chronic inflammation was observed under both treatment regimens. The restoration of serum IgA to normal concentrations in chronic arthritic rabbits by D-penicillamine treatment is of particular importance as the drug has also been shown to decrease the levels of circulating, covalently linked IgA-α_1 antitrypsin complex in the serum of rheumatoid arthritis patients undergoing D-penicillamine therapy (Wollheim *et al.*, 1976). Further, the kinetics of the restoration of normal serum IgA levels in rabbits correlated with the delay observed before the diminution of the monoarticular arthritis became apparent (Hunneyball *et al.*, 1977).

To summarise, our data support the findings of other workers in that D-penicillamine *in vivo* can exert both immunosuppressant and immunostimulant effects by acting on different cell populations; both actions apparently being beneficial in the treatment of rheumatoid arthritis.

ACKNOWLEDGEMENTS

We are grateful to Dr G. A. Stewart and Mr I. Lewin for assistance in this study. Generous financial support from the Medical Research Council is gratefully acknowledged. We are grateful to Dr W. H. Lyle of Dista Products Ltd., Speke, for kindly providing the Distamine used in the study.

Note added in proof The rate of phagocytosis of IgG coated polyvinyl latex particles by polymorphonuclear leucocytes from patients with rheumatoid arthritis has been shown to be reduced when compared to normal healthy individuals, and treatment with D-penicillamine (0.25 g daily) resulted in an increase (mean increment 38 per cent) after 7 days of treatment (Hallgren *et al.*, 1978). These data correlate with the increase in carbon clearance observed in rabbits after treatment with D-penicillamine for 50 days. In addition, recent studies of Cunningham *et al.* (1978) have shown that D-penicillamine treatment of immunised rats (25 mg/kg administered 48, 24 and 1 hour prior to implantation) enhanced leucocyte migration into implanted sponges impregnated with *Bordetella pertussis*. This correlates with the previous studies of Arrigoni-Martelli *et al.* (1976) and Dieppe *et al.* (1976) with pertussis induced pleurisy and paw oedema models of delayed hypersensitivity.

REFERENCES

Altman, K. and Tobin, M. S. (1965). Suppression of the primary immune response induced by D–L-penicillamine. *Proc. Soc. exp. Biol. Med.*, 118, 554

Arrigoni-Martelli, E. (1977). Role of macrophages in D-pencillamine-induced stimulation of DNA synthesis in lymph node cells. In *Perspectives in Inflammation*, (eds. D. A. Willoughby, J. P. Giroud and G. P. Velo), MTP Press, pp. 295–302

Arrigoni-Martelli, E. and Bramm, E. (1975). Investigations on the influence of cyclophosphamide, gold sodium thiomalate, and D-penicillamine on Nystatin oedema and adjuvant arthritis. *Agents and Actions*, 5, 264

Arrigoni-Martelli, E., Bramm, E., Huskisson, E. C., Willoughby, D. A. and Dieppe, P. A. (1976). Pertussis vaccine oedema: an experimental model for the action of penicillamine-like drugs. *Agents and Actions*, 6, 613

Bendixen, G. and Søberg, M. (1969). A leucocyte migration technique for *in vitro* detection of cellular (delayed-type) hypersensitivity in man. *Dan Med. Bull.*, 16, 1

Cunningham, F. M., Ford-Hutchinson, A. W., Oliver, A. M., Smith, M. J. H. and Walker, J. R. (1978). The effects of D-penicillamine and levamisole on leucocyte chemotaxis in the rat. *Br. J. Pharmac.*, 63, 119

Dieppe, P. A., Willoughby, D. A. Huskisson, E. C. and Arrigoni-Martelli, E. (1976). Pertussis vaccine pleurisy: a model of delayed hypersensitivity. *Agents and Actions*, 6, 618

Dumonde, D. C. and Glynn, L. E. (1962). The production of arthritis in rabbits by an immunological reaction to fibrin. *Br. J. exp. Path*, 43, 373

Gibson, T., Huskisson, E. C., Wojtulewski, J. A., Scott, P. J., Balme, H. W., Burry, H. C., Grahame, R. and Hart, F. D. (1976). Evidence that D-penicillamine alters the course of rheumatoid arthritis. *Rheumatol. Rehabil.*, 15, 211

Hällgren, R., Håkansson, L. and Venge, P. (1978). Kinetic studies of phagocytosis. 1. The serum particle uptake by PMN from patients with rheumatoid arthritis and systemic lupus erythematosus. *Arthr. Rheum.*, 21, 107

Hübner, K. F. and Gengozian, N. (1965). Depression of the primary immune response by d-l penicillamine. *Proc. Soc. exp. Biol. Med.*, 118, 561

Hunneyball, I. M., Stewart, G. A. and Stanworth, D. R. (1977). Effect of D-penicillamine on chronic experimental arthritis in rabbits. *Ann. Rheum. Dis.*, 36, 378

Hunneyball, I. M., Stewart, G. A. and Stanworth, D. R., (1978a). The effects of oral D-penicillamine treatment on experimental arthritis and the associated immune response in rabbits I. The effects on humoral parameters. *Immunology*, 34, 1053

Hunneyball, I. M., Stewart, G. A. and Stanworth, D. R. (1978b). The effects or oral D-pencill-amine treatment on experimental arthritis and the associated immune response in rabbits II. The effects on cellular parameters. *Immunology*, 35, 159

Liyanage, S. P. and Currey, H. L. F. (1972). Failure of D-penicillamine to modify adjuvant arthritis or immune response in the rat. *Ann. Rheum. Dis.*, 31, 521

Multicentre Trial Group (1973). Controlled trial of D-penicillamine in severe rheumatoid arthritis. *Lancet*, i, 275

Puschel, W., Rosenkranz, M., Geiler, G., Caffier, B., Stiehl, P. and Richter, V. (1976). Zur Wirkung von D-penicillamin auf die experimentelle allergische Arthritis des Kaninchens. *Z. Rheumatol.*, 35, 201

Schumacher, K., Maerker-Alzer, G. and Schaaf, W. (1975). Influence of D-penicillamine on the immune response of mice. *Arzneim-Forsch. (Drug Research)*, 25, 600

Tobin, M. S. and Altman, K. (1964). Accelerated immune response induced by D–L-penicill-amine. *Proc. Soc. exp. Biol. Med.*, 115, 225

Turk, J. L. (1967). Delayed Hypersensitivity, North-Holland, Amsterdam

Willoughby, D. A. (1976). In *Penicillamine Research in Rheumatoid Disease: Procs. of a Symposium at Spåtind, Norway*, (ed. E. Munthe), p. 49

Wollheim, F. A., Jeppson, J-O. and Laurell, C-B. (1976). Plasma α_1 antitrypsin–IgA complexes, plasma cystine and urinary cysteine–penicillamine disulphide excretion: correlation with responsiveness to penicillamine in rheumatoid arthritis. In *Penicillamine Research in Rheumatoid Disease: Proceedings of a Symposium at Spåtind, Norway*, (ed. E. Munthe), p. 152

5
The effect of drugs on immunological control mechanisms

J. L. Turk and Darien Parker (Department of Pathology, Royal College of Surgeons of England, Lincoln's Inn Fields, London WC2A 3PN, U.K.)

INTRODUCTION

The concept that an immune response is under specific homoeostatic control has been one that has crystallised over the last decade. As a result of increasing dissatisfaction with currently held hypotheses, much recent knowledge has developed from a reassessment of the mechanisms of immunological unresponsiveness. Clarification of the status of certain immunological phenomena that did not conform to current dogma has added to a new understanding of the immune response. This approach has been simplified by the identification of different populations of lymphocytes capable of interaction at various levels in the immune response. The immune response, whether cell-mediated or due to antibody, has in the past been considered as a positive unidirectional force in which the effector mechanism showed a narrow specificity for antigen. Immunological unresponsiveness was considered to be a negative phenomenon as exemplified by terms such as 'tolerance' and 'clone elimination'. The concept that immunological unresponsiveness could be a positive phenomenon developed from the study of 'immunological enhancement' in which the unresponsive state could be transferred by serum and was shown to be dependent on antibody. These studies were the first to indicate a modulatory effect of one form of the immune response on another; in this case of humoral antibody on a cell-mediated immune response.

The phenomenon of the modulation of one limb of the immune response by another is not a new concept. A similar process has been shown to underlie immunological enhancement in which antibody may be shown to modify a tumour graft in such a way that it is no longer susceptible to T-cell rejection (Kaliss, 1958). Antibody may protect the tumour directly by binding to tumour-specific transplantation antigen. It could also act by inhibiting the immune response directed against the tumour and lower the proportion of lymphocytes that can have an inhibitory effect on tumour growth. Sjögren *et al.* (1971) showed that the blocking activity could be due to immune complexes and Baldwin *et al.* (1972) demonstrated that the lymphocyte-blocking activity of immune complexes occurred when these

73

were formed *in vitro* at equivalence.

Early work on the definition of these suppressor cells came mainly from two sources—cancer immunology and the more traditional investigation into chemical contact sensitivity. Populations of suppressor T cells were defined with a regulatory action on both effector T-cell and B-cell functions. Among the systems first studied were the depression of antibody response to sheep erythrocytes in normal mice (Gershon and Kondo, 1971) and prolonged allotypic suppression (Jacobson *et al.*, 1972). In addition, suppressor T cells were shown to play a role as mediators of immunological tolerance in chemical-contact sensitivity in the mouse (Asherson *et al.*, 1971; Zembala and Asherson, 1973). This work was eventually to lead to the definition of populations of specific suppressor cells capable of modulating the action of effector cells.

Both T-cell and B-cell activities can be controlled by suppressor cells or their products. These may be of T cell or B cell origin with the same immunological specificity as the functions that they are modulating. Although it is clear that suppressor functions can control certain aspects of the immune response, it is not clear how extensive this phenomenon might be. Moreover, it is uncertain whether isolated phenomena are being studied or whether these are examples of a general feature of the immune response. Experimentally, the demonstration and definition of these phenomena depended on passive-transfer studies using cells or serum. It was possible to examine models of immunological control in depth after a means was found of blocking the regulatory function. It was discovered that this might be done by the strategic use of the drug cyclophosphamide (CY) given as a single large dose 3 days before immunisation.

THE EFFECT OF CY ON LYMPHOID TISSUE

A single i.p. (intraperitoneal) injection of 300 mg of CY/kg in the mouse and guinea pig has been found to deplete lymphocytes from the lymph follicles and corticomedullary junction of lymph nodes. A similar effect is found on non-thymus-dependent areas of the spleen. The thymus-dependent areas of both lymph nodes and spleen appear to be relatively unaffected (Turk and Poulter, 1972*a*). Maximum depletion occurs 3 days after injection and repopulation may be observed 4 days later. In the mouse there is a proportional increase in θ-antigen-carrying lymphocytes in lymph nodes and spleen, which can be observed after three such injections at intervals of 3 days (Poulter and Turk, 1972). Mice are also found to have a diminished T-lymphocyte response to phytomitogens after CY treatment (Stockman *et al.*, 1973). The effect of CY on lymphocytes labelled with [^{125}I] 5-iodo-2-deoxyuridine compared with those labelled with ^{51}Cr indicated that CY was acting specifically on rapidly dividing cells (Turk and Poulter, 1972*b*). If given after immunisation, CY can be shown to act on T lymphocytes as these cells enter a state of more rapid turnover. This differential effect of CY on more rapidly dividing cells can be used to eliminate effector cells. In the case of certain cell-mediated immune phenomena, effector cells have more slowly turning over pre-cursors that are not sensitive to treatment with CY and this can produce an imbalance in the normal homoeostatic mechanism, as a result of which the cell-mediated immune reactions increase.

Although histologically the effect of CY is mainly on B cells, leaving T cells relatively unaffected, later studies have shown that certain populations of B cells are spared after such treatment. Thus there is no direct parallelism between the effect of CY on suppressor-cell precursors and those involved in humoral antibody production.

THE EFFECT OF CY ON THE PRECURSORS OF SUPPRESSOR CELL POPULATIONS CONTROLLING CELL-MEDIATED IMMUNE REACTIONS

The earliest experiments in this series were on guinea pigs sensitised with chemical-contact agents 2,4-dinitrofluorobenzene (DNFB) and 2-phenyl-4-ethoxy-methylene-5-oxazolone (oxazolone). When treated with CY (300 mg/kg) 3 days before immunisation, animals developed increased skin reactivity when tested 7 days after first contact with the sensitiser. These reactions were not only increased in intensity, but were prolonged in that they could still be detected 8 days after skin testing. This increase in reactivity was not due to an increase in skin irritability as there was no parallel increase in skin reactions to turpentine. Moreover, the increased reactivity in CY-pretreated animals could be partially reversed by an i.p. transplant of spleen fragments from specifically sensitised donors not pretreated with CY (Turk *et al.*, 1972).

Despite these early findings with contact sensitisers, CY pretreatment was not able to increase delayed hypersensitivity to tuberculin in BCG-vaccinated guinea pigs, nor to ovalbumin (OA) in guinea pigs sensitised with OA in Freund's complete adjuvant (FCA). In contrast if animals were sensitised with OA in Freund's in-complete adjuvant (FIA), CY pretreatment produced an increase in skin reactivity similar to that which occurred in animals sensitised by application of a contact sensitiser (Turk and Parker, 1973).

Dvorak *et al.* (1970, 1971) and Richerson *et al.* (1970) have distinguished contact-sensitivity reactions and skin reactions to antigens such as OA in animals sensitised with the antigen in FIA from tuberculin-type reactions by the number of basophilic leucocytes present in the lesions. The stronger tuberculin-type reactions, induced by antigens in FCA, persist for longer than do those induced by immunisation with antigen in FIA and sometimes contain less basophilic leucocytes. The weaker reactions, induced by antigens in FIA, which contain more basophils, are often called Jones–Mote reactions. In our studies we were unable to distinguish between tuberculin-type reactions, Jones–Mote reactions and contact-sensitivity reactions on the basis of the basophil content of the infiltrate (Katz *et al.*, 1974a).

The ability of CY pretreatment to remove the regulator arm of the immune response is not limited to chemical-contact sensitivity and simple antigens such as OA. In animals immunised with a bacterial suspension such as killed tularaemia vaccine in FIA, delayed hypersensitivity can also be potentiated by CY pretreat-ment (Ascher *et al.*, 1977). Moreover, in the mouse enhancement of delayed hypersensitivity to sheep erythrocytes (SRBCs) can be demonstrated by CY pre-treatment even when animals are immunised with SRBCs in FCA (Lagrange *et al.*, 1974; Kerkhaert *et al.*, 1974).

The effect of CY in potentiating the delayed hypersensitivity response is not the same for all soluble protein antigens injected in FIA. In one study (Scheper *et al.*, 1977) the effect on the immune response to five protein antigens was investigated. These were bovine serum albumin (BSA), bovine gamma-globulin

Table 5.1　Skin test reactivity 8 days after immunisation

	BSA	BGG	DNP_5-BGG	DNP_{50}-BGG	OA
FIA	0.6*	1.1	2.2	3.2	1.2
CY/FIA	1.0	2.2	4.1	11.5	5.8

*Increase in skin thickness 48 h after skin test.

(BGG), DNP_5-BGG and DNP_{50}-BGG as well as OA. A spectrum of reactivity was detected depending on the strength of the antigen to stimulate both T cells and B cells. BSA and BGG behaved as relatively weak antigens in which the regulating arm, revealed by CY sensitivity, was poorly stimulated. Thus the effect of CY pretreatment was to cause little enhancement of delayed hypersensitivity (table 5.1). OA and DNP_{50}-BGG behaved as strong antigens and CY pretreatment revealed a strongly developed regulation system. It is noteworthy that the T-cell response to BSA and BGG was easily suppressed if 15 mg of the specific antigen was given intravenously (i.v.) at the same time as the antigen in adjuvant (table 5.2). However, the T-cell response to OA, DNP_5-BGG and DNP_{50}-BGG resisted suppression by soluble antigen. Thus weak antigens showed poor immunoregulation but were easily suppressed by soluble antigen, whereas strong antigens showed strong immunoregulation and could not be suppressed by soluble antigen. A failure to reverse the suppressive effect of the soluble antigens on the immune response by CY suggests that this effect was not produced by a stimulation of regulator cells.

Table 5.2　Skin test reactivity 8 days after immunisation

	BSA	BGG	DNP_5-BGG	DNP_{50}-BGG	OA
FIA	3.2*	3.5	2.1	4.4	4.5
i.v./FIA	0.1	0.4	3.5	11.2†	14.5†
CY/i.v./FIA	0.1	0.8	2.8	2.8	4.0

*Increase in skin thickness 24 h after skin test.
†Increased reactivity due to a residual Arthus reaction.

THE NATURE OF THE SUPPRESSOR-CELL POPULATION THAT IS SUSCEPTIBLE TO CY

On the basis of the previous findings, it was postulated that CY pretreatment removed a population of cells that modulate the expression of delayed hypersensitivity as increased skin reactions occurred without this cell population. It is possible to replace this population by transfer of cells from specifically sensitised donors that have not been pretreated with CY (Katz *et al.*, 1974*b*). The following model was used in such an experiment. Guinea pigs treated with CY 3 days before immunisation with OA in FIA served as cell recipients 8 days later, as they were potentially susceptible to the effect of suppressor cells which they were lacking. Cells that would reduce the skin-test reactions in such animals were found in the

spleen and peritoneal exudate of guinea pigs immunised with OA in FIA 8 and 14
days previously, and in animals immunised with OA in FCA 8 days previously.
This suppression was shown to be antigen specific and to need live cells. In
further experiments (Katz *et al.*, 1974c), the spleen cells from guinea pigs immunised
with OA in FIA 8 days before were passed down columns of plastic beads (Degalan
V26) that had been coated with specifically purified rabbit anti-guinea pig gamma-
globulin. The antisera was purified using cyanogen-bromide-activated Sepharose
beads. After passage of the spleen cells through the coated Degalan bead column,
90–95 per cent of the immunoglobulin-bearing lymphocytes (B cells), as measured
by immunofluorescence, were retained on the column. The population of spleen
cells, depleted of B cells, failed to suppress the skin reactions of animals used for
the detection of suppressor cells (i.e. guinea pigs treated with CY before immunisation with OA in FIA). However, spleen cells that had been passed through columns
coated with normal rabbit serum, and which were therefore not depleted of B cells,
suppressed the delayed reactions of the CY-treated recipients to a degree similar
to that obtained with unseparated cells.

These experiments, together with earlier observations that CY pretreatment has
a preferential effect on B cells rather than on T cells, suggested that the population
of suppressor cells that were susceptible to CY belonged to a conventional B-cell
population. However, attempts to transfer the suppressor effect with fresh serum
from normally sensitised donors consistently proved unsuccessful.

Earlier findings had shown a good correlation between the effects of CY on the
precursors of suppressor cells and B cells making γ_1 homocytotropic antibody.
These findings were in animals contact-sensitised with DNFB and in those sensitised
with OA in FIA. This suggested that the immunoregulatory phenomenon that we

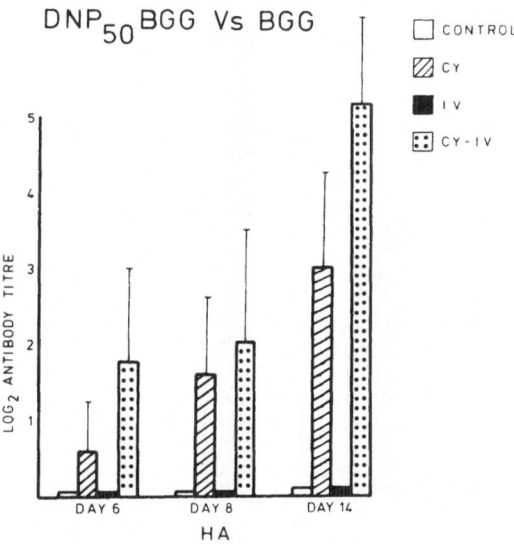

Figure 5.1 Passive haemagglutinating BGG antibody titres in guinea pigs immunised with
DNP$_{50}$-BGG in FIA, 6, 8 and 14 days after immunisation.

were studying was related to the immunological facilitation phenomenon described by Voisin (1971).

A study of the effect of CY pretreatment on precursors of B cells making indirect haemagglutinating antibody (γ_2-globulin) and those making homocytotropic antibody (γ_1-globulin), assayed by passive cutaneous anaphylaxis (PCA-antibody), was therefore initiated by using four antigens: OA, BGG, DNP_5-BGG and DNP_{50}-BGG. Haemagglutinating antibody was studied 6, 8 and sometimes 14 days after immunisation by injection of antigens in either FIA and FCA with or without associated i.v. injection (Noble *et al.*, 1977). Many of the antibody responses were unaffected by CY pretreatment; despite the observation that Arthus reactivity was suppressed by pretreatment with CY. In one case an antibody was detected in the serum of CY-pretreated animals that was not present in the serum of the normally immunised group (figure 5.1). Animals immunised with DNP_{50}-BGG do not make antibody to BGG; however, after CY pretreatment anti-BGG antibodies could be detected. This resistance of antibody precursors to CY pretreatment suggests that long-lived precursors characterise the B-cell lines that produce some haemagglutinating antibody, whereas Arthus reactions are characterised by CY-sensitive precursors. The effect of CY pretreatment in suppressing the PCA antibody at 14 days after immunisation depended on the antigen used (Parker and Turk, 1978). There was little or no correlation between the production of antibody detected by PCA and that detected by haemagglutination (figures 5.2, 5.3 and 5.4). The levels of PCA antibody was increased in some systems and decreased in others by CY pretreatment.

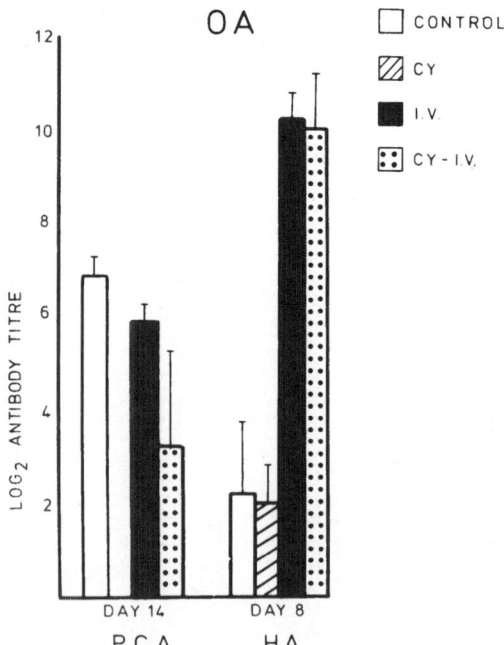

Figure 5.2 Passive cutaneous anaphylactic (PCA) and haemagglutinating (HA) OA antibody titres in guinea pigs immunised with OA in FIA.

In general there was no parallelism with the systems in which haemagglutinating antibody was altered. It was therefore concluded that the B-cell precursors of plasma cells making homocytotropic antibody, haemagglutinating antibody, the antibody involved in the Arthus reaction and the cells modulating T-cell function in delayed hypersensitivity belonged to different cell populations with different susceptibilities to CY.

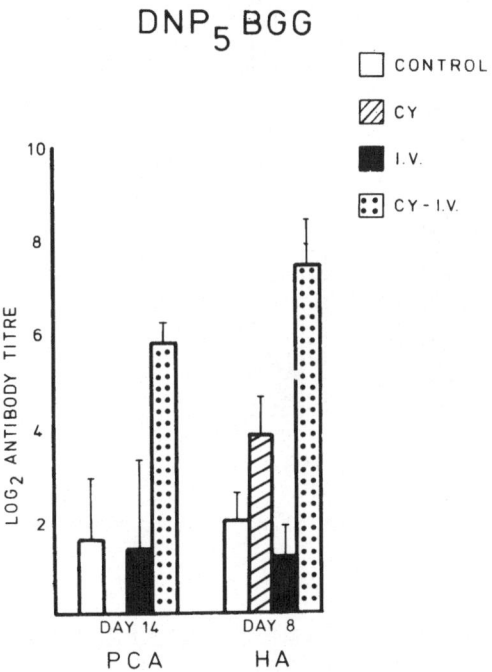

Figure 5.3 Passive cutaneous anaphylactic (PCA) and haemagglutinating (HA) anti-DNP antibody titres in guinea pigs immunised with DNP$_5$-BGG in FIA.

Although it was demonstrated that removal of B cells from spleen suspensions eliminated suppressor cells, it is possible that B cells may not be the actual suppressor elements in peritoneal exudate cell suspensions. Examination of the suspensions used in these transfers shows that approximately 90 per cent of the cells are macrophages and less than 10 per cent are lymphocytes, of which only half are B cells. It could be that the suppressor effect in these preparations is mediated by macrophages carrying a cytophilic antibody that is produced by B cells in the spleen as well as by other central lymphoid tissues. It is thus important to consider the role of macrophages as well as B cells in the mediation of these suppressor effects. In addition the identity of the suppressor cell in the spleen preparation needs further identification, since although it appears that these cells carry surface immunoglobulin, there is no evidence as yet that they do not carry specific T-cell antigens.

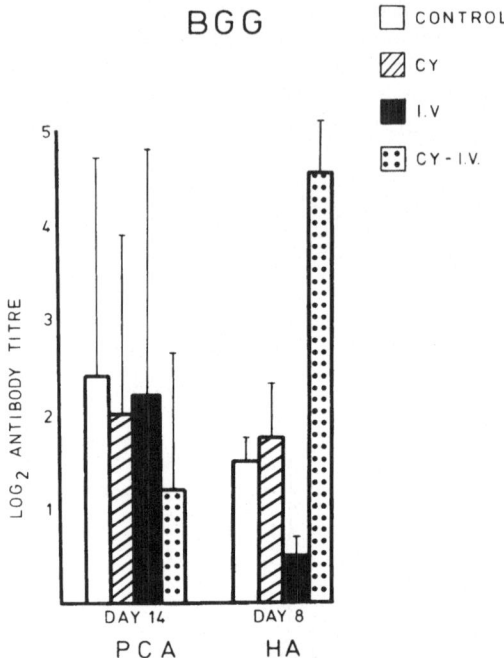

Figure 5.4 Passive cutaneous anaphylactic (PCA) and haemagglutinating (HA) antibody titres in guinea pigs immunised with BGG in FIA.

SPECIFIC RESPONSE *IN VITRO* OF LYMPHOCYTES FROM CY-PRETREATED ANIMALS

Lymph-node lymphocytes from animals treated with CY before immunisation with OA in FIA can be stimulated into DNA synthesis by specific antigen as early as 4 days after sensitisation. However, similar cell suspensions from animals not treated with CY fail to respond (Katz *et al.*, 1975). At 7 and 14 days, cells from all animals treated with CY before immunisation with OA in FIA responded to OA, whereas only half the immunised animals that had not been pretreated with CY responded at these times. Thus in this model CY pretreatment markedly increases the response of sensitised lymphocytes to specific antigen *in vitro*. Similarly, in animals immunised with tularaemia vaccine in FIA, CY pretreatment caused a marked increase in the ability of peripheral blood lymphocytes to respond to the specific antigen. The response could be detected both earlier and with a greater intensity than in animals not treated with CY (Ascher *et al.*, 1977).

ACTION OF CY ON REVERSIBLE TOLERANCE IN THE GUINEA PIG

The demonstration that CY pretreatment could increase contact reactivity and certain forms of delayed-type hypersensitivity by elimination of suppressor cells led to a study of the action of CY in certain models of immunological unresponsiveness. One of the earliest reports of immunological tolerance in experimental animals was the demonstration by Chase (1946) that a state of specific unresponsiveness in contact sensitivity could be induced by feeding 1-chloro-2,4-dinitrobenzene (DNCB) to unsensitised guinea pigs. Another model of unresponsiveness can be induced by two i.v. injections of sodium dinitrobenzenesulphonate ($DNBSO_3$) before attempted sensitisation (Turk and Stone, 1963; Frey *et al.*, 1964). The demonstration that suppressor cells were generated in a similar model of tolerance in the mouse (Zembala and Asherson, 1973) prompted an investigation into the action of CY in these systems.

Guinea pigs, treated with 500 mg of $DNBSO_3$/kg twice at 14-day intervals before attempted sensitisation with DNCB, were completely unresponsive to DNCB. However, if they were treated with CY (250 mg/kg) 3 days before attempted sensitisation, they became responsive (Polak and Turk, 1974). In this model, CY pretreatment was effectively able to reverse the tolerant state. Once tolerance had been shown to be broken, the animals remained responsive. However, if one allowed a 14-day gap between the CY pretreatment and attempted sensitisation, the animals were subsequently found to remain unresponsive. Thus the effect of the CY was a temporary one and after a limited time the population of suppressor cells was able to regenerate.

Guinea pigs made tolerant to DNCB with $DNBSO_3$ failed to show T-cell proliferation in lymph nodes draining the site of sensitisation. One of the effects of CY pretreatment is to allow T-cell proliferation to develop. It seems therefore that CY has a preferential action on the population of suppressor cells, releasing effector cells for proliferation in cell-mediated immunity. CY treatment was able to induce a return of IgG_1 homocytotropic antibody production in this system.

After the demonstration of the reversibility of tolerance induced by i.v. injection of $DNBSO_3$, it was shown that tolerance induced by feeding DNCB could be reversed by CY in a similar manner (Polak *et al.* 1975). However, the tolerance induced by feeding is not so complete as that induced by i.v. injection. When such partially tolerant animals are treated with CY before attempted sensitisation, the resultant sensitivity is far greater than that found after reversal of tolerance induced by $DNBSO_3$. The level reached was that found when normal animals were treated with CY before sensitisation. This could indicate that the tolerance induced by feeding is completely reversible, whereas that induced by i.v. injection might be a combination of reversible suppressor-cell action, with perhaps some degree of irreversibility resulting from clonal elimination.

The reversibility of tolerance induced by feeding is also accompanied by a return of the ability of lymphocytes to proliferate in the draining lymph nodes after sensitisation. In reversal of tolerance induced by i.v. injection, the number of large pyroninophilic cells in the draining lymph nodes 4 days after sensitisation did not return completely to the level found in sensitised controls. The return of sensitivity after treatment with CY in animals made tolerant by feeding was, however, associated with a complete return of T-cell proliferative activity.

EFFECT OF DRUGS OTHER THAN CY ON IMMUNOLOGICAL CONTROL MECHANISMS

An effect similar to that found with CY has been demonstrated in the guinea pig with the alkylating agent melphalan, although chlorambucil and busulphan, in sub-lethal doses, did not potentiate delayed hypersensitivity reactions (Turk and

Parker, 1973). Minimal potentiation was produced with azathioprine; in one series of experiments potentiation was produced. A marked potentiation was found with an original batch of ICRF 159 (4,4-propylene-2,6-di-piperazeinedione) obtained from Dr A. M. Creighton of the Imperial Cancer Research Fund Laboratories, Lincoln's Inn Fields, London. However, subsequent batches of the drug, obtained from I.C.I. Ltd. proved ineffective. So far other drugs used in the same protocol have been ineffective.

Levamisole, although described as an immunopotentiator in other species, was ineffective in the guinea pig when used in the same protocol as CY. However, this agent was a potent skin sensitiser and when incorporated into Freund's adjuvant, together with another antigen, was capable of reversing the effect of CY given 3 days before immunisation. This effect could not be ascribed to antigenic competition. It is possible that under the conditions of the experiment, levamisole acts as a stimulant of suppressor cells rather than as an immunopotentiator.

SUMMARY AND CONCLUSIONS

Lymphocytes involved in all immunological reactions may be divided into effector and suppressor cells. In addition both functional groups have rapidly turning over and slowly turning over precursor cells. Thus for any one antigen and immune response, whether humoral antibody-mediated or cell-mediated, there are four possible combinations (figure 5.5). In only one of these will CY pretreatment result in immunopotentiation. This is the situation in which a rapidly turning over suppressor-cell precursor is regulating a slowly turning over effector-cell population. Where a slowly turning over suppressor-cell population regulates a slowly turning over effector-cell population, CY pretreatment will have no effect. Where the effector-cell precursors are rapidly dividing, CY pretreatment will be immuno-suppressive, whatever the state of the precursors of the suppressor cells. It is interest-

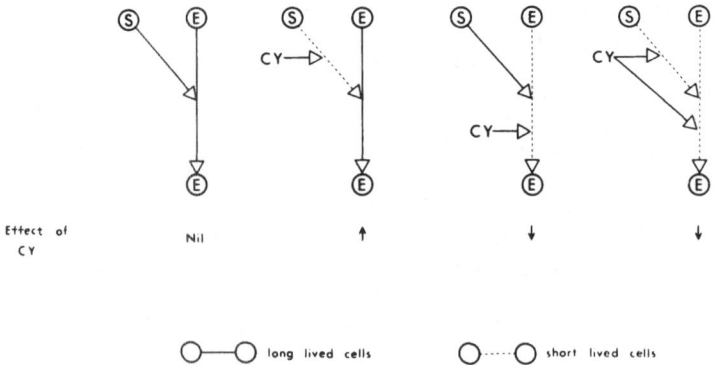

Figure 5.5 The action of cyclophosphamide on immune regulation. (S) suppression cells, (E) effector cells.

ing therefore that potentiation of the immune response by CY is a common event in cell-mediated immune reactions. However, this phenomenon does not occur with the same frequency in humoral antibody responses. Susceptibility of a cell to CY does not appear to depend on whether the cell is a T cell or a B cell. However, the strength of the suppressor response appears to be related to the strength of the antigen as an immunogen.

The role of the basophil in delayed hypersensitivity responses appears to be related to suppressor-cell action in the periphery. Wherever there is a strong suppressor element, basophils may be found in the lesion. However, these cells are not needed for effector mechanisms as their precursors are eliminated by CY at the same time as the delayed hypersensitivity reactions are increased. The role of these cells is conjectural but it would appear that suppressor-cell action must result in the local release of basophil chemotactic factors.

REFERENCES

Ascher, M. S., Parker, D. and Turk, J. L. (1977). Modulation of delayed-type hypersensitivity and cellular immunity to microbial vaccines: Effects of cyclophosphamide on the immune response to tularaemia vaccine. *Infection and Immunity*, 18, 318

Asherson, G. L., Zembala, M. and Barnes, R. M. R. (1971). The mechanism of immunological unresponsiveness to picryl chloride and the possible role of antibody mediated depression. *Clin. exp. Immun.*, 9, 111

Baldwin, R. W., Price, M. R. and Robbins, R. A. (1972). Blocking of lymphocyte-mediated cytotoxicity for rat hepatoma cells by tumour-specific antigen-antibody complexes. *Nature New Biol.*, 238, 185

Chase, M. W. (1946). Inhibition of experimental drug allergy by prior feeding of the sensitizing agent. *Proc. Soc. exp. Biol. Med.*, 61, 257

Dvorak, H. F.,Dvorak, A. M., Simpson, B. A., Richerson, H. B., Leskowitz, S. and Karnovsky, M. J. (1970). Cutaneous basophil hypersensitivity II A light and electron microscopic description. *J. exp. Med.*, 132, 558

Dvorak, H. F., Simpson, B. A., Bast, R. C. and Leskowitz, S. (1971). Cutaneous basophil hypersensitivity. III Participation of the basophil in hypersensitivity to antigen–antibody complexes, delayed hypersensitivity and contact allergy. passive transfer. *J. Immun.*, 107, 138

Frey, J. R., De Weck, A. L. and Geleick, H. (1964). Immunological unresponsiveness in allergic contact dermatitis to dinitrochlorobenzene in guinea pigs. *J. invest. Dermat.*, 42, 41

Gershon, R. K. and Kondo, K. (1971). Infectious immunological tolerance. *Immunology*, 21, 903

Jacobson, E. B., Herzenberg, L. A., Riblet, R. and Herzenberg, L. A. (1972). Active suppression of immunoglobulin allotype synthesis. II Transfer of suppressing factor with spleen cells. *J. exp. Med.*, 135, 1163

Kaliss, N. (1958). Immunological enhancement of tumour homografts in mice: a review. *Cancer Res.*, 18, 992

Katz, S. I., Heather, C. J., Parker, D. and Turk, J. L. (1974a). Basophilic leukocytes in delayed hypersensitivity reactions. *J. Immun.* 113, 1073

Katz, S. I., Parker, D., Sommer, G. and Turk, J. L. (1974b). Suppressor cells in normal immunization as a basic homeostatic phenomenon. *Nature*, 248, 612

Katz, S. I., Parker, D. and Turk, J. L. (1974c). B-cell suppression of delayed hypersensitivity reactions. *Nature*, 281, 550

Katz, S. I., Parker, D. and Turk, J. L. (1975). Mechanisms involved in the expression of Jones–Mote hypersensitivity. II Lymph node morphology and *in vitro* correlates. *Cell. Immun.*, 16, 404

Kerckhaert, J. A. M., Berg, G. J. von den and Willers, J. M. N. (1974). Influence of cyclophosphamide on the delayed type hypersensitivity of the mouse. *Annls Immun. (Inst. Pasteur)*, 125c, 415

Lagrange, P. H., Mackaness, G. B. and Miller, T. E. (1974). Potentiation of T-cell mediated immunity by selective suppression of antibody formation with cyclophosphamide. *J. exp. Med.*, 139, 1529

Noble, B., Parker, D., Scheper, R. J. and Turk, J. L. (1977). The relation between B-cell stimulation and delayed hypersensitivity. The effect of cyclophosphamide pretreatment on antibody production. *Immunology*, 32, 885

Parker, D. and Turk, J. L. (1978). The effect of cyclophosphamide pretreatment on B-cell stimulation: dissociation of action on homocytotropic antibody and other B-cell functions. *Immunology*, 34, 115

Polak, L. and Turk, J. L. (1974). Reversal of immunological tolerance by cyclophosphamide through inhibition of suppressor cell activity. *Nature*, 249, 654

Polak, L., Geleick, H. and Turk, J. L. (1975). Reversal of tolerance in contact sensitization by cyclophosphamide: tolerance induced by prior feeding with DNCB. *Immunology*, 28, 939

Poulter, L. W. and Turk, J. L. (1972). Proportional increase in the θ carrying lymphocytes in peripheral lymphoid tissue following treatment with cyclophosphamide. *Nature. New Biol.*, 238, 17

Richerson, H. B., Dvorak, H. F. and Leskowitz, S. (1970). Cutaneous basophil hypersensitivity. I A new look at the Jones–Mote reaction, general characteristics. *J. exp. Med.*, 132, 546

Scheper, R. J., Parker, D., Noble, B. and Turk, J. L. (1977). The relation of immune depression and B-cell stimulation during the development of delayed hypersensitivity to soluble antigens. *Immunology*, 32, 265

Sjögren, H. O., Hellström, T., Bonsal, S. C. and Hellström, K. E. (1971). Suggestive evidence that 'blocking antibodies' of tumour bearing individuals may be antigen–antibody complexes. *Proc. natn. Acad. Sci.*, 68, 1372

Stockman, G. D., Heim, L. R., South, M. A. and Trentin, J. J. (1973). Differential effects of cyclophosphamide on the B- and T-cell compartments of adult mice. *J. Immun.*, 110, 277

Turk, J. L. and Parker, D. (1973). Further studies on B-lymphocyte suppression in delayed hypersensitivity indicating a possible mechanism for Jones–Mote hypersensitivity. *Immunology*, 24, 751

Turk, J. L. and Poulter, L. W. (1972a). Selective depletion of lymphoid tissue by cyclophosphamide. *Clin. exp. Immun.*, 10, 285

Turk, J. L. and Poulter, L. W. (1972b). Effects of cyclophosphamide on lymphoid tissues labelled with 5-Iodo-2-deoxyuridine-^{125}I and ^{51}Cr. *Int. Archs Allergy*, 43, 620

Turk, J. L. and Stone, S. H. (1963). Implication of the cellular changes in lymph nodes during the development and inhibition of delayed type hypersensitivity in cell bound antibodies. (eds. B. Amos and H. Koprowski), Wistar Institute Press, Philadelphia, p. 51

Turk, J. L., Parker, D. and Poulter, L. W. (1972). Functional aspects of the selective depletion of lymphoid tissue by cyclophosphamide. *Immunology*, 23, 493

Voisin, G. A. (1971). Immunological facilitation, a broadening of the concept of the enhancement phenomenon. *Prog. Allergy*, 15, 328

Zembala, M. and Asherson, G. L. (1973). Depression of the T-cell phenomenon of contact sensitivity by T-cells from unresponsive mice. *Nature*, 244, 227

6

Immunological profile of levamisole and its clinical application in man

J. De Cree* and J. Symoens[+] (*Clinical Research Unit St. Bartholomeus,
B-2060 Merksem, Belgium and [+]Department of Clinical Research,
Janssen Pharmaceutica, B-2340 Beerse, Belgium.)

IMMUNOLOGICAL PROPERTIES

Immunological spectrum of activity

The immunological effects of levamisole have been extensively studied on isolated cells, on experimental animals, on healthy volunteers and on patients.

The early literature was conflicting for several reasons. Levamisole was indiscriminately tested at physiological and supraphysiological doses on cellular and humoral immune functions of healthy and compromised hosts.

A careful analysis of the literature with these variables in mind, shows a consistent dual pattern of levamisole. The drug restores immunocompetence in compromised hosts and induces T-cell maturation. These effects have been described in detail by Symoens and Rosenthal (1977), whose review article should be consulted for references, and can be summarised as follows.

Restoration of effector-cell functions

Levamisole, added to cell cultures or given *in vivo*, is able to increase the major functions of cells involved in cell-mediated immune responses. It increases random migration, chemotaxis, antibody and complement receptor activity, adherence, phagocytosis, NBT reduction, peroxidase activity and intracellular killing of polymorphonuclear cells, monocytes and macrophages. It also increases spontaneous and mitogen- or antigen-induced proliferation of T cells, active and total E-rosette formation, cytotoxicity, lymphokine (MIF) production, suppressor activity and plaque-cell formation. Levamisole does not directly stimulate B cells. It does not increase their proliferative response to mitogens and it has no direct effect on anti-body production. If B cell activity is pathologically increased, it is returned to normal level as shown by reduced numbers of Ig-bearing or EAC-rosette-forming cells and by the normalisation of antibody levels. Excessive null cell numbers are also reduced.

The effects of levamisole are most pronounced and consistent in compromised hosts in whom lymphocyte or phagocyte functions are below normal. At physiological concentrations, levamisole restores immunocompetence but does usually not mount an adequate immune response. The net effect on leucocytes is to restore to normal cellular responses to antigens. Stimulation above normal may be observed with doses of levamisole that largely exceed physiological concentrations (for example 1 mM), or by using special test systems, such as suboptimal concentrations of antigen.

Studies in animals and patients to measure the overall immune reactivity show restoration of delayed skin hypersensitivity in anergic patients and an increase of delayed hypersensitivity reactions to various antigens in animals. The graft-*versus*-host reaction to splenic cells in mice, the blood clearance of colloidal particles in animals and man, and macrophage migration in skin wounds — all models in which responsiveness depends on T cell or macrophage functions — may be increased. When an effect of levamisole is seen in these models it is generally moderate and not higher than that of properly responding control animals. At therapeutic doses the drug is inactive in models designed to measure stimulation of immunity, such as skin-graft rejection time or induction of experimental allergic encephalomyelitis and adjuvant arthritis in rats.

Maturation of T cells and granulocytes
In vivo, but not *in vitro*, levamisole is capable of inducing early precursor cells to mature into functioning T lymphocytes. It induces thymic antigens in nude and thymectomised mice splenocytes (Van Ghinckel and Hoebeke, 1976; Renoux and Renoux, 1977a), inhibits autologous rosette formation in nude mice (Van Wauwe and Van Nijen, 1977), stimulates lymphocyte proliferation in nude and thymectomised mice (Merluzzi *et al.*, 1976) and stimulates IgG plaque-cell formation in nude mice (Renoux and Renoux, 1977a). Indirect evidence for T-cell maturation is the property of levamisole to restore cell-mediated immune functions in NZB mice (Zulman *et al.*, 1978), in children with primary immune deficiencies (Griscelli *et al.*, 1978), and to temper autoimmune disease in NZB/NZW mice (Russell, 1976).

Levamisole also enhances release of colony-stimulating factor, resulting in increased granulopoiesis (Mahmood and Robinson, 1977).

Mechanism of action
Evidence has accumulated during the last few years that the cyclic nucleotides adenosine and guanosine monophosphate (AMP and GMP) mediate at least in part the actions of diverse hormones and hormone-like substances acting at the cell surface. These nucleotides appear to participate in the regulation of cells involved in the immune and inflammatory responses. Agents that cause an elevation of cyclic GMP levels in lymphocytes and phagocytes (for example cholinergic agents) promote the proliferative and secretory functions of these cells, probably by sustaining microtubular assembly. Substances that induce an augmentation in intracellular concentrations of cyclic AMP (for example, β-adrenergic agents) reduce such leucocyte functions (table 6.1). By contrast, cyclic AMP-inducing agents have the ability to differentiate precursor lymphocytes into fully mature T or B lymphocytes (Goldstein *et al.*, 1977).

Table 6.1 Influence of cyclic nucleotide inducers and levamisole on leucocyte functions

Effector functions	Cyclic GMP inducers	Cyclic AMP inducers	Levamisole	References
EAC-rosette formation	↑	↑	↑	1
E-rosette formation	↑	↓	↑	2, 3
Lymphocyte proliferation	↑	↓	?	4, 5
Granulocyte-macrophage proliferation	↑	↓	↑	6, 7
Plaque-cell formation	↑	↓	↑	8
Cytotoxicity	↑	↓	↑	9, 10
Spontaneous motility	↑	↓	↑	11, 12
Chemotaxis	↑	↓	↑	11, 13
Migration inhibition	↑	↓	↑	14
Granulocyte adhesiveness	↑	↓	↑	15
Phagocytosis	↑	↓	↑	16, 17
Lysosomal enzyme release	↑	↓	↑	16
Intracellular killing	↑	↓	↑	18

Cyclic GMP inducers are cholinergic agents, levamisole; cyclic AMP inducers are adrenergic agents, theophylline, histamine, etc. ↓, Decrease; ↑, increase. References: 1, Ferreira *et al.*, 1976; 2, Galant and Remo, 1975; 3, Galant *et al.*, 1976; 4, De Rubertis *et al.*, 1974; 5, Weinstein *et al.* 1974; 6, Kurland *et al.*, 1977; 7, Oshita *et al.*, 1977; 8, Watson *et al.*, 1973; 9, Lichtenstein *et al.*, 1973; 10 Ström *et al.*, 1973; 11, Estensen *et al.*, 1973; 12, Schreiner and Unanue, 1975; 13, Hatch *et al.*, 1977; 14, Koopman *et al.*, 1973; 15, Bryant and Sutcliffe, 1973; 16, Ignarro and Cech, 1976; 17 Oliveira Lima *et al.*, 1974; 18, Bourne *et al.*, 1971.

Drugs and Immune Responsiveness

The immune responses are also influenced by several polypeptide hormones, such as thymic hormones secreted in the thymus, bursapoietin secreted in the Bursa of Fabricius and ubiquitin, which can be found in virtually any cell (Bach *et al.*, 1975; Bach, 1977; Goldstein *et al.*, 1977; Scheid *et al.*, 1975). These agents augment cyclic AMP in precursor lymphocytes (Yakir *et al.*, 1977) and are potent inducers of lymphocyte maturation. Ubiquitin, like cyclic AMP-inducing agents, is unspecific in its action and induces differentiation of both B and T cells. Bursapoietin induces differentiation of B cells only. Thymopoietin and the other so-called thymic hormones induce differentiation of T cells only. Ubiquitin and thymopoietin also induce granulocyte differentiation (Kagan *et al.*, 1977). In addition, thymopoietin appears to stimulate certain effector functions of phagocytes and lymphocytes (table 6.2).

Table 6.2   Comparative testing of levamisole and 'thymic hormone'

	Levamisole	'Thymic hormone' (TH)	Reference
Maturation effects			
Autologous rosettes (*in vivo*)	↗	↗	1
Peripheral effects			
T lymphocytes			
Azathioprine sensitivity (*in vitro*)	↗	↗	2
Low total E-rosettes (*in vitro*)	↗	↗	2
Active E-rosettes (*in vitro*)	↗	↗	2
Granulocytes			
Phagocytosis of neutrophils (*in vitro*)	↗	↗	3
Macrophages			
Carbon clearance (*in vivo*)	↗	↗	4

↗ , Decrease; ↗ , increase. References: 1, Van Wauwe and Van Nijen, 1977; 2, Verhaegen *et al.*, 1978; 3, De Cock *et al.*, 1978*b*; 4, Van Ghinckel and De Brabander, 1978.

Levamisole seems to influence host defense mechanisms in a manner that is similar to that of other immune modulators. It has inducing properties on precursor T lymphocytes with thymic hormones. It also strangely mimics the effects of cyclic GMP-inducing agents on effector leucocytes. The drug, which has cholinergic properties, increases cyclic GMP but lowers cyclic AMP concentrations in T-cell-enriched mouse spleen cells (Hadden *et al.*, 1975; Woods *et al.*, 1977). It increases cyclic GMP concentrations in polymorphonuclear cells during the early phase of chemotaxis (Anderson *et al.*, 1976; Hogan and Hill, 1977; Wright *et al.*, 1977). Further, it counteracts the inhibition of E-rosette formation by cyclic AMP inducers such as histamine, dibutyryl-cyclic AMP and adenosine (De Cock *et al.*, 1977; De Cock *et al.*, 1978*c*; Di Perri *et al.*, 1977). This suggests that levamisole promotes the expression of receptors on T-lymphocytes, which seems to be mediated through changes in intracellular nucleotides.

Intracellular nucleotides regulate, at least in part, microtubular assembly (editorial, 1978). The morphological and functional integrity of microtubuli are essential to the motility and to the secretory functions of cells (editorial, 1978). A recent study has shown that the major thiol metabolite of levamisole (OMPI), unlike the parent compound, enhances the polymerisation rate of tubulin. This effect mimics that of thiols such as glutathione, indicating that OMPI probably interacts with microtubule formation by interference with critical -SH groups on the tubulin molecule. The effects of levamisole on host defense mechanisms might at least partially be due to the formation of OMPI, which could enhance microtubule integrity and function in leucocytes (De Brabander *et al.*, 1978).

The dual effect of levamisole on peripheral T lymphocytes, whose function it restores, and on precursor T lymphocytes, which it stimulates to differentiate into mature T cells, seems not to be unique to the drug. Evidence is accumulating that the thymic hormone thymopoietin behaves similarly. Comparative studies between levamisole and thymopoietin, or its active pentapeptide moiety, show a striking parallellism in tests designed to study maturation of T lymphocytes, or effector functions of T lymphocytes, polymorphonuclear neutrophils and macrophages (table 6.3). This parallellism is further shown in clinical studies in which both levamisole and thymic hormones restore immune functions without elevating them above normal values (Bliznakov *et al.*, 1978; Rossio and Goldstein, 1977; Zaizov *et al.*, 1977).

Levamisole thus seems to behave as a thymomimetic agent. It is conceivable that it interacts at the thymic-hormone receptor sites on lymphocytes, polymorphonuclear neutrophils and macrophages, and influences cell metabolism by altering the cyclic GMP/AMP ratio in the cell. There is, however, no direct evidence for common receptor sites so far.

In conclusion, there are several mechanisms by which levamisole may interfere with host defense mechanisms. They are not mutually exclusive and it is still not clear which are the more important mechanisms for its therapeutic actions. Its likely immunoregulatory mode of action is by mimicry of the thymic hormone thymopoietin.

IMMUNOTHERAPEUTIC PROPERTIES

This spectrum of immunological activities provides a useful basis to explore rationally the immunotherapeutic potential of levamisole. One can advance the working hypothesis that the drug is, in principle, indicated whenever hypofunction of T lymphocytes, polymorphonuclear cells or macrophages causes immunopathology.

Such possible mechanisms are schematically shown in figure 6.1.

The elimination and degradation of foreign antigens is a primary function of the immune system. This function is accomplished by a cascade of immune processes which include the recognition of foreign materials as non-self, the production of mediators of inflammation and the accumulation and activation of immune effector cells at the sites of immunological reaction. Failure of any component of this complicated network may allow disease-producing antigen to persist as in recurrent or chronic infections and cancer. Or, for reasons that are poorly understood, it may

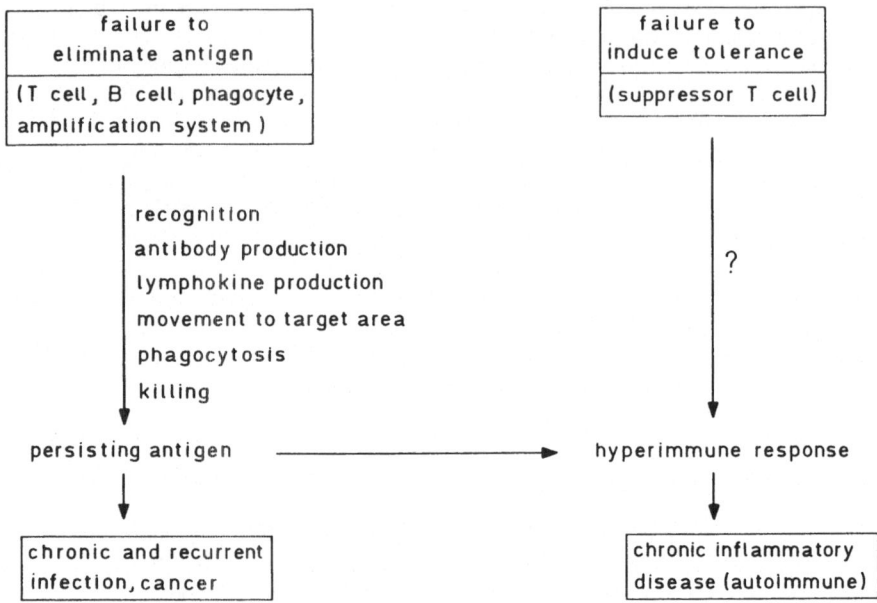

Figure 6.1   Possible mechanisms of immunopathology

lead to chronic inflammatory and hyperimmune conditions characterised by reduced T-cell and increased B-cell activities and frequently by immune-complex
formation.

Levamisole favourably influences the course of a considerable number of apparently unrelated diseases of which all are chronic or recurrent. Infection predomi-
nates in some, lymphoid inflammation in others. The underlying immune defects
have rarely been recognised but this may be more related to our lack of understanding of the mechanisms leading to immunopathology, than to the absence of
such an immune defect.

Immunodeficiency and allergic diseases
The immunodeficiency and allergic diseases in which levamisole was tested are
listed in table 6.3.

Immunodeficiency diseases
Patients with immunodeficiency disorders are highly susceptible to infections by
viruses, bacteria, fungi or protozoa, including sometimes organisms normally of
low virulence. The patients have frequently recurring or chronic infections of the
skin, the lungs, the upper respiratory tract or other organs from early life. Eczema
may be present.

Levamisole was given to children with immunodeficiency diseases in an attempt
to reduce the frequency and severity of infectious episodes and to restore immune
functions.

(a) T- or B-cell deficiency diseases. Levamisole was given to 36 children with T- or B-cell deficiency diseases for periods of 1 month to 2 years (table 6.3). The frequency and severity of infections decreased significantly in approximately two-thirds of the patients. Some became symptom-free. Patients with Wiskott-Aldrich syndrome, who were unresponsive to transfer factor, had a regression of skin lesions (Nadal Ortega *et al.*, 1977; Spitler *et al.*, 1977*a*). Patients with chronic mucocutaneous candidosis did not improve. Delayed skin hypersensitivity reactions and T-cell functions (E-rosette formation, lymphocyte proliferation) improved in a majority of cases; B-cell functions were not influenced. According to Griscelli (1976), levamisole treatment does not substitute for anti-infectious, anti-allergic or gammaglobulin treatments in patients with immune deficiency disorders; it reduces the need for such treatments by opposing a state of increased susceptibility to infection.

(b) Phagocytic dysfunctions. Chronic granulomatous disease: levamisole treatment reduced the number of infections in two patients with chronic granulomatous disease and was without effect in two others (Griscelli, 1976).

Hyper-immunoglobulinaemia E syndrome (HIE): six children received levamisole for periods ranging from 6 months to 3 years (De Cree *et al.*, 1978*a*; Vanheule *et al.*, 1976; Weening *et al.*, 1977). In five, the number of infectious episodes and their severity gradually decreased in the course of the first 6 months of treatment. Two patients became free of infections after 1 year of treatment. Eczematous lesions were not influenced. Clinical improvement was parallelled by a gradual recovery of neutrophil chemotaxis and by other parameters of cell-mediated immunity such as delayed skin hypersensitivity, E-rosette formation, lymphocyte proliferation and phagocytosis (De Cree *et al.*, 1978*a*; Vanheule *et al.*, 1976). IgE levels remained high. Neutrophil chemotaxis was restored by physiological concentrations of levamisole *in vitro* (Wright *et al.*, 1977).

Allergic diseases
Patients with allergic diseases (asthma, atopic dermatitis) are immunologically characterised by type-I reactions, but T-lymphocyte and granulocyte dysfunctions have also been described. Levamisole was given to 70 patients for periods of 1 to 6 months; 51 had asthma and 40 had atopic dermatitis or eczema (table 6.3). A subjective improvement of skin lesions was reported in 13 of 36 patients with — generally severe — atopic dermatitis. Levamisole was ineffective in asthma. Only one study was controlled and showed no difference between levamisole and placebo in 10 asthmatic patients (Bruninx, 1973).

Tests of E-rosette formation or delayed skin hypersensitivity in a few patients were inconclusive. IgE was reported to decrease after 2 months of treatment in seven patients with asthma, rhinitis, atopic dermatitis and eczema (Halpern, 1978).

Infectious diseases
Patients with specific or overall defects of lymphocyte or phagocyte function are highly susceptible to recurrent and chronic infections. Such infections also occur in patients in whom no underlying immune defects have been recognised. It is probable that defects exist but that they are not recognised during routine immunological evaluations. For example, T lymphocytes of patients with recurrent herpes

Table 6.3   Levamisole in immunodeficiency and allergic diseases

	References
Immunodeficiency diseases	
(a) *T- or B-cell deficiency diseases*	
X-linked hypogammaglobulinaemia (Bruton type)	1
Acquired hypoglobulinaemia	1
Selective IgA deficiency	2, 3
Selective IgM deficiency	1
Chronic mucocutaneous candidosis	4, 5, 6, 7
Severe combined immunodeficiency disease	1
Immunodeficiency with ataxia-telangiectasia	1, 3
Wiskott–Aldrich syndrome	1, 4, 8
(b) *Phagocytic dysfunctions*	
Chronic granulomatous disease	1
Hyper-immunoglobulinaemia E syndrome (HIE)	9, 10, 11, 12
Allergic diseases	
Asthma	13, 14, 15, 16
Atopic dermatitis	3, 5, 14, 15, 16

References: 1, Griscelli, 1975; 2, De Cree *et al.*, 1975; 3, Verhaegen *et al.*, 1977*a*; 4, Spitler *et al.*, 1977*a*; 5, Allen *et al.*, 1978; 6, Wells, 1975; 7, Valdimarsson, 1975; 8, Nadal Ortega *et al.*, 1977; 9, Vanheule *et al.*, 1976; 10, Weening *et al.*, 1977; 11, De Cree *et al.*, 1978*a*; 12, Wright *et al.*, 1977; 13, Bruninx, 1973; 14, Halpern, 1978; 15, De Loore, 1974; 16, Samsoen *et al.*, 1977.

respond normally to the usual mitogens or antigens such as PHA (phytohaemagglutinin) or PPD (purified protein derivative). They fail to respond to the herpes antigen during infectious episodes but respond to it between episodes.

Some infectious agents can temporarily depress immune responses, a phenomenon called immune repulsion. Prolonged immune repulsion has been held responsible for the protracted convalescence of some patients after influenza, measles, hepatitis or other infections.

Levamisole was tested in a variety of recurrent or chronic infections caused by bacteria, viruses, fungi and protozoa. Acute infections were not treated because experiments in animals had shown that levamisole did not influence the course of an acute infection in an immunologically competent animal.

Recurrent infections
Recurrent labial or genital herpes: 151 patients with severe, long-lasting, frequently relapsing and therapy-resistant labial or genital herpes were treated with levamisole for at least 3 months (De Queiroz Carvalho *et al.*, 1976; Grupper, 1976; Jarish and Sandor, 1977; Kint *et al.*, 1974; O'Reilly *et al.*, 1977; Racz, 1977; Runne and Aulepp, 1975; Symoens and Brugmans, 1974). The frequency, duration and intensity of episodes decreased in 110 patients. Some patients became symptom-free

during the whole observation period. There was no apparent difference in response between treatment at fixed intervals (for example, two consecutive days each week) or treatment at the start of each disease episode only (Kint *et al.*, 1974). In the 10 placebo-controlled studies, in which individual responsiveness was evaluated, 107 out of 172 patients (62 per cent) improved with levamisole and 86 of 194 (44 per cent) with placebo. There is thus a considerable placebo-effect, but the number of patients who improved with levamisole is significantly higher than with placebo ($P = 0.0009$, χ^2 test) (Fanta, 1978; Krupp, 1977*a*; Bierman, 1976; Gier *et al.*, 1977*a*; Chang and Fuimara, 1978; Carr, 1978; Barrett-Connor, 1978; Pinnell *et al.*, 1978; Russell *et al.*, 1978; Spruance *et al.*, 1978).

Two investigators found a correlation between immunological and clinical responses (Jarish and Sandor, 1977; O'Reilly *et al.*, 1977). Patients with recurrent herpes seem to be able to mount a cell-mediated immune response to the herpes antigen, but the response is temporarily depressed during infectious episodes. Patients who responded clinically to levamisole had considerably higher herpes-induced lymphocyte proliferation during levamisole treatment, than before. Lymphocyte proliferation was not improved in non-responders (O'Reilly *et al.*, 1977). Similarly, herpes-induced migration inhibition, which is strongly reduced or absent in patients with frequent recurrence, was restored to normal in patients who responded clinically to levamisole but remained low in non-responders (Jarish and Sandor, 1977). Levamisole corrected defective chemotactic response of neutrophils from herpes patients *in vitro* and *in vivo* (Rabson *et al.*, 1977).

Recurrent systemic infections in children: levamisole was studied in very young children (under 4 years of age) with relapsing or chronic rhinitis, and in older children (over 4 years of age) with recurrent febrile infections of ear, nose, throat, lung or urinary tract. Levamisole was compared with placebo in three double-blind trials.

Levamisole was superior to placebo in reducing the frequency, duration and severity of febrile episodes in 70 children who had frequently relapsing infections of the adenoids, tonsils or upper respiratory tract. The children were treated for 6 months during winter time (Van Eygen *et al.*, 1976). Two open studies with 37 children came to similar conclusions (Griscelli, 1976; La Jouanine, 1975). Delayed skin hypersensitivity was restored and spontaneous NBT reduction was increased in one patient who also responded clinically to levamisole (De Cree *et al.*, 1975). Children with recurring febrile infections of the urinary tract had a significantly reduced relapse rate when they received levamisole (one relapse in 14 children), as compared to children who received placebo (six relapses in 13 children). Treatment lasted 8 months (Lubetkin *et al.*, 1977).

Eight of nine children with continuously relapsing or chronic rhinitis of non-allergic origin had their symptoms improved after 1 to 3 weeks of treatment with levamisole. Of the 14 placebo-treated patients, only seven improved (De Loore, 1977).

In conclusion, long-term treatment with levamisole seems to reduce the rate of infections in children with recurrent febrile illnesses. Antibiotics have no influence on the frequency of recurrences. In most cases these infections are not life-threatening and disappear spontaneously after a few years. They may, however, seriously hamper the social and scolar life of these children. In infants with chronic rhinitis, levamisole seems to interrupt the pathological process. No side-effects or

toxicity due to the drug were observed in any of the children treated with
levamisole.

Chronic infections

(a) *Infections of the skin. Pyogenic infections*: patients with localised pyogenic
infections of the skin, clinically diagnosed as acne conglobata and/or pustulosa
(27 patients), furunculosis (six patients), folliculitis (three patients) or pyoderma
(seven patients), were treated with levamisole for periods ranging from 1 to 18
months (Allen *et al.*, 1978; Balogh and Szabolscy, 1976; De Cree *et al.*, 1975,
1978*b*; Grupper, 1976; Haneke and Meinhof, 1977; Ippen and Qadripur, 1975;
Kaslik *et al.*, 1978; Lods, 1976; Spitler *et al.*, 1977*a*; Thornes, 1975; Verhaegen
et al., 1977*a*; Zilko, 1975). All cases were chronic or recurrent, and several had
become resistant to antibiotic treatment. Phagocytosis and T-lymphocyte
function are frequently impaired in such patients.

Marked clinical improvement or cure was reported in 42 of 52 patients treated.
The patients generally started to respond after only 2 or 3 weeks of treatment.
One patient with antibiotic-resistant folliculitis was cured after 3 weeks, relapsed
after discontinuation of treatment and responded again to a new course of levamisole. The phagocytic index was restored in 15 patients (Ippen and Qadripur,
1975; Kaslik *et al.*, 1978) and E-rosettes were restored in 19 patients (Balogh and
Szabolscy, 1976; De Cree *et al.*, 1978*b*). There was a good correlation between
immunological and clinical responses in most patients.

Mycotic infections: five patients with continuously relapsing and therapy-
resistant vaginal candidosis became virtually free of relapses during treatment with
levamisole which lasted 3 to 8 months (Vandervellen, 1978).

Two of four patients with chronic candidosis of the skin had their lesions
cleared during levamisole treatment which lasted 1 to 4 months (Grupper, 1976;
La Jouanine, 1975; Penny, 1976).

Levamisole had no influence on the lesions of three patients with chronic tri-
chophytosis (La Jouanine, 1975; Allen *et al.*, 1978; Spitler *et al.*, 1978). One
patient had improved cell-mediated immune responses to PPD and DNCB (dinitrochlorobenzene) during levamisole treatment but failed to respond to trichophytin
(Touraine *et al.*, 1975).

Superinfected skin lesions: levamisole or placebo was given together with
topical therapies to 59 patients with varicose ulcers (ulcus cruris). After 5 months
of treatment the cure rate was significantly higher in the levamisole-treated
patients than in those who received placebo (Morias *et al.*, 1977). Somewhat
paradoxal to this finding is the delayed healing of a varicose ulcer during levamisole treatment reported in a patient with rheumatoid arthritis (El-Ghobarey *et
al.*, 1977*a*).

In a controlled study with 19 patients, levamisole monotherapy significantly
improved the healing of the skin lesions of patients with intertrigo inguinalis
without affecting the skin flora. Patients who received placebo did not improve
(De Cree, 1974).

In conclusion, levamisole seems to promote wound healing by a mechanism
independent of the flora present in the wound.

Levamisole increased neutrophil and macrophage migration and giant cell formation on s.c. (sub-cutaneous) coverslips in mice (Dieppe *et al.*, 1976) and

markedly enhanced the phagocytosis of staphylococci from a skin lesion in rats (Moese, 1974; Fischer *et al.*, 1975). In air-exposed surgical incisions in guinea pigs, levamisole significantly enhanced the course of repair as shown by gross observation, histological examination and mechanical testing (Linsky, 1975).

Warts: 245 patients with common warts of hands, feet or other localisations, including patients with plane warts, received levamisole for periods ranging from 1 to 18 months (Hellin and Bergh, 1974; Grupper, 1976; Krupp, 1977*b*; Krupp and Jolly, 1977; Moncada *et al.*, 1977; Racz, 1977; Sutton, 1977; Allen *et al.*, 1978). Over 50 per cent of the patients were claimed to improve during treatment. Four placebo-controlled studies, however, showed that a similar rate of improvement can be obtained with placebo as with levamisole (De Peuter, 1975; Puissant, 1976; Schou and Hellin, 1977). A suggestion in one study that plantar warts are more sensitive to levamisole treatment than other warts (Puissant, 1976) was not confirmed by others (Schou and Hellin, 1977).

A double-blind study in 50 patients failed to show any difference between levamisole and placebo in patients with veneral warts (condylomata accuminata) (Schou and Hellin, 1977).

(*b*) *Infections of the eye*. A few open studies in patients with herpes corneae (Lods, 1976; Spitler *et al.*, 1977*a, b*), zona ophthalmica (Lods, 1975; Spitler *et al.*, 1978) and ocular toxoplasmosis (Spitler *et al.*, 1977*a*) suggest that there is an effect but they are not conclusive.

(*c*) *Pulmonary infections*. The majority of 29 patients with chronic bronchitis superinfected with *Pseudomonas aeruginosa, Pneumocystis carinii, Aspergillus fumigatus* or an unidentified flora, experienced a marked relief of their pulmonary symptoms after a few weeks of treatment with levamisole. The cultures became sterile in some cases but were unchanged in others (La Jouanine, 1975; De Leeuw-Delvigne, 1976; Roge and Lods, 1976; Griscelli, 1976). Marked improvement was also claimed for two children with mucoviscidosis (La Jouanine, 1975).

(*d*) *Chronic or protracted systemic infections. Leprosy*: lepromatous leprosy is characterised by the virtual absence of a specific cellular immune response to *Mycobacterium leprae* and by widespread bacillary invasion. There is no granuloma formation. Borderline disease is characterised by clinical and immunological instability.

In an open study, ten patients with lepromatous leprosy and four patients with borderline disease received levamisole in monotherapy for 18 months. The patients started to improve within a few weeks, as judged by clinical, histological and bacteriological criteria. Neurological symptoms did not deteriorate but regressed or remained unchanged (Saint-André and Louvet, 1976).

In a controlled study, 12 patients with nodular lepromatous or nodular dimorphic leprosy received dapsone as a basic treatment. Six of these patients also received levamisole for 6 months. These six patients had a better clinical evolution than those who received dapsone alone (Martinez and Zaias, 1976).

As a rule, delayed skin hypersensitivity to the usual antigens such as candidin or PPD increased during levamisole treatment. Skin tests with lepromin were not improved (Meyers *et al.*, 1975; Saint-André and Louvet, 1976; Nelson *et al.*, 1978).

Brucellosis: patients with chronic brucellosis have suppression of their cellular immune system. The patients present with a variety of unspecific symptoms, such as chronic fatigue, depression, bouts of chills and fever, sweating and flu-like symptoms.

Remission of all symptoms was reported in 43 of 55 patients with chronic brucellosis, treated with levamisole for 1 to 6 months. Some patients also received antibiotics or other immunotherapeutic agents. Patients who responded, usually developed an acute exacerbation of symptoms within the first month. There was a fair correlation between clinical response to treatment and restoration of immune functions as measured by E-rosette formation, lymphocyte proliferation and, to a lesser extent, delayed skin hypersensitivity to DNCB (Renoux and Renoux, 1977*b*; Thornes, 1977*a, b*). Apart from exacerbation of symptoms, side-effects to leva-misole were confined to nausea and vomiting in four cases and skin rash in one (Thornes, 1977*a, b*).

Influenza: some patients recover very slowly from an outbreak of influenza and have prolonged physical and psychic asthenia. Host defenses are reduced during acute influenza but spontaneously recover as the infection subsides. Prolonged anergy caused by the virus has been held responsible for the protracted course of the disease in certain patients.

Levamisole reversed depression of monocyte chemotaxis induced by the influenza virus *in vitro* (Snyderman *et al.*, 1978) and prevented the depression of delayed skin hypersensitivity to PPD that normally occurs after influenza vaccination (Van Hooren, 1976). Levamisole thus seemed to abolish post-viral anergy.

In the assumption that recovery could be accelerated by abolishing anergy, leva-misole or placebo was given to 50 patients during a severe outbreak of clinically diagnosed 'flu'. Levamisole significantly hastened recovery compared with placebo, as measured by body temperature, pulmonary symptoms, muscle and joint pain and the ability to return to work (Kromer, 1977). No differences were shown between levamisole and placebo in a similar trial performed during a mild epidemic, when symptoms persisted for only 1 week (J. Symoens, unpublished work).

Australia antigen hepatitis: levamisole or placebo was given to 25 patients with Australia antigen-positive hepatitis during the second and third week of the acute disease. The patients who received levamisole showed a transient rise in transaminases but recovered more quickly from the acute disease than those who received placebo, as judged by transaminases, antigen titre and/or histology (Par *et al.*, 1977).

Patients with chronic Australia antigen hepatitis had increased transaminases, increased total haemolytic complement and increased or reduced antigen titres during levamisole treatment. These changes returned to control values when the drug was withdrawn and occurred again each time the drug was restarted (De Cree *et al.*, 1973; Chadwick *et al.*, 1977). Prolonged treatment with levamisole in nine patients with chronic Australia antigen hepatitis resulted in an early increase of transaminases followed by a gradual decrease to normal values in four patients. Antigen titre persisted. After 18 months, liver biopsies showed no further signs of chronic inflammation (J. De Cree, unpublished work).

Immunological tests showed restoration of E-rosettes to normal values in leva-misole-treated patients (Chadwick *et al.*, 1977; Verhaegen *et al.*, 1977*a*) and stimulation of null cells to form E-rosettes under the influence of levamisole *in vitro*. Thymosin had similar effects *in vitro* (Thomas *et al.*, 1976).

In conclusion, levamisole seems to hasten recovery of acute hepatitis, and to inactivate disease in chronic cases. The first effect is reminiscent of a reversal of post-viral anergy. The second effect is reminiscent of the induction of tolerance to the antigen, a phenomenon in which suppressor T cells are thought to be involved.

Measles: deficient cell-mediated immunity owing to undernourishment or chronic disease is held responsible for the high morbidity and mortality caused by measles in African children.

During a severe outbreak of measles, 22 African children received levamisole for 1 week and 18 were left untreated. All patients received symptomatic treatments and antibiotics if necessary. One patient died and two suffered from infectious complications in the levamisole group. Three died and eight presented complications in the control group (Barbaix, 1976). A similar, though not significant, trend in favour of levamisole was seen in another trial involving 103 African children of whom 48 received levamisole and 55 received placebo (N. Gernier, unpublished work). No difference between levamisole and placebo was shown in 136 children studied during a relatively mild epidemic of measles (M. Jancloes, unpublished work).

Other diseases: a therapeutic benefit has been claimed in a few patients with mononucleosis (Thornes, 1975), systemic herpes or varicella infections (Cullen, 1977; La Jouanine, 1975; Lods, 1975; Ramot and Biniaminov, 1977), paracocci-dioidomycosis (Musatti *et al.*, 1976) and toxoplasmosis (Fegies and Guerrero, 1977). A double-blind study in otherwise healthy individuals suffering from an acute outbreak of herpes zoster failed to show any difference in healing time between levamisole and placebo (De Donder, 1976).

Chronic inflammatory diseases

Chronic inflammatory diseases are often characterised by lymphoid infiltration, granuloma formation and by an imbalance of humoral and cellular immune mechanisms. In some of these diseases a preferential defect of suppressor T cells is suspected. Auto-immune phenomena are common. Levamisole was tested in these diseases in an attempt to restore immune homoeostasis.

Rheumatic diseases

(a) *Rheumatoid arthritis. Clinical and biological effects*: the effectiveness of levamisole in rheumatoid arthritis has been studied in 12 controlled and 21 open trials involving 1037 patients (table 6.4). The largest controlled study (Eular study) involved 16 study centres with 110 control patients and 253 patients receiving two different treatment regimens of levamisole. The vast majority of the patients were severely affected and in need of basic therapy. Many had already been treated with gold, D-penicillamine, antimalarials or immunosuppressive agents. Most patients were said to have classic or definite rheumatoid arthritis by the ARA criteria and active disease that responded poorly to anti-inflammatory drugs.

Levamisole or the control drug (placebo, gold, D-penicillamine) were usually given in addition to the anti-inflammatory agents that the patients were already taking, including low doses of corticosteroids. With a few exceptions (Franchimont *et al.*, 1976; Veys and Mielants, 1977a), the concomitant use of basic antirheumatics was excluded. A few patients received levamisole without any other drug (Lequesne and Floquet, 1976; Franchimont *et al.*, 1978; Multicenter Study Group, 1978a). The usual dose of levamisole was 150 mg, either daily, on 2 to 5 consecutive days each week or once weekly. Most patients were treated for at least 6 months.

The longest observation time was 36 months (table 6.4).

Criteria to measure clinical disease activity included assessments such as the number of tender and swollen joints, technetium index, pain, duration of morning stiffness, grip strength, proximal interphalangeal joint circumference, walking time and the functional index of Lee.

All well-documented controlled studies showed significant clinical improvement over placebo by each of the criteria used. All open studies confirmed the efficacy of the drug. One poorly documented controlled study claimed that levamisole was ineffective (Dinai and Pras, 1975).

The effects were usually apparent between 6 weeks and 3 months of treatment, sometimes earlier (Di Perri *et al.*, 1978*a*; Szpilman *et al.*, 1977) or later (Michel, 1978). A mild flare-up of inflammatory symptoms may precede improvement (Basch, 1978; Michel, 1978). An optimal effect was usually reached between 6 and 12 months of treatment, after which no further improvement was observed (Schuermans, 1975; Veys and Mielants, 1977*a*; Basch, 1978; Kalfa, 1978; Michel, 1978). Flare-ups may occur despite continuation of treatment but they seemed to be of shorter duration and lesser severity compared with previous episodes (Basch, 1978). Deterioration usually occurred a few weeks or months after cessation of treatment depending on exposure time, but long-term remissions have also been observed (Schuermans, 1975; Veys and Mielants, 1977*a*; Michel, 1978). Relapsing patients generally responded again if levamisole treatment was re-instituted.

The clinical improvement was accompanied by biological modifications: reduction or normalisation of erythrocyte sedimentation rate (ESR) (Multicenter Study Group, 1978*a*), reduction of acute-phase reactants such as CRP, C3, α_1-antitrypsin, α_2-haptoglobin (Verhaegen *et al.*, 1977*b*; Veys and Mielants, 1977*b*; Foroozanfar *et al.*, 1978; Multicenter Study Group, 1978*a*), reduction or negation of rheumatoid factor titres (Michel, 1978), reduction of immune-complex concentrations (Foroozanfar *et al.*, 1977; Rosenthal *et al.*, 1977; Franchimont *et al.*, 1978; Multicenter Study Group, 1978*a*), increase in haemoglobin and haematocrit concentrations (Alcalay *et al.*, 1977; Multicenter Study Group, 1978*a*). Anti-nuclear antibody (ANA) concentrations did not show consistent changes (El-Ghobarey *et al.*, 1977*b*; Runge and Pinals, 1977; Michel, 1978; Taube, 1978).

The levels of immunoglobulins G, M and A (Hodinka *et al.*, 1977*a*; Szpilman *et al.*, 1977; Veys and Mielants, 1977*c*; Michel, 1978; Multicenter Study Group, 1978*a*) and total haemolytic complement (Verhaegen *et al.*, 1977*b*), and the total leucocyte, lymphocyte and neutrophil counts (Gallice, 1977; Hodinka *et al.*, 1977*a*; Kalfa, 1978; Multicenter Study Group, 1978*a*) have a tendency to decrease within normal range after 3 to 6 months of treatment. An increased eosinophil count was coincident with erythema in two of four cases (Hodinka *et al.*, 1977*b*).

The biological modifications during levamisole treatment thus tended towards normalisation and indicated reduced inflammatory activity. The changes were most pronounced in those patients whose values were most aberrant before levamisole treatment. They are slow in onset and are usually significant between 3 and 6 months of treatment. There is no evidence of development of auto-antibodies (Rosenthal *et al.*, 1976*a*; Multicenter Study Group, 1978*a*), although Browning (1977) reports a higher incidence of cold lymphocytotoxic antibodies during treatment. A reduction of para-articular manifestations of the disease such as subcutaneous nodules, was reported after prolonged treatment (Basch, 1978), whereas in the Eular study levamisole seemed to prevent the new development of such manifestations (Multicenter Study Group, 1978*a*).

Table 6.4   Studies with levamisole in rheumatoid arthritis

References	Levamisole				
	No. of patients (start)	Daily dose (mg)	Schedule doses/week	Duration (months)	Reference drug
Controlled studies					
Dinai and Pras, 1975	14	150	7	3	P
Huskisson et al., 1976	12	150	7	6	P, Pen
Franchimont et al., 1976	28	150	7→2	6	P
Basch et al., 1977b	22	150	3	3	Px
Miller et al., 1977	20	150	7	4	Px
Runge et al., 1977	14	150	4	4	P
Myers and Schimmer, 1977	6	150	7	6	P
Taube, 1978	13	150	4	6	P
El-Ghobarey et al., 1977	15	150	7	2	P
El-Ghobarey et al., 1978	20	150	7	12	Gold
Multicenter, 1978a	253	150	3–7	6	P
Multicenter, 1978b	86	50–150	1	6	—
Open studies					
Verhaegen et al., 1977b	16	150	7	3–8	
Schuermans, 1975	33	150	3–7	4–20	
Gallice, 1977	32	150	3–7	12	
Alcalay et al., 1977	8	150	3–7	3–11	
Michel, 1978	23	60–150	4–7	7–15	
Kalfa, 1978	24	150	3–7	3–23	
Runge and Pinals, 1977	21	100	4	15	
Franchimont et al., 1976	57	100–150	3–7	6–28	
Roig et al., 1977	16	150	3–7	3–9	
Rave et al., 1978	18	150	3–4	?	
Lequesne and Floquet, 1976	8	150	7	1–6	
Leca et al., 1976	20	150	3–7	6	
Guaydier et al., 1977	30	2 mg/kg	2–7	?	
Hodinka et al., 1977a	17	150	3–7	6	
d'Anglejan et al., 1977	26	150	2–7	6	
Davatchi et al., 1977	30	150	3–7	3–10	
Basch, 1978	49	100–150	3–7	3–36	
Rosenthal et al., 1976a	9	150	3–7	2–5	
Di Perri et al., 1977b	20	150	1–2	6	
Szpilman et al., 1977	25	150	7	1	
Veys and Mielants, 1977b	70	150	4	6–36	

Abbreviations: P, placebo; Pen, penicillamine; x, cross-over.

As a result of the clinical and biological improvement, the number of concomitant medications and their dosage can be reduced in certain patients (d'Anglejan *et al.*, 1977; Davatchi *et al.*, 1977; Basch, 1978). In the Eular study, 20 per cent of the patients had discontinued all concomitant medications after 6 months of treatment with levamisole (Multicenter Study Group, 1978*a*).

The treatment schedule does not influence responsiveness. Clinical and biological responses are identical with a standard dose of 150 mg on 1, 3 or 7 consecutive days each week (Multicenter Study Group, 1978*a, b*). The earlier onset of responses with daily treatment, suggested by Kalfa (1978) is not confirmed in the Eular study (Multicenter Study Group, 1978*a*). In patients receiving a standard dose of 150 mg, there is no correlation between response and body weight. However, 150 mg once weekly is definitely superior to 50 mg once weekly. A threshold dose thus exists but it is not critically dependent on body weight (Symoens and Lewi 1978).

Most investigators claim that 50-70 per cent of patients improve on levamisole, with responses varying from clinical remission to marked or moderate improvement. One-third or more of patients remain unchanged. A few deteriorate.

Using a new mathematical model to express the degree of individual responsiveness, the responses of the patients in the Eular study can be classified as deterioration, moderate improvement or marked improvement (Lewi and Symoens, 1978). Significantly more control patients deteriorated than patients on levamisole, and significantly more levamisole-treated patients improved markedly than controls. The number of patients who improved moderately was similar in both groups. Levamisole is thus beneficial to at least 50 per cent of the patients by preventing deterioration or inducing marked improvement (Symoens and Lewi, 1978). Disease stabilisation as a response to treatment has not been recognised in the literature. However, several investigators have observed patients who apparently did not improve on levamisole, discontinued treatment, and soon thereafter had a flare-up of their disease which subsided again when levamisole was reinstituted (Meyers and Schimmer, 1977). The number of patients whose disease is stabilised by levamisole is as large as the number of patients whose condition is markedly improved (Symoens and Lewi, 1978).

Levamisole is thus definitely superior to anti-inflammatory agents. The clinical and biological effects are similar to those of gold and D-penicillamine (Huskisson *et al.*, 1976; El-Ghobarey *et al.*, 1977*b*), with which levamisole shares the delayed onset, the variable therapeutic action and the relatively prolonged remissions after treatment is discontinued.

Immunological effects: during treatment, several immunological abnormalities were corrected. Delayed skin hypersensitivity to DNCB, PPD and other antigens was reconstituted in anergic patients and in patients with reduced reactivity (Basch *et al.*, 1977*a*; Di Perri *et al.*, 1978*a*; Szpilman *et al.*, 1977). Reduced E-rosette numbers (Basch *et al.*, 1977*a*; Di Perri *et al.*, 1978*a*; Massoud *et al.*, 1977; Roux *et al.*, 1977; Verhaegen *et al.*, 1977*b*), excessive EAC-rosette numbers (Massoud *et al.*, 1977) and excessive null cell numbers (Massoud *et al.*, 1977; Rosenthal *et al.*, 1976*b*) were usually normalised, whereas no changes were seen in patients in whom these numbers were normal before treatment. Restoration of E-rosette formation lasted 5-6 days after two doses of levamisole (Di Perri *et al.*, 1978*a*). This effect is thought to be due to the shedding of an immunorepulsive blocking substance from the lymphocyte surface by levamisole (Del Giacco, 1977; Moroz *et al.*, 1977).

Restored lymphocyte proliferation in response to PHA and various antigens was reported in some studies, especially when suboptimal concentrations of antigens were used (Levy and Miller, 1976; Scheinberg *et al.*, 1978). No consistent change was seen in other studies (Basch *et al.*, 1977*a*; Merryman and Jaffe, 1977; Szpilman *et al.*, 1977). Neutrophil chemotaxis rose substantially after 2 days of treatment with levamisole and this effect was maintained for 5 days (Mowat, 1978*a*, *b*). The phagocytic activity of blood neutrophils was activated, but no such effect was seen on synovial phagocytes (Wynne *et al.*, 1977). Migration inhibition of leucocytes was also enhanced (Huskisson *et al.*, 1976).

Although there was considerable variation in the immunological responses in any group of patients treated with levamisole, the trend was towards a restoration to normal values. Immunological restoration was usually prompt, within days. Trends towards decreasing response have been described after a few months of treatment (Levy and Miller, 1976; Spitler *et al.*, 1977*c*).

Correlations between immunological normalisation and clinical responsiveness have been observed (Basch *et al.*, 1977*a*; Di Perri *et al.*, 1978*a*; Massoud *et al.*, 1977), but most studies report no such relationship. None of the immunological tests could reliably predict clinical responsiveness or act as immunological markers for clinical improvement.

(*b*) *Other rheumatic diseases. Juvenile rheumatoid arthritis*: ten patients with juvenile rheumatoid arthritis were treated with levamisole for 1 to 3 months. Three patients developed agranulocytosis within 5 weeks after the start of treatment. Two of these patients were on high doses of steroids and died of infection (Ruuskanen *et al.*, 1976). The third patient recovered within 1 week and was in complete remission of all symptoms of juvenile rheumatoid arthritis for at least 6 months thereafter (Clara and Germanes, 1977). Of the remaining seven patients, two improved and five did not (Griscelli, 1976; La Jouanine, 1975).

Lupus erythematodes: 31 patients with SLE were treated with levamisole for 3 to 20 months. Three had renal involvement. Levamisole reduced the number of symptoms in patients with active disease (Gordon and Keenan, 1975; Gordon and Yanagihara,1977), had a steroid-sparing effect (Gordon and Keenan, 1975; Gordon and Yanagihara, 1977; Smolen *et al.*, 1977) and reduced circulating immune complexes (Berenyi *et al.*, 1976). One patient with severe renal involvement became asymptomatic after 14 months of treatment (Ores *et al.*, 1977). Another patient had a temporary worsening of nephrotic syndrome (Gordon and Yanagihara, 1977). Of five patients with discoid lupus erythematodes, two improved (Baart de la Faille, 1977).

When tests of cell-mediated immunity, such as delayed skin hypersensitivity or lymphocyte proliferation, were low before treatment, they were increased during treatment (Attias, 1976; Gordon and Keenan, 1975; Gordon and Yanagihara, 1977). Effects on E-rosettes were variable (Berenyi *et al.*, 1976; Gordon and Keenan, 1975; Gordon and Yanagihara, 1977). *In vitro*, levamisole restored phagocytosis by PMNs (polymorphonucleocytes), from patients with SLE (Molnar *et al.*, 1976) and seemed partially to prevent the inhibition of E-rosette formation by SLE serum. These studies showed no evidence that levamisole would be detrimental to patients with SLE.

Sjögren's syndrome: of eleven patients who were evaluated clinically, nine improved after 2 to 4 months of treatment with levamisole. None of four placebo-treated patients improved (Racz, 1976; Talal and Michalski, 1977). In another study, eight of nine patients were withdrawn because of pruritic rash (Balint *et al.*, 1977).

Progressive systemic sclerosis (scleroderma): the skin changes observed in progressive systemic sclerosis improved in three of seven patients who were treated for less than 2 months (Racz, 1976; Allen *et al.*, 1978).

Polymyositis - dermatomyositis: two patients who had active disease with a 50-fold increase in CPK, had a virtual normalisation of their clinical and biochemical tests after 3 months of treatment (Gordon, 1977). Another patient was withdrawn after 1 week because of disease exacerbation (Tennstedt and Lachapelle, 1977).

Ankylosing spondylitis: in a double-blind cross-over study with 18 patients levamisole induced a significant improvement of joint index, spondylometry, morning stiffness and pain. This was parallelled by a reduction of IgM and antilymphocyte antibody levels and by an increase of migration inhibition (Goebel *et al.*, 1977). In an open study with 13 patients, 11 improved objectively or subjectively. Null cells decreased but this did not correlate with clinical response (Rosenthal *et al.*, 1976*a*, *b*).

Reiter's syndrome: four patients treated by three investigators were claimed to be cured by levamisole (Ippen and Qadripur, 1975; Rosenthal *et al.*, 1976*a*; Allen *et al.*, 1978). In two of these patients, phagocytosis was normalised (Ippen and Qadripur, 1975). The clinical efficacy of levamisole in Reiter's syndrome was confirmed in a double-blind cross-over study with 14 patients (Goebel *et al.*, 1977).

Psoriatic arthritis: no clinical benefit was observed in eight patients treated for 3 to 6 months (Rosenthal and Trabert, 1976).

Neurological diseases

Multiple sclerosis: in a long-term controlled study, neurological functions and the disability status significantly deteriorated in 31 patients who received placebo but remained unchanged in 22 patients who received levamisole. Levamisole thus seemed to delay progression of the disease (Gonsette *et al.*, 1977). In two other long-term studies, levamisole-treated patients had reduced CNS IgG synthesis (Oakley *et al.*, 1977) and reduced concentrations of basic myelin protein (Camenga, 1977). The results of small uncontrolled short-term studies (Dau *et al.*, 1976; Cendrowski and Czlonkowska, 1977) should be interpreted carefully, owing to the slow progression of the disease and the spontaneous fluctuations of disease activity.

Levamisole did not consistently increase cell-mediated immune responses (delayed skin hypersensitivity, lymphocyte proliferation, E-rosette formation, migration inhibition), which usually were within normal range (Dau *et al.*, 1976; Camenga, 1977; Cendrowski and Czlonkowska, 1977; Gonsette *et al.*, 1977; Myers *et al.*, 1977).

Subacute sclerosing panencephalitis: levamisole seemed to induce delayed progression or stabilisation of neurological symptoms in six of 23 patients. In the majority of these patients, the number of recurrent infections decreased (J. De Cree, personal communication; La Jouanine, 1975; Verhaegen *et al.*, 1977*a*).

Amyotrophic lateral sclerosis: levamisole increased lymphocyte proliferation to various antigens, except for polio in eight patients with amyotrophic lateral sclerosis (Cunningham-Rundles *et al.*, 1977).

Gastro-intestinal diseases

Recurrent aphthous ulceration: of 246 patients with severe, frequently relapsing oral ulceration, 72 per cent were said to improve during levamisole treatment for 3 months or more. The frequency, severity and duration of disease episodes were reduced to a variable degree, some patients becoming relapse-free (Allen *et al.*, 1978;

De Meyer *et al.* 1977; Fanta, 1978; Grupper, 1976; Lods and Dujardin, 1976; Olson *et al.*, 1976; Penny, 1976; Symoens and Brugmans, 1974; Van de Heyning, 1978; Verhaegen *et al.*, 1973).

In nine controlled studies with 318 patients (180 levamisole, 166 placebo), 61 per cent of the levamisole-treated patients improved against 23 per cent of the controls ($P \leqslant 0.0001$, χ^2 test) (Lehner *et al.*, 1976; De Meyer *et al.*, 1977; Drinnan and Fischman, 1977; Gier *et al.*, 1977b; Olson and Silverman, 1977; De Cree *et al.*, 1978c; Fanta, 1978; Van de Heyning, 1978). Six studies showed significant improvement of levamisole over placebo. Levamisole was not better than placebo in three studies in which patients with a relatively low relapse rate were selected.

Gingivitis: in a placebo-controlled study, levamisole increased the degree of clinical inflammation in 34 patients with chronic gingivitis. This exacerbation was associated with increased lymphocyte stimulation *in vitro* by antigens from oral bacteria (Ivanyi and Lehner, 1977).

Crohn's disease: levamisole was claimed to be effective in four long-term studies (treatment up to 1 year) involving 26 patients. In eight of these patients it seemed to maintain the remission induced by an elemental diet (Bertrand *et al.*, 1974). In the other patients, who had chronic active disease, it induced clinical, biochemical and immunological improvement (Bertrand *et al.*, 1974; Asquith *et al.*, 1976; Verhaegen *et al.*, 1977a). The results of short-term studies should be interpreted carefully because of the spontaneous fluctuations of the disease (Barbier, 1976; Wesdorp *et al.*, 1977).

Ulcerative colitis: levamisole showed no effect in seven patients with ulcerative colitis (Bertrand *et al.* 1974).

Pulmonary diseases
Idiopathic interstitial fibrosis (Hamman–Rich syndrome): one child showed radiological evidence of improvement of its syndrome after 5 weeks of treatment with levamisole, when it died of a complication of agranulocytosis (Clara and Germanes, 1977).

Dermatological diseases
Two investigators treated 81 patients with a variety of dermatological diseases for periods ranging from 2 to 12 months. A significant improvement was claimed in a majority of 81 patients with *dermatitis herpetiformis* (Morbus Dühring), *psoriasis pustulosa*, *vitiligo*, *keloid*, *lichen ruber*, *erythema multiforme*, *erythema nodosum*, *erythema indurata* and *rosacea*. In vitiligo and keloid, the association with low doses of corticosteroids was said to be superior to either treatment alone. Diseases in which levamisole does not seem to be effective are *psoriasis vulgaris* and *pemphigus vulgaris* (Racz, 1976; Allen *et al.*, 1978).

Renal diseases
Open studies in a few patients with chronic renal failure (Bansal and Robinson, 1976) glomerulonephritis (Goldberg, 1977) or on maintenance haemodialysis (Bansal and Robinson, 1976; Prinzen, 1977) were inconclusive.

Other inflammatory diseases
Sarcoidosis: treatment with levamisole for 1 to 6 months does not seem to influence the clinical course or delayed skin hypersensitivity of 38 patients with active chronic sarcoidosis of whom 16 had skin lesions only (Rosenthal *et al.*, 1976c; Veien, 1977).

Angio-immunoblastic lymphadenopathy: two patients, who had an imbalance of their cellular and humoral immune functions, recovered clinically and had their immune functions normalised (Bensa *et al.*, 1976; Ellegaard and Boesen, 1976).

Burns: a favourable effect of levamisole was claimed in a few patients (Greco and Dhennin, 1975).

Cancer

Animal studies have shown that levamisole may prolong the remission induced by classical anti-cancer treatment, but has little effect when used alone in the treatment of advanced cancer (Amery *et al.*, 1977; Symoens and Rosenthal, 1977). Prolongation of remission was related to the effectiveness of the anti-cancer treatment (Chirigos *et al.*, 1978). This principle of adjuvant therapy, first described by Chirigos *et al.*(1973), is the basis of all controlled studies with levamisole in human cancer (Amery, 1977). The controlled studies for which interim reports are available, are listed in table 6.5. Seventeen of the 23 studies showed either statistical significance or a trend in favour of levamisole. Two studies showed no difference from control, but follow-up time is relatively short. Four could not be evaluated. Levamisole was never detrimental.

The duration of remission and the survival time are the major criteria used to evaluate treatment regimens. A number of factors seem to influence the response to levamisole.

The response to the primary cytoreductive treatment

In three studies in which this effect was evaluated, only patients whose tumour load was reduced by the primary anti-cancer treatment, had a prolonged survival with levamisole. Patients whose tumour kept growing in spite of cytoreductive treatment did not benefit from the drug. There is no evidence that this type of anti-cancer treatment influences responsiveness to levamisole, provided that the cancer proves susceptible to it.

The timing of levamisole treatment

It seems advisable to start levamisole before or as soon as possible after the start of remission-inducing therapy. The concomitant administration of levamisole and cytotoxic treatment may, however, be deleterious (Woods *et al.*, 1975; Willoughby *et al.*, 1977; Chang *et al.*, 1978). In patients receiving aggressive cytotoxic treatment, levamisole is therefore started as soon as this treatment is completed and in patients receiving cyclic maintenance treatment with cytostatics, levamisole is given between courses of chemotherapy. The drug may enhance bone-marrow reconstitution in such patients (Lods *et al.*, 1976).

Dosage of levamisole

In one study where the significance of the dose was evaluated, patients receiving approximately 2.5 mg/kg had prolonged survival, whereas those who received less than 2 mg/kg did not respond.

Absolute lymphocyte count

In two studies, patients who responded to levamisole had a low absolute lymphocyte count at the start in contrast to non-responders who had a high count at the start (Amery, 1977; Verhaegen, 1977). It is possible that the lymphocyte count

Table 6.5   Controlled clinical studies with levamisole as an adjuvant in cancer treatment

Cancer	Basic therapy	*n*	Effect	References
Breast	Radiotherapy	20	+	Rojas *et al.*, 1978
	Cytostatics	49	+	Klefström, 1977
	Cytostatics	127	+	Hortobagyi *et al.*, 1978
	Cytostatics	29	+	Stephens, 1978
Lung	Surgery	96	+	Amery, 1978
	Surgery	46	?	Wright *et al.*, 1978
	Radiotherapy	33	?	Pines, 1977
	Cytostatics	24	−	Chahinian *et al.*, 1978
Head and neck	Surgery	26	+	Wanebo *et al.*, 1978
Larynx	Surgery + Rx	12	+	Mussche *et al.*, 1977
Gastro-intestinal	Surgery	143	+	Miwa *et al.*, 1978
Colo-rectal	Surgery	30	+	Verhaegen, 1977
	Cytostatics	19	−	Valdivieso *et al.*, 1977
Melanoma	Surgery	103	+	Gonzalez *et al.*, 1978
	Cytostatics	60	(+)	Hall *et al.*, 1977
Brain	Surgery + Rx	31	?	Takakura *et al.*, 1977
Bladder	Surgery + Rx	33	(+)	Smith *et al.*, 1978
Various	Radiotherapy	186	(+)	Debois, 1978
AML + ALL	Cytostatics	31	+	Vuopio, 1978
AML	Cytostatics	12	(+)	Brincker *et al.*, 1976
ALL	Cytostatics	111	+	Pavlovsky *et al.*, 1978
ANLL	Cytostatics	30	(+)	Chang *et al.*, 1978
NH lymph.	Cytostatics	35	?	Cabanillas *et al.*, 1977

n is the number of patients receiving levamisole. +, statistically significant difference in favour of levamisole; (+), trend in favour of levamisole;−, no difference between levamisole and control; ?, could not be evaluated.

is a marker of a subpopulation with a high risk of recurrence which profits most from levamisole treatment.

Two other factors must be taken into consideration when analysing the data. *The stage of the disease*: patients in an early stage have a relatively good prognosis. Prolongation of survival by immunotherapy can be apparent only after years (figure 6.2). Advanced though still potentially curable patients seem to profit most from levamisole treatment. *The duration of follow-up*: remission time and the mortality rate are often comparable between groups during the first months of study, after which a trend is seen in favour of levamisole, followed by statistical significance if treatment groups are sufficiently large (figure 6.2).

A few studies have evaluated levamisole when used alone in patients with advanced cancer and it had little or no effect. It is now clear that levamisole should not be used as a remission-inducing agent. It is, however, particularly useful as an adjuvant in patients who are known to be at risk of developing recurrent disease after they have undergone clinically effective anti-cancer treatment. The effect ob-

tained by the primary treatment will be maintained for a significantly longer time
than if no further treatment is given. An early start of levamisole at an adequate
dose level is particularly critical for those patients who show early relapse. Levamisole thus consolidates the effects obtained by other anti-cancer therapies. Its
effects in one study are comparable with those of BCG (Hortobagyi *et al.*, 1976).

Cancer patients who are immunocompetent have a better prognosis than those
who are not (Klefström, 1977; Smith *et al.*, 1978), and patients with advanced
cancer are more often immunosuppressed than those in an early stage of disease.
Often no immune deficiencies are found in patients with early cancers. If immune
defects are found, their relevance to the clinical situation is uncertain.

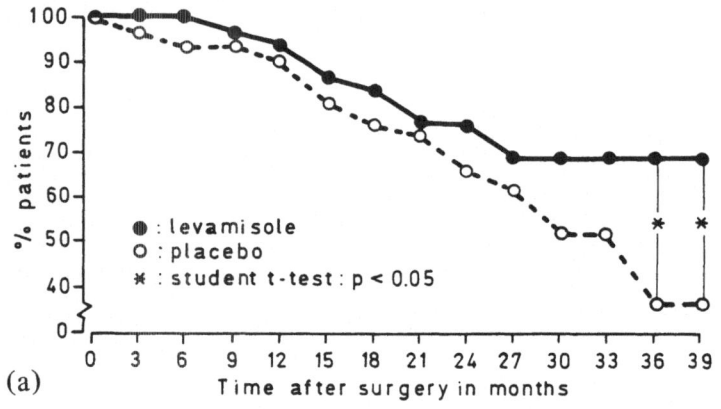

(a)

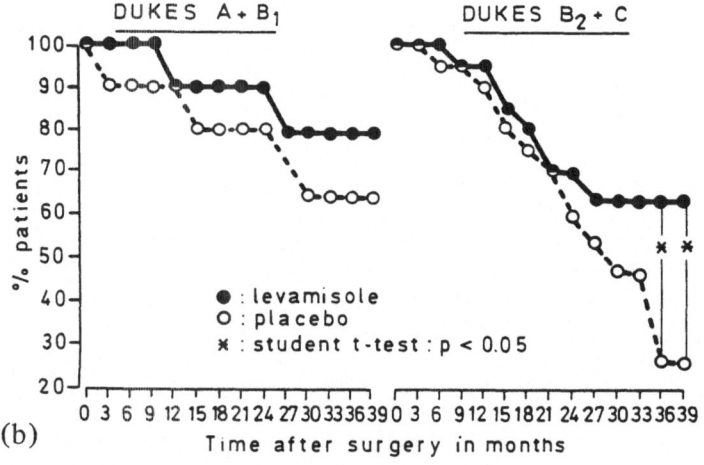

(b)

Figure 6.2(a) Actuarial analysis of survival in patients with colo-rectal carcinoma after surgery
and during treatment with levamisole or placebo. (b) Actuarial analysis of survival in patients
with colo-rectal carcinoma after surgery and during treatment with levamisole or placebo, subdivided according to the Dukes' classification. See Verhaegen (1977).

The immunological effects of levamisole in cancer patients have usually been investigated in short-term studies not exceeding 3 months of treatment. The most consistent effect was a restoration of cutaneous delayed hypersensitivity to various antigens (Tripodi *et al.*, 1973; Levo *et al.*, 1975; Ramot *et al.*, 1976; Berenyi *et al.*, 1977; Heath, 1977; Klefström, 1977; Pavlovsky *et al.*, 1978). Other studies concerned lymphocyte proliferation (Heath, 1977; Klefström, 1977; Miwa and Orita, 1977; Holmes and Golub, 1978), lymphocyte cytotoxicity (Jerry *et al.*, 1977; Urist *et al.*, 1977), E- or EAC-rosette formation (Levo *et al.*, 1975; Ramot *et al.*, 1976; Berenyi *et al.*, 1977; Jerry and Shea, 1977), monocyte chemotaxis (Smith *et al.*, 1978) and levels of immune complexes (Berenyi *et al.*, 1977). In the majority of these studies, heterogeneous groups of patients with variable immunocompetence were used. Very often no effect was seen by grouping the data, whereas restorative effects of levamisole could more readily be shown by analysing individual responses. Correlations with responsiveness are difficult to evaluate because study periods were relatively short. In conclusion there is today no single immunological parameter that is of undeniable use to monitor levamisole treatment in cancer patients.

Adverse reactions
A single intake of a therapeutic dose of levamisole (2.5 mg/kg) is practically devoid of side-effects, as shown in controlled studies where levamisole was used as an antihelminthic (Moens *et al.*, 1978). Repeated administration, which is needed for immunotherapy, may cause severe adverse reactions in certain patients. These reactions (skin rash, febrile illness, mouth ulceration and agranulocytosis) are idiosyncratic and may necessitate discontinuation of treatment. These patients constitute a susceptible subpopulation. It is evident from controlled studies that levamisole is well tolerated by 80–95 per cent of the patients. Occasional reports on a higher incidence of adverse reactions are not confirmed in controlled studies.

All adverse reactions to levamisole mentioned in the literature are listed in table 6.6. Those that occur in at least 1 per cent of the patients are shown in table 6.7.

Idiosyncratic adverse reactions are significantly more frequent in patients with rheumatic disorders than in patients with other diseases. Gastrointestinal side effects predominate in cancer patients. Febrile illness, neurological side effects and gastrointestinal intolerance occur in all patients, irrespective of the disease.

Placebo-controlled studies have shown that the idiosyncratic reactions are definitely related to levamisole treatment. Neurological excitement is slightly more frequent with levamisole than with placebo but rarely necessitates discontinuation of treatment. Gastrointestinal intolerance is as frequent with placebo as with levamisole, even in cancer where the observed incidence is the highest.

Agranulocytosis (a selective fall of the number of neutrophils below 25 per cent) is the only potentially dangerous side-effect of levamisole. It is most frequent in patients with rheumatic diseases, in women and in HLA B27 genotypes. It is caused by a peripheral destruction of neutrophils and may occur at any time after an initial sensitisation period. The bone marrow remains intact and recovery occurs always within 1 or 2 weeks after discontinuation of treatment. Agranulocytosis should be differentiated from leucopenia, which is drug-related but not allergic. In contrast to agranulocytosis, leucopenia recovers spontaneously during treatment.

Full details on agranulocytosis and other adverse reactions to levamisole are available in a recent review by Symoens *et al.* (1978).

Table 6.6   Qualitative survey of adverse reactions to levamisole mentioned in the literature

(A) *Haematological*	(D) *Neurological*
Agranulocytosis/leucopenia	Sensory stimulation (hyperosmia, dysgeusia, . . .)
Thrombocytopenia	Hyper alert state
Agammaglobulinaemia	Insomnia
	Psychic confusion
(B) *Skin and mucosae*	Tremor
Rash	
Vasculitis	(E) *Gastro-intestinal*
Mouth ulcers	Nausea
Erythema nodosum leprosum	Gastric intolerance
Lichen planus	Anorexia
	Vomiting
(C) *Flu-like illness*	Diarrhoea
Febrile illness	Constipation
Shiverings, chills	
Sore throat	(F) *Various*
Myalgia, arthralgia	Proteinuria
Excessive perspiration	Hyperazotaemia
Dizziness	Allergic shock
Malaise	Increased transaminases
Headache	Ocular symptoms, iridocyclitis
Apathy	Skin ulceration
Fatigue	Polyuria

Dosage and treatment schedule

The highest well-tolerated dose in man (2.5 mg/kg) happens to be the therapeutic dose in the antihelminthic and immunotherapeutic indications. A single dose is effective against worms and restores immune functions for at least 5 days (De Cock *et al.*, 1978*a*; Di Perri, 1978*b*; Mowat, 1978). Repeated pulse treatment is needed for immunotherapy. A single pulse once weekly is effective in recurrent upper-respiratory-tract infections of children and in rheumatoid arthritis. This dose regimen is currently being tested in other indications as well. It is preferred to more intensive regimen, because the risk of agranulocytosis is considerably lessened by not repeating treatment on consecutive days.

Levamisole is effective *in vitro* in concentrations similar to those found after administration of a therapeutic dose of 150 mg to man (10^{-5} to 10^{-9} M). One may question the relevance of effects obtained at higher concentrations *in vitro*.

DISCUSSION

The clinical efficacy of levamisole is now well established in a number of recurrent or chronic diseases such as respiratory-tract infections of children, herpes, aphthous ulceration and rheumatoid arthritis in which it reduces disease activity. This list is

Table 6.7 Quantitative survey of adverse reactions to levamisole and, in parentheses, withdrawal rate because of side effects*

Type of adverse reaction	Cancer (n = 1179)	Infectious diseases (n = 888)	Inflammatory diseases (n = 601)	Rheumatic diseases (n = 989)	Various (n = 243)
Idiosyncratic					
Skin rash	2.6 (0.9)	1.5 (0.3)	1.7 (0.2)	14.8 (7.0)	2.1 (0.4)
Leucopenia/agranulocytosis	2.0 (1.4)	0.2 (0.3)	1.0 (0.3)	4.9 (4.5)	0.8 (0)
Febrile illness	4.8 (1.4)	1.9 (0.5)	2.8 (1.5)	3.9 (1.5)	0.4 (0)
Mouth ulcers	0.3 (0)	0.1 (0)	0.0 (0)	1.9 (0.3)	0.0 (0)
Neurological					
Sensory stimulation	3.0 (0.1)	6.1 (0)	4.8 (0)	6.2 (0.5)	0.4 (0)
Hyper alert state	1.2 (0)	1.2 (0)	0.2 (0)	1.8 (0)	0.0 (0)
Insomnia	2.5 (0.1)	0.3 (0)	0.3 (0)	1.4 (0)	0.0 (0)
Headache	2.1 (0)	2.3 (0)	2.2 (0)	1.3 (0.2)	0.0 (0)
Dizziness	1.2 (0)	0.5 (0)	0.3 (0)	2.9 (0)	4.5 (0)
Fatigue	4.4 (0)	1.5 (0.1)	0.8 (0)	0.9 (0)	0.0 (0)
Gastro-intestinal					
Nausea	13.1 (0.4)	5.0 (0.5)	4.8 (0.3)	5.0 (1.3)	5.8 (0)
Gastric intolerance	4.8 (0.4)	4.2 (0.3)	3.5 (0.2)	5.7 (0.8)	2.5 (0)
Anorexia	2.8 (0)	0.0 (0)	0.2 (0)	2.7 (0)	0.0 (0)
Vomiting	7.2 (0)	2.3 (0)	0.8 (0)	2.1 (0.2)	0.4 (0.4)
Diarrhoea	2.6 (0)	0.5 (0)	0.8 (0)	0.3 (0.1)	0.0 (0)
Miscellaneous (†)	4 (0.3)	6 (0.7)	5 (0.8)	16 (1.6)	0 (0)
Total discontinued	(4.9)	(2.6)	(3.3)	(18.0)	(2.5)

* Numbers indicate percentage of patients with side effect.
† Various isolated instances of less relevant conditions.

likely to be extended as new controlled studies appear. In cancer, levamisole is able to prolong survival time when properly used.

Treatment may last a few weeks only in self-limiting diseases but is long-lasting in chronic progressive diseases. In a number of diseases, a clinical exacerbation frequently occurs during the first 2 months of treatment, preceding marked clinical improvement. These clinical phenomena reflect on the one hand the complex network of immune reactions involved in immunopathology, and on the other hand the possible sequential action of levamisole on these different functions. Indeed, shortly after the start of levamisole therapy, one might expect an activation of the effector cells to eliminate a possible persisting antigen, activating the inflammatory response and resulting in temporary exacerbation. The more subtle immunological interactions, involving feed-back mechanisms, probably need more time to be restored, leading to the induction of tolerance and tempering of the chronic disease process.

Levamisole in all likeliness restores a basic immunological impairment in each of the diseases in which it is effective. However, the lack of correlation between the restoration of immunological functions and clinical responsiveness in most diseases, suggests that the available immunological assessments do not always reflect the underlying defect responsible for the disease.

Our understanding of the mechanism of action of levamisole grows in parallel with an increased knowledge of the mechanisms leading to immunopathology. Future studies should aim at finding those immunological features that are specific for the disease and the interaction with levamisole.

REFERENCES

Alcalay, M., Alcalay, D., Reboux, J. F., Devries, M. and Bontous, D. (1977). *Nouv. Presse Méd.,* **6.** 1959
Allen, D. E., Kaplan, B. and Pinnell, S. R. (1978). *Int. J. Dermatol.,* 17, 287
Amery, W. K. (1977). *Symposium on Immunotherapy of Malignant Diseases,* Vienna, Austria
Amery, W. K. (1978). 4th *Conference on Immune Modulation and Control of Neoplasia by Adjuvant Therapy,* Bethesda, Maryland
Amery, W. K., Spreafico, F., Rojas, A. F., Denissen, E. and Chirigos, M. A. (1977). *Cancer Treat. Rev.,* 4, 167
Anderson, R., Glover, A., Koornhof, H. J. and Rabson, P. (1976). *J. Immun.,* **117,** 428
Asquith, P., Ross, I. N., Montgomery, R. D. and Thompson, R. A. (1976). Unpublished Report
Attias, M. R. (1976). *National Scientific Meeting of the American Rheumatism Association,* Miami, Florida, U.S.A.
Baart de la Faille, H. (1977). Unpublished Report
Bach, J. F. (1977). *A. Rev. Pharmac. Tox.,* 17, 281
Bach, M. A., Fournier, C. and Bach, J. F. (1975). *Ann. N. Y. Acad. Sci.,* 249, 316
Balint, G., El-Ghobarey, A., Capell, H., Madkour, M., Dick, W. C., Ferguson, M. M. and Anwar-Ul-Hoq, M. (1977). *Br. med. J.,* 2, 1386
Balogh, E. and Szobolscy, M. (1976). Unpublished Report
Bansal, V. K. and Robinson, J. A. (1976). *Kidney Int.,* 10, 538
Barbaix, E. (1976). Unpublished Clinical Research Report No. 53
Barbier (1976). Unpublished Report
Barrett-Connor, E. (1978). Unpublished Clinical Research Report
Basch, C. M. (1978). Unpublished Report
Basch, C. M., Spitler, L. E., Engleman, E. P. and Engleman, E. (1977*a*). *J. Rheumat.,* 4, 377
Basch, C. M., Spitler, L. E. and Engleman, E. P. (1977*b*). XIVth *International Congress of Rheumatology,* San Francisco, California, U.S.A.

Bensa, J. -Cl., Faure, J., Martin, H., Sutto, J. -J. and Schaerer, R. (1976). *Lancet*, i, 1081
Berenyi, E., Kavai, M., Palkovi, E., Paloczi, K., Sonkoly, I., Szabolcsi, M. and Szegedi, G. (1976). In *Proceedings of current problems of immunology and their dermatological aspects*, (ed. I. Racz,), Budapest, Hungary, p. 206
Berenyi, E., Sonkoly, I., Kavai, M., Szabolsci, M. and Szegedi, Gy. (1977). *New Engl. J. Med.*, 296, 941
Bertrand, J., Renoux, G., Renoux, M. and Palat, A. (1974). *Nouv. Presse Méd.*, 3, 2265
Bierman, S. M. (1976). Unpublished Report
Bliznakov, E. G., Wan, Y. P., Chang, D. and Folkers, K. (1978). *Biochem. Biophys. Res. Commun.*, 80, 631
Bourne, H. R., Lehrer, R. I., Clein, M. J. and Melmon, K. L. (1971). *Clin. Invest.*, 50, 920
Brincker, H., Thorling, K. and Jensen, K. B. (1976). *Spring Meeting of Scandinavian Haematologists*, Arhus
Browning, J. D. (1977). *Lancet*, ii, 820
Bruninx, M. (1973). Unpublished Report
Bryant, R. E. and Sutcliffe, M. (1973). *Clin. Res.*, 21, 594
Cabanillas, F., Rodriguez, V., Hersh, E. M., Mavdigit, G., Bodey, G. P. and Middleman, E. L. (1977). *Proc. Am. Ass. Cancer Res. Am. Soc. clin. Oncol.*, 18, 328
Camenga, D. L. (1977). 11th *World Congress of Neurology*, Amsterdam, The Netherlands
Carr, M. C. (1978). Unpublished Clinical Research Report No. 82
Cendrowski, W. and Czlonkowska, A. (1977). In *Immunosuppressive Treatment in Multiple Sclerosis*, Chapter XI, European Press, Gent, Belgium, p. 148
Chadwick, P. D., Jain, S., Thomas, H. C. and Sherlock, S. (1977). *Gut*, 18, A979
Chahinian, A. P., Mandel, E. M., Jaffrey, I. S.., Teirstein, A. S. and Holland, J. F. (1978). *World Conference on Lung Cancer*. The International Association for the Study of Lung Cancer, Palmetto Dunes, South Carolina, U.S.A.
Chang, I. and Fuimoura, N. (1978). *Antimicrob. Agents Chemother.*, 13, 809
Chang, P., Wiernik, P. H., Schiffer, C. A. and Lichtenfeld, J. L. (1978). *ASCO meeting*, U.S.A.
Chirigos, M. A., Pearson, J. W. and Pryor, J. (1973). *Cancer Res.*, 33, 2615
Chirigos, M. A., Schultz, R. M. Pavlidis, N., Feingold, D. S. and Youngner, J. S. (1978). *Cancer Treat. Rep.*, (in press)
Clara, R. and Germanes, J. (1977). *Lancet*, i, 47
Cullen, S. I. (1977). Unpublished Report
Cunningham-Rundles, S., Dupont, B., Posner, J. B., Hansen, J. A. and Good, R. A. (1977). *Fedn. Proc.*, 36, 1190
d'Anglejan, G., Guedj, D., Debeyre, N., Lermusiaux, J. -L and Ryckewaert, A. (1977). *Rev. Rhum.*, 44, 633
Dau, P. C., Johnson, K. P. and Spitler, L. E. (1976). *Clin. exp. Immun.*, 26, 302
Davatchi, F., Chafizadeh, A., Massoud, A. and Jalili, M. (1977). *International Seminar on Treatment of Rheumatic Diseases*, Petah-Tiqva, Israel
Debois, J. M. (1978). Unpublished Clinical Research Report No. 69
De Brabander, M., Aerts, F., Geuens, G., Van Ghinckel, R., Van de Veire, R. and Van Belle, H. (1978). *Chem-Biol. Interactions*, 23, 45
De Cock, W., De Cree, J. and Verhaegen, H. (1977). *Int. Archs. Allergy appl. Immun.*, 54, 176
De Cock, W., Vogels, O., De Cree, J., Verhaegen, H. and Brugmans, J. (1978a). Unpublished Clinical Research Report No. 74
De Cock, W., Van der Veken, L., De Cree, J. and Verhaegen, H. (1978b). Unpublished Report
De Cock, W., De Cree, J. and Verhaegen, H. (1978c). *J. Immunopharmac.* (in press)
De Cree, J. (1974). Unpublished Clinical Research Report No. 14
De Cree, J., Verhaegen, H., De Cock, W. and Brugmans, J. (1973). *Memorial Sloan-Kettering Cancer Center Meeting*, New York, U.S.A.
De Cree, J., Verhaegen, H. and De Cock, W. (1975). Unpublished Clinical Research Report No. 23
De Cree, J., Emmery, L., Timmermans, J., Eeckels, R., De Cock, W. and Verhaegen, H. (1978a). *Archs. Dis. Child.*, 53, 144
De Cree, J., De Cock, W. and Verhaegen, H. (1978b). Unpublished Report
De Cree, J., Verhaegen, H., De Cock, W. and Verbruggen, F. (1978c). *Oral Surg.*, 45, 378
De Donder, C. (1976). Unpublished Report

De Leeuw-Delvigne, C. (1976) Unpublished Report
Del Giacco, G. S. (1977). Unpublished Report
De Loore, F. (1974). Unpublished Report
De Loore, F. (1977). Unpublished Clinical Research Report No. 66
De Meyer, J., Degraeve, M., Clarysse, J., Deloose, F. and Peremans, W. (1977). *Br. J. Med.*, 1, 671
De Peuter, M. (1975). Unpublished Report
De Queiroz Carvalho, C. Á., Kinue Otoki, T., Poli, M. E., Nogueira, J. L. and Guerrero, J. (1976). *An. Bras. Derm.*, **51**, 115
De Rubertis, F. R., Zenser, T. V., Adler, W. H. and Hudson, T. (1974). *J. Immun.*, **113**, 151
Dieppe, P. A., Willoughby, D. A., Stevens, C., Kirby, J. D. and Huskisson, E. C. (1976). *Rheumat. Rehabil.*, **15**, 201
Dinai, Y. and Pras, M. (1975). *Lancet*, **ii**, 556
Di Perri, T., Auteri, A., Laghi Pasini, L., Mattioli, F. and Volpi, L. (1977). *Symposium on Immunotherapy of Malignant Diseases*, Vienna, Austria
Di Perri, T., Auteri, A., Laghi Pasini, F. and Mattioli, F. (1978*a*). *Eur. J. Rheum. Inflam.* 1, 155
Di Perri, T. (1978*b*). Unpublished Clinical Research Report No. 79
Drinnan, A. J. and Fischman, S. L. (1977). Unpublished Report.
Editorial (1978). *Lancet*, **i**, 697
El-Ghobarey, A. E., Mavrikakis, M., Morgan, I. and Mathieu, J. P. (1977*a*). *Br. med. J.*, 1, 616
El-Ghobarey, A. E., Mavrikakis, M., Macleod, M., Raynaulds, P., Cappel, H., Spencer, D., Mathiew, J. P., Dick, W. C., Watson, Buchanan, W., Macalister, T. and Cooney (1977*b*). *Q. Jl. Med.*, 47, 385
Ellegaard, J. and Boesen, A. M. (1976). *Scand. J. Haemat.*, **17**, 36
Estensen, R. D., Hill, H. R., Quie, P. G., Hogan, N. and Goldberg, N. D. (1973). *Nature*, **245**, 458
Fanta, D. (1978). Unpublished Report
Fegies, M. and Guerrero, J. (1977). *Trans. R. Soc. Trop. Med. Hyg.*, **71**, 178
Ferreira, G. G. R., Massuda Brascher, H. K., Javierre, M. Q., Sassine, W. A. and Lima, A. O. (1976). *Experientia*, **32**, 1594
Fischer, G. W., Podgore, J. K., Bass, J. W., Kelley, J. L. and Kobayashi, G. Y. (1975). *J. infect. Dis.*, **132**, 578
Foroozanfar, N., Zandieh, T., Davatchi, F. and Ala, F. (1977). *International Seminar on Treatment of Rheumatic Diseases*, Petah-Tiqva, Israel
Foroozanfar, N., Tuft, S., Davatchi, F. and Ala, F. (1978). 4th *European Immunology Meeting*, Budapest, Hungary
Franchimont, P., Berghs, H., Remans, J. and Vroninks, Ph. (1976). Unpublished Clinical Research Report No. 52
Franchimont, P., Hauwaert, C., Heynen, G., Denis, F. and Betz-Rigaux, Ch. (1978). *Eur. J. Rheumat.* (in press)
Galant, S. P. and Remo, R. A. (1975). *J. Immun.*, **114**, 512
Galant, S. P., Lundak, R. L. and Eaton, L. (1976). *J. Immun.*, **117**, 48
Gallice, R. (1977). *Mémoire de Rhumatologie*, Marseille, France
Gier, R., George, B., Wilson, T., Hart, J., Quaison, F., Rueger, A., Hardman, P. and Sakumura, J. (1977*a*). *International Association for Dental Research and American Association for Dental Research*,
Gier, R. E., George, B., Wilson, T., Rueger, A., Hart, J. H., Quaison, F. and Hardman, P. K. (1977*b*). *NIH Etiology and Treatment of aphthous stomatitis and Behcet syndrome Workshop*,
Goebel, K. M., Goebel, F. D., Schubotz, R., Hahn, E. and Neurath, F. (1977). *Lancet*, **ii**, 214
Goldberg, B. (1977). Unpublished Report
Goldstein, G., Scheid, M., Boyse, E. A., Brand, A. and Gilmour, D. G. (1977). *Cold Spring Harb. Symp. Quant. Biol.*, 41, 5
Gonsette, R., Demonty, L., Delmotte, P., De Cree, J., De Cock, W., Verhaegen, H. and Symoens, J. (1977). Unpublished Clinical Research Report No. 61
Gonzalez, R. L., Spitler, L. E. and Sagebiel, R. (1978). 4th *Conference on Immune Modulation and Control of Neoplasia by Adjuvant Therapy*, Bethesda, Maryland

Gordon, B. L. (1977). Unpublished Report
Gordon, B. L. and Keenan, J. P. (1975). *Ann. Allergy*, 35, 343
Gordon, B. L. and Yanagihara, R. (1977). *Ann. Allergy*, 39, 227
Greco, J. and Chennin, Ch. (1975). *J. Chir. (Tours)*, 9, 155
Griscelli, C. (1976). Unpublished Report
Griscelli, C. Prieur, A. M. and Da Guillard F. (1978). In *Immune Modulation and Control of Neoplasia by Adjuvant Therapy*, (ed. M. A. Chirigos), Raven Press, New York, U. S. A. p. 165
Grupper, Ch (1976). Unpublished Report
Guaydier, G., Loyau, J. F. G., Dumas, M., Lehman J. Heron. J. F. and L'Hirondel, J. L. (1977). *Nouv. Presse Méd.*, 6, 3332
Hadden, J. W., Coffey, R. G., Hadden, E. M., Lopez-Corrales, E. and Sunshine, G. H. (1975). *Cell Immun.*, 20, 90
Hall, S. W., Benjamin, R. S., Heilbrun, L. K., Lewinski, U., Gutterman, J. U. and Mavligit, G. (1977). Unpublished Report
Halpern, G. M. (1978). Unpublished Report
Haneke, E. and Meinhof, W. (1977). *Z. Hautkr.*, 52, 688
Hatch, G. E., Nichols, W. K. and Hill, H. (1977). *J. Immun.*, 119, 450
Heath, T. (1977). Unpublished Report
Hellin, P. and Bergh, M. (1974). *New Engl. J. Med.*, 291, 1311
Hodinka, L., Meretey, K. and Bozsoky, S. (1977a). XIVth *World Congress of Rheumatology*, San Francisco, California, U.S.A.
Hodinka, L., Meretey, K. and Bozsoky, S. (1977b). Unpublished Report
Hogan, N. A. and Hill, H. R. (1977). *Clin. Res.*, 25, 181A
Holmes, E. C. and Golub, S. H. (1978). In *Immune Modulation and Control of Neoplasia by Adjuvant Therapy*, (ed. M. A. Chirigos), Raven Press, New York, U.S.A.
Hortobagyi, G. N., Gutterman, J. U., Blumenschein, G. R., Tashima, C. K., Buzdar, A. U. and Hersh, E. M. (1978). In *Immune Modulation and Control of Neoplasia by Adjuvant Therapy*, (ed. M. A. Chirigos), Raven Press, New York, U.S.A., p. 131
Huskisson, E. C., Dieppe, P. A., Scott, J., Trapnell, G., Balma, H. W. and Willoughby, D. A. (1976). *Lancet*, i, 393
Ignarro, L. J. and Cech, S. Y. (1976). *Proc. Soc. exp. Biol. Med.*, 151, 448
Ippen, H. and Qadripur, S. A. (1975). *Dtsch. Med. Wochenschr.*, 100, 1710
Ivanyi, L. and Lehner, T. (1977). *Scand. J. Immun.*, 6, 219
Jarish, P. and Sandor, I. (1977). *Archs dermat. Res.*, 258, 151
Jerry, L. M. and Shea, M. (1977). *Meeting of the Canadian Society for Clinical Investigation*
Jerry, L. M., Shibata, H. R., Lewis, M. G., Mansell, P. W., Capek, A. and Marquis, G. (1977). VIIIth *Symposium of Cancerology*, Quebec City, Canada
Kagan, W. A., O'Neill, G. J., Incefy, G. S., Goldstein, G. and Good, R. A. (1977). *Blood*, 50, 275
Kalfa, G. (1978). Thèse, Montpellier, France
Kaslik, J., Vanek, I., Haskova, V. and Hatala, M. (1978). 4th *European Immunology Meeting*, Budapest, Hungary
Kint, A., Coucke, C. and Verlinden, L. (1974). *Archs belg. Derm. Syph.*, 30, 167
Klefström, P. (1977). *Symposium on Immunotherapy of Malignant Diseases*, Vienna, Austria
Koopman, W. J., Gillis, M. H. and David, J. R. (1973). *J. Immun.*, 110, 1609
Kromer, K. (1977). Unpublished Clinical Research Report No. 65
Krupp, I. M. (1977a). *Meeting of the Southwest Health Association*,
Krupp, I. M. (1977b). Unpublished Clinical Research Report
Krupp, I. M. and Jolly, H. W. (1977). Unpublished Clinical Research Report
Kurland, J. I., Hadden, J. W. and Moore, M. A. S. (1977). *Cancer Res.*, 37, 4534
La Jouanine (1975). Unpublished Report
Leca, A. P., Crouzet, J., Prier, A., Camus, J. -P. (1976). *Nouv. Presse Méd.*, 5, 89
Lehner, T., Wilton, J. M. A. and Ivanyi, L. (1976). *Lancet*, ii, 926
Lequesne, M. and Floquet, J. (1976). *Nouv. Presse, Méd.*, 5, 358
Levo, Y., Rotter, V. and Ramot, B. (1975). *Biomedicine*, 23, 198
Levy, J. and Miller, B. (1976). *American Rheumatism Association Annual Scientific Meeting*, Chicago, Illinois
Lewi, P. J. and Symoens, J. (1978). *J. Rheumat.*, 5 (suppl. 4), 17

114   *Drugs and Immune Responsiveness*

Lichtenstein, L. M., Henney, C. S., Bourne, H. R. and Greenough, W. B. (1973). *J. clin. Invest.*, **52**, 691
Linsky, C. B. (1975). Unpublished Report
Lods, J. C. (1975). Unpublished Report
Lods, J. C. and Dujardin, P. (1976). *Med. Hyg.*, **34**, 53
Lods, J. C., Dujardin, P. and Halpern, G. M. (1976). *Lancet*, **i**, 548
Lods, M. F. (1975). *Bull. Soc. Ophtalmol. Fr.*, **75**, 37
Lods, M. F. (1976). *Nouv. Presse Méd.*, **5**, 148
Lubetkin, A. M. Remedi, R., Granero, M., Brarda, O. (1977). XVth *International Congress of Pediatrics*, New Delhi
Mahmood, T. and Robinson, W. A. (1977). *Proc. Soc. exp. Biol. Med.*, **156**, 359
Martinez. E. and Zaias, N. (1976). *Lancet*, **ii**, 209
Massoud, A., Davatchi, F., Emadi, H. and Ala, F. (1977). *International Seminar on Treatment of Rheumatic Diseases*, Petah-Tiqva, Israel
Mehr, K. A. and Albano, L. (1977). *Lancet*, **ii**, 773
Merluzzi, V. J., Kaiser, C. W. and Cooperband, S. R. (1976). *Fedn Proc.*, **35**, 334
Merryman, P. and Jaffe, I. A. (1977). *Biochem. Pharmac.*, **26**, 1350
Meyers, A. R. and Schimmer, B. M. (1977). *International Seminar on Treatment of Rheumatic Diseases*, Petah-Tiqva, Israel
Meyers, W. M., Kvernes, S. and Staple, E. M. (1975). *Am. J. trop. Med. Hyg.*, **24**, 857
Michel, A. P. M. (1978). Thèse, Strasbourg, France
Miller, B., Srinivasan, R., Fan, P., Levy, J., Clements, P. J. and Paulus, H. E. (1977). XIVth *International Congress of Rheumatology*, San Francisco, California, U.S.A.
Miwa, H. and Orita, K. (1977). *Acta med. Okayama*, **31**, 325
Miwa, H., Orita, K. and Tanaka, S. (1978). *Acta med. Okayama*, 32, 239
Moens, M., Dom, J., Burke, W., Schlossberg, S. and Schuermans, V. (1978). *Am. J. Trop. Med. Hyg*, 27 897
Moese, J. R. (1974). Unpublished Report
Molnar, I., Horvath, A. and Racz, I. (1976). In *Proceedings of current problems of immunology and their dermatological aspects*, (ed. I. Racz), Budapest, Hungary, p. 218
Moncada, B., Rodriquez, M. L., Cepeda, M. and Ceballos, R. (1977). Unpublished Report
Morias, J., Peremans, W., Campaert, H. and Mertens, R. L. J. (1977). Unpublished Report
Moroz, C., Lahat, N., Biniaminov, M. and Ramot, B. (1977). *Clin. exp. Immun.*, **29**, 30
Mowat, A. G. (1978*a*). *Ann. Rheum. Dis.*, **37**, 1
Mowat, A. G. (1978*b*). *J. Rheumat.*, **5** (suppl. 4), 55
Multicenter Study Group (1978*a*). *Lancet*, **ii**, 1007
Multicenter Study Group (1978*b*). *J. Rheumat.*, **5**(suppl. 4), 5
Musatti, C. C., Rezkallah, M. T., Mendes, E. and Mendes, N. F. (1976). *Cell. Immun.*, **24**, 365
Mussche, R. A., Plum, J., De Smedt, M. and Kluyskens, P. (1977). *Acta otorhinolaryngol. belg.*, **31**, 1977
Myers, L. W., Ellison, G. W., Levy, J., Holevoet, M., Ma, B. I. and Tourtelotte, W. W. (1977). 11th *World Congress of Neurology*, Amsterdam, The Netherlands
Nadal Ortega, J. M., Gonzales-Moro Prats, L. and Rodriguez Lopez, F. (1977). Unpublished Report
Nelson, K. E., Pagels, G. A., Batt, M. D. and Vithaysai, V. (1978). *Clin. Res.*, (in press)
Oakley, G. A., Hogarth-Scott, R. S. and Symoens, J. (1977). *World Association for the Advancement of Veterinary Parasitology*, Sydney, Australia
Oliveira Lima, A., Javierre, M. G., Dias da Silva, W. and Sette Camara, D. (1974). *Experientia*, **30**, 945
Olson, J. A. and Silverman, S. (1977). *Aphthous Stomatitis Behcet's Syndrome Workshop at the National Institutes of Health*, Bethesda, Maryland, U.S.A.
Olson, J. A., Nelms, D. C., Silverman, S. and Spitler, L. F. (1976). *Oral Surg.*, **41**, 588
O'Reilly, R. J., Chibbaro, A., Wilmot, R. and Lopez, C. (1977). *Ann. N. Y. Acad. Sci.*, **284**, 161
Ores, R. D., Schwartz, J. V. and Cuti, A. J. (1977). VIth *International Congress of Lymphology*, Prague, Czechoslovakia
Oshita, A. K., Rothstein, G. and Lonngi, G. (1977). *Blood*, **49**, 585
Par, A., Barna, K., Hollos, I., Kovacs, M., Miszlai, Zs., Patakfalvi, A. and Javor, T. (1977). *Lancet*, **i**, 702
Pavlovksy, S., Garay, G., Giraudo, C., Sackmann, F., Hayes, A. and Svarch, E. (1978). Sixty-ninth *Annual Meeting of the American Association for Cancer Research*

Penny, R. (1976). Unpublished Interim Data
Pines, A. (1977). Unpublished Report
Pinnell, S. R., Tindall, J., Allen, D. E., Kaplan, B. and Carolarelli, C. H. (1978). Unpublished Clinical Research Report No. 86
Prinzen, F. (1977). Unpublished Report
Puissant, A. (1976). Unpublished Report
Rabson, A. R., Whiting, D. A., Anderson, R., Glover, A. and Koornhof, H. J. (1977). *J. infect. Dis.*, **133**, 113
Racz, I. (1976). (ed). In *Proceedings of Current Problems of Immunology and their Dermatological Aspects*, Budapest, Hungary, p. 188
Racz, I. (1977). IV *Arzneimittel Symposium*, Berlin, Germany
Ramot, B. and Biniaminov, M. (1977). In *Control of Neoplasia by Modulation of the Immune System*, (ed. M. A. Chirigos), Raven Press, New York, U. S. A. p. 239
Ramot, B., Biniaminov, M., Shoham, Ch. and Rosenthal, E. (1976). *New Engl. J. Med.*, **294**, 809
Rave, O., Albrecht, H. J. and Vorlaender, K. O. (1978). *Z. Rheumatol.*, **37**, 12
Renoux, G. and Renoux, M. (1977a). *J. exp. Med.*, **145**, 466
Renoux, G. and Renoux, M. (1977b). *Lancet*, i, 372
Roge, J. and Lods, J. C. (1976). Unpublished Report
Roig Escofet, D., Valverde, G. J., Arnal Guimera, C., Sans Valeta, X., Arsra Fava, J., Graell Massana, J. and Ribas Subiros, R. (1977). *Rev. Esp. Reum.*, **4**, 23
Rojas, A. F., Feierstein, J. N., Glait, H. M. and Olivari, A. J. (1978). In *Immunotherapy of Cancer: Present Status of Trials in Man*, (eds. W. D. Terry and D. Windhorst), Raven Press
Rosenthal, M. and Trabert, U. (1976). *New Engl. J. Med.*, **295**, 1204
Rosenthal, M., Trabert, U. and Müller, W. (1976a). *Scand. J. Rheum.*, **5**, 216
Rosenthal, M., Trabert, U. and Müller W. (1976b). *Clin. exp. Immun.*, **25**, 493
Rosenthal, M., Trabert. U., Müller, W., Müller, S. and Wurm, K. (1976c). *New Engl. J. Med.*, **294**, 112
Rosenthal, M., Graf, U. and Müller, W. (1977). *Dtsch. Med. Wochenschr.*, **102**, 415
Rossio, J. L. and Goldstein, A. L. (1977) *World J. Surg.*, **1**, 605
Roux, H., Mercier, P., Jeandel, Y., Gabriel-Brouillet, M. T. and Serratrice, G. (1977). In *Perspectives in Inflammation*, (eds. D. A. Willoughby, J. P. Giroud and G. P. Velo), MTP Press Limited, Lancaster, p. 585
Runge, L. A. and Pinals, R. S. (1977). Unpublished Report
Runge, L. A., Pinals, R. S., Lourie, S. H. and Tomar, R. H. (1977). *Arthritis. Rheum.*, **20**, 1445
Runne, U. and Aulepp, H. (1975). *Dtsch. Med. Wochenschr.*, **100**, 2510
Russell, A. S. (1976). *J. Rheumat.*, **3**, 380
Russell, A. S., Brisson, E. and Grace, M. (1978). Unpublished Report
Ruuskanen, O., Remes, M., Maelelae, A. -L., Isomaeki, H. and Toivanen, A. (1976). *Lancet*, ii, 958
Saint-André, P. and Louvet, M. (1976). *Med. Armees*, **4**, 223
Samsoen, M., Heid, E., Schlachter, A., Grosshans, F. and Basset, A. (1977). *Ann. Derm. Venerol.*, **104**, 365
Scheid, M. P., Goldstein, G., Hammerling, U. and Boyse, E. A. (1975). *Ann. N. Y. Acad. Sci.*, **249**, 531
Scheinberg, M. A., Santos, L., Mendes, N. F. and Musatti, C. (1978). *Arthritis Rheum.*, **21**, 326
Schou, M. and Hellin, P. (1977). *Acta Derm. Venerol.*, **57**, 449
Schreiner, G. F. and Unanue, E. R. (1975). *J. Immun.*, **114**, 802
Schuermans, Y. (1975). Unpublished Report
Smith, R. B., Dekernion, J., Lincoln, B., Skinner, D. G. and Kaufman, J. J. (1978). Unpublished Report
Smolen, J., Scherak, O., Menzel, J., Kojer, M. and Kolarz, G. (1977). *Arthritis Rheum.*, **20**, 1558
Snyderman, R., Daniels, C. A. and Pike, M. C. (1978). In *Immune Modulation and Control of Neoplasia by Adjuvant Therapy*, (ed. M. A. Chirigos), Raven Press, New York, U.S.A. p.29
Spitler, L. E., Glogau, R. G., Nelms, D. C., Basch, C. M., Olson, J. A. Silverman, S. and Engleman, E. P. (1977a). In *Control of Neoplasia by Modulation of the Immune System*, (ed. M. A. Chirigos), Raven Press, New York, p. 217

Spitler, L. E., Glogau, R., Nelms, D., Silverman, S., Olson, J., O'Connor, R., Ostler, H., Smolin, G., Basch, K., Wong, P., Engleman, E. P. and Brugmans, J. (1977*b*). In *Modulation of Host Immune Resistance in the Prevention or Treatment of Induced Neoplasias*, Fogarty International Center Proceedings No. 28, U.S. Government Printing Office, Washington, U.S.A., p. 71

Spitler, L. E., Basch, C. M. and Engleman, E. P. (1977*c*). Unpublished Report

Spitler, L. E., Glogau, R., Nelms, D., Olson, J., Silverman, S., O'Connor, G. R., Ostler, H. B., Smolin, G., Kimura, S., Hogan, M., Miller, J. and Brugmans, J. (1978). *Am. J. Med.*, (in press)

Spruance, S. L., Krueger, G. G., MacCalman, J., Overall, J. C. and Klauber, M. (1978). Unpublished Report

Stephens, E. (1978). *4th Conference on Immune Modulation and Control of Neoplasia by Adjuvant Therapy*, Bethesda, Maryland, U.S.A.

Ström, T. B., Carpenter, C., Garovoy, M. R., Austen, K. F., Merrill, J. P. and Kaliner, M. (1973). *J. exp. Med.*, **138**, 381

Sutton, J. D. (1977). *Archs Dermat.*, **113**, 521

Symoens, J. and Brugmans, J. (1974). *Br. med. J.*, **4**, 592

Symoens, J. and Rosenthal, M. (1977). *J. Reticuloendothel. Soc.*, **21**, 175

Symoens, J. and Lewi, P. J. (1978). *J. Rheumat.*, (in press)

Symoens, J., Veys, E., Mielants, H. and Pinals, R. (1978). *Cancer Treat. Rep.*, (in press)

Szpilman, H., Drajozowska-Fischer, W., Luft, S., Glinska-Urban, D., Pomianowska, L., Fazdur, J., Kubasiewicz, E., Kopec, M. and Plachecka-Gutowska, M. (1977). XIVth *International Congress of Rheumatology*, San Francisco, California, U.S.A.

Takakura, K., Shitara, N. and Kohno, T. (1977). *Excerpta Medica*, International Congress Series No. 418, p. 32

Talal and Michalski (1977). Unpublished Report

Taube, H. (1978). *Z. Rheumaforsch.*, (in press)

Tennstedt, D. and Lachapelle, J. -M. (1977). *Ann. Derm. Vener.*, **104**, 98

Thomas, H. C., Freni, M., Sanchez-Tapias, J., De Villiers, D., Jain, S. and Sherlock, S. (1976). *Clin. exp. Immun.*, **26**, 222

Thornes, R. D. (1975). Unpublished Report

Thornes, R. D. (1977*a*). *Vet. Rec.*, **101**, 27

Thornes, R. D. (1977*b*). *J. Irish med. Ass.*, **70**, 480

Touraine, R., Sayag, J., Roujeau, J. -C., Revuz, J., Bussone, A. and Wechsler, J. (1975). *Bull. Soc. fr. Derm. Syph.*, **82**, 235

Tripodi, D., Parks, L. C. and Brugmans, J., (1973). *New Engl. J. Med.*, **289**, 254

Urist, M. M., Boddie, A. W., Townsend, C. M. and Holmes, E. C. (1977). *J. Thorac. Cardiovasc. Surg.*, **73**, 189

Valdimarsson, H. (1975). Unpublished Report

Valdivieso, M., Bedikian, A., Burgess, M. A., Rodriguez, V., Hersh, E. M., Bodey, G. P. and Mavligit, G. M. (1977). *Cancer*, **40**, 2731

Van de Heyning, J. (1978). *Laryngoscope*, **88**, 522

Vandervellen, R. (1978). Unpublished Clinical Research Report No. 72

Van Eygen, M., Znamensky, P. Y., Heck, E. and Raymaekers, I. (1976). *Lancet*, **i**, 382

Van Ghinckel, R. and Hoebeke, J. (1976). *Eur. J. Immun.*, **6**, 305

Van Ghinckel, R. and De Brabander, M. (1978). Unpublished Report

Van Heule, R., De Cree, J., Adriaenssens, K. and De Hauwere, R. (1976). *Acta paediat. scand.*, **29**, 41

Van Hooren, J. (1976). *Lancet*, **i**, 44

Van Wauwe, J. and Van Nijen, G. (1977). *Clin. exp. Immun.*, **30**, 465

Veien, N. (1977). *Dermatologica*, **154**, 185

Verhaegen, H. (1977). *Symposium on Immunotherapy of Malignant Diseases*, Vienna, Austria

Verhaegen, H., De Cree, J. and Brugmans, J. (1973). *Lancet*, **ii**, 842

Verhaegen, H., De Cree, J., De Cock, W. and Verbruggen, F. (1977*a*). *Clin. exp. Immun.*, **27**, 313

Verhaegen, H., De Cree, J., De Cock, W., Schuermans, Y., Engels, M. and Sonck, W. (1977*b*). *Biomedicine*, **26**, 283

Verhaegen, H., De Cock, W., De Cree, J. and Goldstein, G. (1978). Unpublished Report

Veys, E. M. and Mielants, H. (1977*a*). In *Perspectives in Inflammation*, (eds. D. A. Willoughby, J. P. Giroud and G. P. Velo), MTP Press Limited, Lancaster, U.K. p. 599

Veys, E. M. and Mielants, H. (1977*b*). *International Seminar on Treatment of Rheumatic Diseases*, Petah-Tiqva, Israel
Veys, E. M. and Mielants, H. (1977*c*). *J. Rheumat.*, **4**, 27
Vuopio, P. (1978). Unpublished Clinical Research Report No. 71
Wanebo, H. J., Hilal, E., Strong, E. W., Pinsky, C., Oettgen, H. F. and Hirshaut, Y. (1978). 4th *Conference on Immune Modulation and Control of Neoplasia by Adjuvant Therapy*, Bethesda, Maryland, U.S.A.
Watson, J., Epstein, R. and Cohn, M. (1973). *Nature*, **246**, 405
Weening, R. S., Stricker, L., Roos, D., Molenaar, J. L., Dooren, L. J. and Schuurman, R. K. B. (1977). In *Perspectives in Inflammation*, (eds. D. A. Willoughby, J. P. Giroud and G. P. Velo), MTP Press Limited, Lancester, U.K., p. 445
Weinstein, Y., Chambers, D. A., Bourne, H. R. and Melmon, K. L. (1974). *Nature*, **251**, 352
Wells, R. S. (1975). Unpublished Report
Wesdorp, E., Schellekens, P. T. A., Weening, R., Meuwissen, S. G. M. and Tytgat, G. N. J. (1977). *Gut*, **18**, A971
Willoughby, M. L. N., Baird, G. M. and Campbell, A. M. (1977). *Lancet*, **i**, 657
Woods, W. A., Papas, T. S. and Chirigos, M. A. (1977). In *Modulation of Host Immune Resistance in the Prevention or Treatment of Induced Neoplasias*, Fogarty International Center Proceedings No. 28, U.S. Government Printing Office, Washington, U.S.A. p. 23
Wright, D. G., Kirkpatrick, C. H. and Gallin, J. I. (1977). *J. clin. Invest.*, **59**, 941
Wright, P. W., Hill, L. D., Peterson, A. V., Pinkham, R., Johnson, L., Ivey, T., Bernstein, I., Bagley, C. and Anderson, R. (1978). 4th *Conference on Immune Modulation and Control of Neoplasia by Adjuvant Therapy*, Bethesda, Maryland, U.S.A.
Wynne, K. M., Dieppe, P. A., Huskisson, E. C., Willoughby, D. A. (1977). *Proceedings of Heberden Society Meeting*,
Yakir, Y., Kook, A. I., Schlesinger, M. and Trainin, N. (1977). *Isr. J. Med. Sci.*, **13**, 1191
Zaizov, R., Vogel, R., Cohen, I., Varsano, I., Shohat, B., Rotter, V. and Trainin, N. (1977). *Biomedicine*, **27**, 105
Zilko, P. J. (1975). Unpublished Report
Zulman, J., Michalski, J., McCombs, C., Greenspan, J. and Talal, N. (1978). *Clin. exp. Immun.*, **31**, 321

7

Effect of levamisole *in vivo* and *in vitro* on lymphocytes from patients with Behcet's syndrome and recurrent oral ulceration

T. Lehner and J. M. A. Wilton (Department of Oral Immunology
and Microbiology, Guy's Hospital Medical and Dental Schools,
London SE1 9RT, U.K.)

Levamisole (1-2, 3, 5, 6-tetrahydro-6-phenylimidazo [2, 1-b] -thiazol mono-hydrochloride) is an antihelminthic drug that can modulate immune responses in man both *in vivo* and *in vitro* (Tripodi *et al*., 1973; Pabst and Crawford, 1975; Huskisson *et al*., 1976; Ivanyi and Lehner, 1977) and in animals (Renoux and Renoux, 1973; Fischer *et al*., 1975). Enhancement of lymphocyte proliferation *in vitro* by mitogens or the mixed leucocyte culture reaction has been reported when levamisole was added to lymphocyte cultures (Hadden *et al*., 1975; Sampson and Lui, 1976).

The drug may influence some of the most common oral diseases; gingivitis (Ivanyi and Lehner, 1977), recurrent oral ulcers (ROU; Lehner, *et al*, 1976; Olson *et al*., 1976; De Meyer *et al*., 1977) and recurrent herpes labialis (Kint and Verlinden, 1974). It is of particular interest that these diseases share one common feature, that the pathogenesis appears to be strongly associated with the host immune response. The aetiological agents, however, differ greatly; recurrent herpes labialis is caused by herpes simplex virus (HSV), gingivitis is induced by dental bacterial plaque, consisting of a great variety of bacteria and their products. ROU shows predominantly immunological manifestations consistent with autoimmunity or some as yet undiscovered microbial agent. A common interpretation of the therapeutic effect of levamisole on the different oral diseases is based on the influence of levamisole on the host immune response. An immunological rationale will have to account not only for the beneficial effects of levamisole in ROU and recurrent herpes labialis, but also for the increased severity of gingivitis and of a proportion of patients with ROU.

The aims of this paper are to present some of our investigations on the proliferative response of peripheral blood lymphocytes when levamisole was given *in vivo* or *in vitro*. An attempt will be made to relate the data to a double-blind trial of levamisole in ROU. The effects of the drug on Behcet's syndrome will also be considered.

Table 7.1   Clinical analysis of the effect of

Type	Patient nos.	Mouth						Genitals			
		Res	Det	Nil	(% Res)	Cor. no. Res‡	(% Cor. Res)	Res	Det	Nil	(% Res)
Muco-cutaneous	9*	3	2	4	(33)	2	(22)	4	0	5	(44)
Arthritic	8	6	0	2	(75)	2	(25)	2	0	1	
Ocular	6	5	0	1	(83)	4	(67)	2	0	1	
Total	23	14	2	7	(61)	8	(35)	8	0	7	(53)

Abbreviations: Res, responders; Det, deteriorated; Nil, non-responders.
* 1 patient developed flu-like syndrome and was excluded.
† Also treated with prednisolone and azathioprine.
‡ Corrected number of responders as initial improvement was not sustained with subsequent treatment.
N.B. two patients had pustular skin lesions that cleared.

EXPERIMENTAL

Patients and dosage of levamisole

The investigation was carried out in 47 patients with ROU. Patients received either 150 mg of levamisole in three divided doses daily for 2 days weekly, or placebo, for 2 months and were then crossed-over to the alternative medication. Details of the trial have been fully described elsewhere (Lehner et al., 1976). Blood was taken for lymphocyte transformation tests before the start of administration of levamisole and again at the end of the 2 month period of medication in 32 patients.

Clinical assessment of the same dose of levamisole given for up to 1 year was made in 24 patients with Behcet's syndrome (BS). These were further subdivided into four types (Table 7.1) by the following criteria: (1) muco-cutaneous (M-C) type involves oral, genital and/or skin manifestations, (2) arthritic (A) type with joint involvement and some or all of the M-C manifestations, (3) neurological (N) type with brain involvement and some or all of the lesions found in the M-C and A types; (4) ocular (Oc) type with uveitis and some or all of the M-C, A and N manifestations. The presence of vascular lesions, such as thrombosis or aneurysm and intestinal disease can be found in any one of the four types of BS. Patients with rheumatoid arthritis and osteoarthritis have been excluded from the A type of BS. One patient with the M-C type developed a 'flu-like syndrome', so that administration of levamisole was discontinued and the patient withdrawn from the series. The response to levamisole was divided into three groups; those who improved, those who deteriorated and those patients showing no change. Improvement was defined as a decrease in the number of ulcers by more than 50 per cent over the period of observation and included patients whose ulcers cleared completely. In arthritis, responders were patients whose pain and swelling decreased or cleared and in uveitis there was an objective improvement in visual acuity.

Levamisole was administered *in vitro* in doses of 1 μg to 500μg per culture of 10^6 lymphocytes to control, as well as PHA (phytohaemagglutinin)-and PPD (purified protein derivative)-stimulated cultures.

levamisole in patients with Behcet's syndrome

		Joints						Eyes					
Cor. no. Res‡	(% Cor. Res)	Res	Det	Nil	(% Cor. Res)	no. Res‡	(% Cor. Res)	Res	Det	Nil	(% Cor. Res)	no. Res‡	(% Cor. Res)
4	(44)												
1		3	0	5	(37)	0							
1		2	0	0		1		1‡	2	3	(17)	1	(17)
6	(40)	5	0	5	(50)	1	(10)	1	2	3	(17)	1	(17)

Lymphocyte transformation test

Mononuclear cells were isolated from peripheral blood by using Ficol–Hypaque gradients (Boyum, 1968). Duplicate or triplicate cultures were set up in round-bottom plastic tubes (Falcon 3033, Oxnard, CA, U.S.A.) and consisted of 1×10^6 viable cells in tissue culture medium (TC199, Wellcome Reagents, Beckenham, Kent U.K.), containing 10 per cent autologous serum, penicillin 10 units/ml and streptomycin $1 \mu g/ml$. Stimulants were added in volumes of 0.1 ml and the cultures were then incubated for 72 h in humidified air with 5 per cent CO_2. They were then labelled with 1 μCi of [*methyl-*^{3}H] thymidine (1mCi/ml, Amersham, U.K.) for a further 24h and the cells were placed on filter-paper discs (Whatman Reeve Angel, U.K.), using an automated multi-sample harvester. After extensive washing with saline, the discs were dried in a hot-air oven, placed in scintillation fluid and the radioactivity was measured in a Wallac 81000 liquid-scintillation counter (LKB, Sweden), by the external-standard channels-ratio method. The results are expressed as Δc.p.m. $\pm$ s.e.m./10^6 cells, which is the mean radioactivity (counters per minute) of antigen- or mitogen-stimulated cultures minus the mean counts per minute of unstimulated cultures.

Lymphocyte stimulants

All stimulants were diluted in medium TC199 containing 10 per cent autologous serum and were prepared from stock by previously determined optimal dilutions. Pokeweed mitogen (PWM; Gibco, N.Y., U.S.A.) was used at a final dilution of 1:100 per culture. Streptokinase–streptodornase (SKSD-Varidase, Eli Lilly, U.K.) at 10 units per culture, preservative-free purified protein derivative from *Mycobacterium tuberculosis* (PPD; Weybridge, U.K.) at $10 \mu g$ per culture and herpes simplex virus type 1 (HSV; Public Health Laboratory Service, Colindale, London) at 1:1000 dilutions per culture. The same batch of each of the stimulants was used for all the experiments. All control cultures received 0.1ml of medium TC199 in place of the stimulant.

ADMINISTRATION OF LEVAMISOLE *IN VIVO*

The results of the spontaneous [³H] thymidine incorporation are shown in figure 7.1. The mean baseline incorporation was 1036 ± 110 c.p.m. and this increased to 1638 ± 186 after 2 months of levamisole ($P < 0.01$; $n = 32$, $t = 2.9795$). When the post-levamisole lymphocytes were cultured in baseline serum, incorporation was 1508 ± 191 but this failed to reach the 5 per cent level of significance ($P < 0.1$; $n = 28$, $t = 2.036$) when compared with the proliferation of lymphocytes before the drug was administered.

When lymphocytes were cultured with PWM at the start of the trial, the mean incorporation was 44492 ± 3988c.p.m. (figure 7.2) and this rose to 67508 ± 6563 c.p.m. when cells and serum collected after 2 months of drug therapy were cultured together ($P < 0.01$; $n = 35$, $t = 2.7444$). Post-levamisole lymphocytes and baseline serum cultured together incorporated 58895 ± 6170 c.p.m. and this was not significantly different when compared either with the cells cultured in post-levamisole

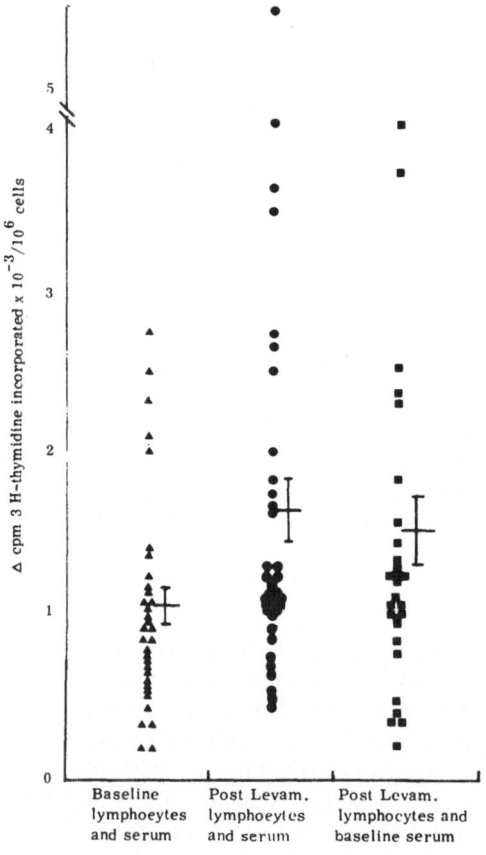

Figure 7.1 [³H] Thymidine uptake by unstimulated lymphocytes from patients before and after levamisole treatment

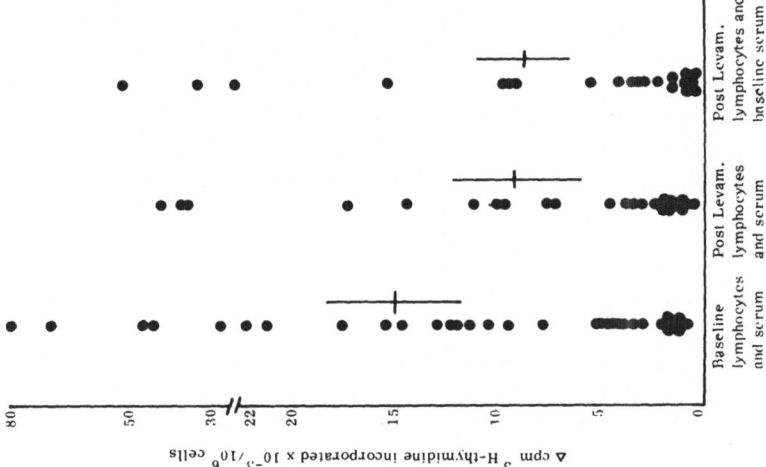

Figure 7.3 [³H] Thymidine uptake by lymphocytes stimulated with PPD from patients before
and after levamisole treatment

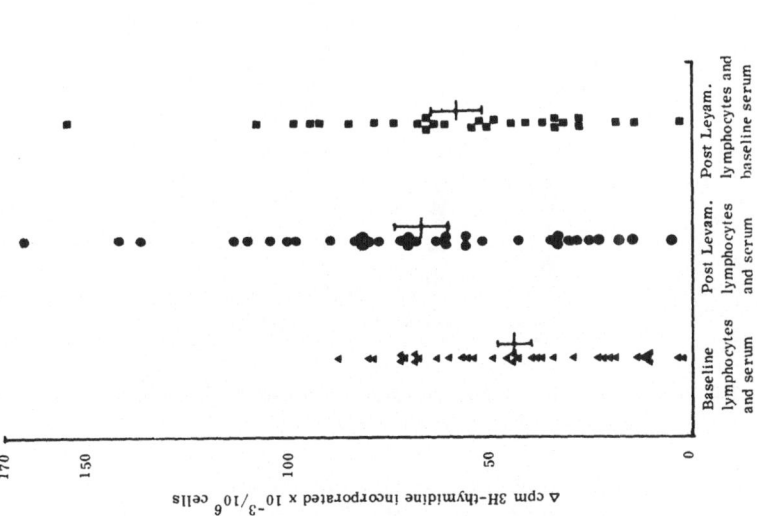

Figure 7.2 [³H] Thymidine uptake by lymphocytes stimulated with PWM from patients before
and after levamisole treatment

serum ($P < 0.1; n = 28, t = 1.5462$) or with lymphocytes cultured before commencement of the study ($P < 0.1; n = 26, t = 1.3341$).

PPD-induced lymphocyte transformation at the start of the study was 15 193 ± 3175 c.p.m. and this fell to 9090 ± 2454 c.p.m. after levamisole treatment (figure 7.3). The decrease was not significant ($P < 0.1; n = 24, t = 1.7114$) and when baseline serum was substituted, lymphocytes incorporated 8704 ± 2885 c.p.m.

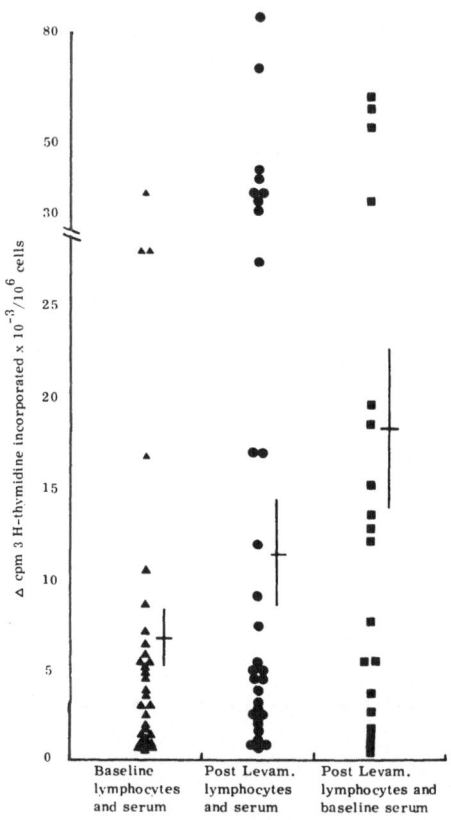

Figure 7.4 [³H] Thymidine uptake by lymphocytes stimulated with SKSD from patients before and after levamisole treatment

Thymidine incorporation induced by SKSD before treatment was 6770 ± 1629 c.p.m. (figure 7.4) and this increased significantly after levamisole to 11 504 ± 3004 c.p.m. ($P < 0.05; n = 32, t = 2.3091$). This again rose when baseline serum and post-drug lymphocytes were cultured, the mean incorporation being 18 287 ± 4260 c.p.m. This was significantly different from the thymidine incorporation before the trial ($P < 0.01; n = 20, t = 3.4912$) but not from the incorporation when both the lymphocytes and the serum were taken after the 2 month period of medication ($P < 0.2; n = 22, t = 1.2578$).

HSV type 1 stimulated thymidine incorporation in lymphocytes taken from patients before the start of the trial, the mean being 5654 ± 876 c.p.m. (figure 7.5). After levamisole treatment this rose significantly to 9039 ± 1512 c.p.m. ($P < 0.02$; $n = 20$, $t = 2.6538$). When the lymphocytes were cultured in baseline serum they incorporated 8781 ± 1568 c.p.m. which was also significantly greater than the base-line value ($P < 0.05$; $n = 14$, $t = 3.160$). PHA-stimulated lymphocytes showed a

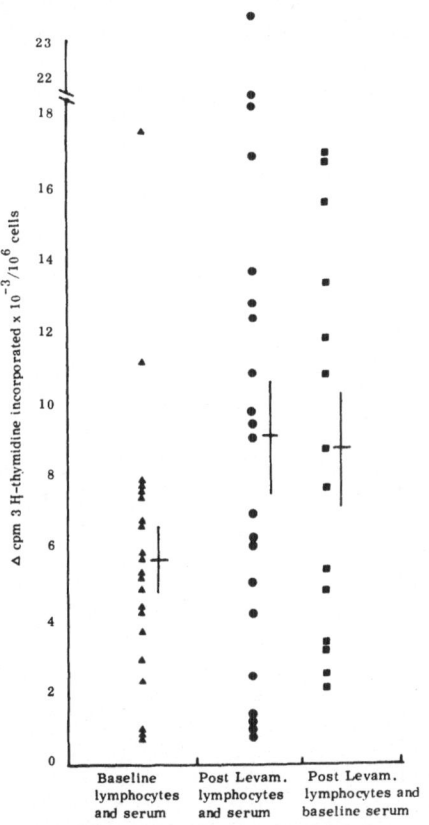

Figure 7.5 [^{3}H] Thymidine uptake by lymphocytes stimulated with HSV from patients before and after levamisole treatment

slight but not significant decrease in the uptake of [^{3}H] thymidine from a mean value of 105 883 (± 16 482) c.p.m. before, to 102 308 (± 12 585) c.p.m. after levamisole. Culture of lymphocytes after levamisole treatment in the presence of baseline serum resulted in a further decrease in the mean uptake of [^{3}H] thymidine (87 798 ± 9585 c.p.m.) but this again was not significant.

ADMINISTRATION OF LEVAMISOLE *IN VITRO*

A negative correlation was found (figure 7.6) between the dose of levamisole and the uptake of [^{3}H] thymidine in control cultures. From Δc.p.m. it can be seen that at the highest concentrations of levamisole there is a depression in the uptake of [^{3}H] thymidine with negative values, and at the lowest concentrations of levamisole there is a net increase in the uptake of [^{3}H] thymidine; regression analysis showed this to be very significant ($P < 0.001$, $n = 87$, $t = -5.81$). Similar, though less significant correlations were observed with PHA ($P < 0.05$, $n = 78$, $t = -2.06$) but not with PPD.

Viability of lymphocytes was determined at the end of the 4 days of incubation by the Trypan Blue exclusion test, and this failed to show any difference in viability between lymphocytes with 500μg and those with 1μg of levamisole added to 10^6 lymphocytes.

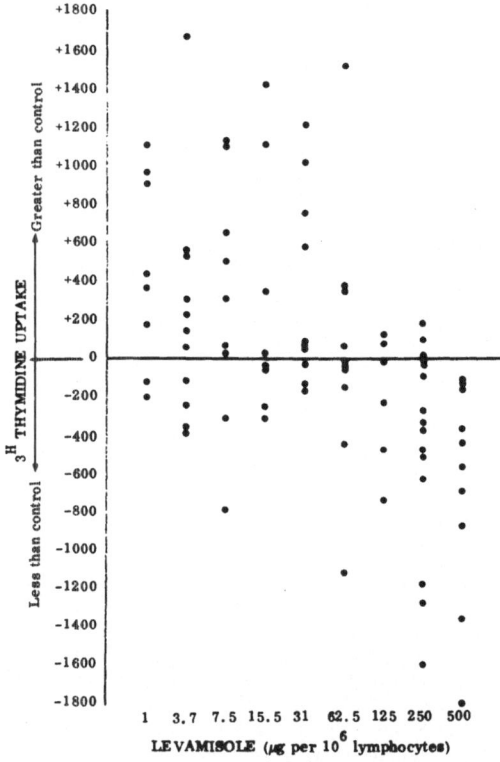

Figure 7.6 The effect of dose of levamisole on thymidine uptake of unstimulated cultures of lymphocytes.

CORRELATION BETWEEN THE UPTAKE OF [^{3}H] THYMIDINE AND CLINICAL CHANGES IN ROU

In the double-blind cross-over trial of levamisole in 47 patients with ROU a significant decrease in the number of ulcers was found after 2 months of administration of levamisole in 64 per cent of patients (Lehner *et al.*, 1976). In 23 per cent of the patients there was an increased number of ulcers. An attempt to correlate the change in the [^{3}H] thymidine uptake with the clinical manifestations has failed.

BEHCET'S SYNDROME

The results of the clinical assessment (Table 7.1) show that ROU responded in 62 per cent, genital ulcers in 53 per cent, arthritis in 55 per cent, but uveitis in only 20 per cent of patients. Correcting these figures for patients in whom recurrence of clinical manifestations failed to respond to further administration of levamisole, there is a substantial decrease in the percentage of responders, most evident in those with arthritis. As only one patient with uveitis was controlled with levamisole, after he had failed to respond to immunosuppressive treatment, and two patients deteriorated, this drug is unlikely to be helpful in the ocular type of BS. Although the arthritic manifestations responded well initially, this was not sustained on giving the drug for recurrences of arthritis. A convincing therapeutic effect was found only in the M-C type of BS, with sustained improvement or clearance of both oral (8/23) and genital (6/15) ulcers in about 40 per cent of patients.

DISCUSSION

This study has shown that lymphocytes from patients with ROU gave enhanced proliferative responses *in vitro* after 2 months of administration of therapeutic doses of levamisole *in vivo*. The rate of spontaneous incorporation of thymidine was significantly increased and stimulation of lymphocytes with PWM, SKSD and HSV type 1 yielded an increased uptake of thymidine by lymphocytes after administration of levamisole, compared with those before the drug was given. Levamisole administered *in vivo* in man appears to have induced a significantly augmented response of lymphocytes *in vitro*, both in the presence and absence of mitogens or antigens. The effect of the mitogens and antigens could not be accounted for by the increase in thymidine uptake of the control cultures, as the former was expressed as Δc.p.m. Stimulation with PPD was an exception for which there is no obvious interpretation. There has been little work reported on the proliferative response of lymphocytes that have been exposed to levamisole *in vivo*. An enhanced response of lymphocytes to PHA was recorded in patients with nasopharyngeal carcinoma (Chan and Simons, 1975) but not in those with other carcinomas (Verhaegen *et al.*, 1973). Our results are consistent with the enhanced skin delayed hypersensitivity after treatment with levamisole *in vivo* (Tripodi *et al.*, 1973; Huskisson *et al.*, 1976).

The potentiating effect of levamisole was observed within 1 week of the last dose of levamisole being taken orally in a 2 month course of treatment. The possibility that active levamisole may have been retained in the blood at the time of establishing the culture is unlikely, as the drug is virtually eliminated from the body within 2 days (Symoens and Rosenthal, 1977). However, the possibility of a drug-induced serum factor was explored because an enhanced immune response to sheep erythrocytes and tumour antigens was transferable by sera from levamisole-treated animals (Renoux *et al.*, 1974), and the thymidine uptake of lymphocytes stimulated with *Veillonella alcalescens* was enhanced by serum factors (Ivanyi and Lehner, 1977). A study of the effect on lymphocytes of serum taken after treatment compared with that taken before the levamisole treatment was started, has shown a small increase in thymidine uptake with the former serum in unstimulated cultures and those stimulated with PWM. A serum factor can not therefore be excluded from playing a part in enhanced lymphoproliferative responses in man. However, the most likely effect of levamisole is directly on the lymphocytes or indirectly on the macrophages as will be discussed below.

The direct effect of adding levamisole (1–500μg per 10^6 lymphocytes) *in vitro* has also been studied. The maximum dose of levamisole was selected so as not to impair the viability of lymphocytes. A significant negative correlation was found between the dose of levamisole and thymidine uptake of unstimulated lymphocytes ($P < 0.001$) and those stimulated with PHA ($P < 0.05$). Thus low doses of levamisole enhance, whereas high doses depress the proliferative response of lymphocytes in man. This confirms previous reports of a dose-dependent effect of levamisole, with enhancement usually being found with low concentrations and suppression with high concentrations of the drug (Pabst and Crawford, 1975; Sampson and Lui, 1976; Al-Ibrahim *et al.*, 1977). The doses used in some studies were one-tenth or less than those used in the present work, but the number of lymphocytes were 10^5 in the former, compared with 10^6 per culture in this investigation. We have extended the doses beyond what might be assumed to be the therapeutic range, but within the viability of lymphocytes, as there is some evidence that monocytes may take up an increased amount of levamisole (Fischer *et al.*, 1976).

The critical nature of the dose of levamisole needs to be emphasised. The lymphoproliferative response is augmented at low concentrations of up to $5\mu g$ of levamisole per 10^5 cells but at greater concentrations the response is suppressed. This is in contrast to the increased chemotaxis at high doses of levamisole, maximum at $100\mu g$ (Pike and Snyderman, 1976) and augmented phagocytosis at doses between 2.5 and $10\mu g$ of levamisole (Al-Ibrahim *et al.*, 1977). Although the optimum concentration of levamisole for the three functions varies, with the macrophage function being augmented at a higher dose than lymphocyte functions, this may be interpreted on the basis of a greater uptake of ^{3}H-labelled levamisole by monocytes than by lymphocytes (Fisher *et al.*, 1976). There is therefore the possibility of an increased concentration of levamisole in an inflammatory focus. The inverse effects of low and high doses of levamisole might also be one interpretation of the paradoxical clinical effects sometimes resulting from levamisole.

The enhanced lymphoproliferative effect of levamisole could be due to a direct effect on lymphocytes or on the macrophages or on both cell types. The drug probably acts on T lymphocytes as shown in mice by the increased graft-*versus*-host reaction (Renoux and Renoux, 1973), by accelerated rejection of isogeneic skin grafts (Chirigos *et al.* 1973; Renoux *et al.*, 1976), by enhancing the skin delayed hypersensitivity reactions (Renoux *et al.*, 1976) and by the effect of mitogens on mouse T- or B-enriched cells *in vitro* (Merluzzi *et al.*, 1975; Hadden *et al.*, 1975). Levamisole is apparently capable of augmenting suppressor T-cell activity of spleen and thymus cells in man *in vitro* (Sampson and Lui, 1976). It can also induce T-cell differentiation from precursor spleen cells *in vivo* and induce a significant number of IgG plaque-forming cells in immunised nude mice (Renoux and Renoux, 1977). However, LPS induced a significant increase in the response of unfractionated lymphocytes from subjects taking intermittent doses of levamisole for 2 months (Ivanyi and Lehner, 1977).

Levamisole may affect the function of monocytes both by enhancing their chemotactic response (Pike and Snyderman, 1976) and phagocytosis (Hoebeke and Franchi, 1973; Lima *et al.*, 1974). As macrophages bind levamisole preferentially they may regulate the dose of the drug made available to the T-lymphocyte subsets. At low doses levamisole-bound macrophages may induce increased proliferation of lymphocytes, whereas at high doses macrophages are activated (Schultz *et al.*, 1977) and these may suppress lymphocyte proliferation (Keller, 1974).

Significant decreases in the number of ulcers and ulcer days were found after

2 months of intermittent administration of levamisole in patients with ROU. About 64 per cent of patients responded to the drug by a decrease in the number of ulcers of more than 50 per cent, for 2 or more months. The remaining 36 per cent of patients failed to respond to levamisole and 23 per cent of these had an increased number of ulcers. A double-blind trial of levamisole in BS was not thought to be justifiable and the results of treatment were assessed in an open trial. It was rather surprising that the proportion of patients who showed a greater than 50 per cent decrease in the number of ulcers was 62 per cent and this was almost identical with that found in the double-blind trial of ROU. A beneficial effect was also found with genital ulcers (in 53 per cent) and arthritis (in 55 per cent) but only in one out of five patients with uveitis (Table 7.1). The beneficial effect was, however, not found on repeated administration of levamisole for recurrence of arthritis and responders fell to 22 per cent. A useful therapeutic effect was retained only in the muco-cutaneous type of BS, with sustained improvement or clearance of both oral (8/21) and genital (6/15) ulcers in about 40 per cent of patients. The effect on cutaneous manifestations could not be assessed as only two patients had skin lesions, though in both the lesions cleared. It should be noted that vaginal ulceration in four of these patients was severe and failed to respond to topical steroids and antibiotics and in three of these to systemic steroids; these patients found relief from vaginal ulcers for the first time after several years of troublesome ulceration.

None of the 47 patients with ROU or 24 patients with BS developed neutropenia, but a 'flu-like syndrome' developed in one patient in each series and urticaria also in one patient in each series. However, the patient with BS and urticaria felt so unhappy about the vaginal ulcers that she persevered with levamisole treatment and both the urticaria and vaginal ulcers cleared. A relationship between the clinical improvement and enhanced lymphoproliferative response *in vitro* could not be established. This is perhaps not entirely surprising as a specific stimulant of lymphocytes was not used in the diseases under investigation. It remains therefore an assumption that the therapeutic effect is brought about by the immunopotentiating effect of levamisole.

The best relationship between the action of levamisole, the clinical manifestations and lymphoproliferative responses *in vitro* in man is the effect on gingival inflammation (Ivanyi and Lehner, 1977). Administration of levamisole for a period of 2 months in 31 patients with ROU, but otherwise healthy subjects, revealed a significant increase in the index of gingival inflammation. This was associated with an increased lymphoproliferative response stimulated by oral bacteria, but no effect on the antibody titres to the same antigens. Thus an effect of levamisole *in vivo* was observed on gingival inflammation and this was correlated with a corresponding increase in the lymphoproliferative response to oral bacterial antigens. These results are consistent with the increase in gingival inflammation and the lymphoproliferative responses to oral bacteria in experimental gingivitis in man (Lehner *et al.*, 1974).

The two apparently diverse clinical effects of levamisole, of increased gingival inflammation and decreased number of ulcers in the mouth share the increased lymphoproliferative response to oral and unrelated bacterial antigens, as well as mitogens. There is no demonstrable defect in cell-mediated immunity in ROU, but an abnormal cellular response to oral epithelial antigens (Lehner, 1967; Dolby, 1969; Donatsky, 1976; Rogers *et al.*, 1974). However, gingivitis is associated with increased cell-mediated immunity to a variety of antigens and mitogens. It is suggested that the effect of levamisole might be on different subsets of T lymphocytes and this may be mediated by macrophages. The promoting effect of the drug on gingivitis might be mediated by augmenting the effector lymphocytes, whereas the reduction of ulcers in patients with ROU and BS might be associated with augmenting the suppressor lymphocytes.

ACKNOWLEDGEMENTS

We thank Mr R. G. Ward for his technical help and Janssen Pharmaceutica Ltd., Beerse, Belgium, for the supply of levamisole.

REFERENCES

Al-Ibrahim, M. S., Holzman, R. S. and Lawrence, H. S. (1977). *J. infect. Dis.*, 135, 517
Boyum, A. (1968). *Scand. J. clin. Lab. Invest.*, 21, (Suppl. 97), 77
Chan, S. H. and Simons, M. J. (1975). *Lancet*, i, 1246
Chirigos, A., Pearson, J. W. and Pryor, J. (1973). *Cancer Res.*, 33, 2615
De Meyer, J., Degraeve, M., Clarysse, J., De Loose, F. and Peremans, W. (1977). *Brit. Med. J.*, 1, 671
Dolby, A. E. (1969). *Immunology*, 17, 709
Donatsky, O. (1976). *Acta Path. Micro. Scand., Sec. C*, 84, 227
Fischer, G. W., Podgore, J. K., Bass, J. W., Kelley, J. L. and Kobayashi, G. Y. (1975). *J. infect. Dis.*, 132, 578
Fischer, G. W., Crumrine, M. H., Balk, M. W., Chang, S. P., Hokama, Y., Heu, P. and Chou, S. C. (1976). *Proc. 3rd Con. Modulation of Host Resistance in the Prevention of Treatment of Induced Neoplasias*, Bethesda, MD
Hadden, J. W., Coffey, R. G., Hadden, E. M., Lopez-Corrales, E. and Sunshine, G.H. (1975). *Cell. Immunol.* 20, 98
Hoebeke, J. and Franchi, G. (1973). *J. reticuloendothel. Soc.*, 14, 317
Huskisson, E. C., Scott, J., Balme, H. W., Dieppe, P. A., Trapnell, J. and Willoughby, D. A. (1976). *Lancet*, i, 393
Ivanyi, L. and Lehner, T. (1977). *Scand. J. Immunol.*, 6, 219
Keller, R. (1974). *Immunology*, 27, 285
Kint, A. and Verlinden, L. (1974). *New Eng. J. Med.*, 291, 308
Lehner, T. (1967). *Immunology*, 13, 159.
Lehner, T., Wilton, J. M. A., Challacombe, S. J. and Ivanyi, L. (1974). *Clin. exp. Immunol.*, 16, 481
Lehner T., Wilton, J. M. A. and Ivanyi, L. (1976). *Lancet*, ii, 926
Lima, A. O., Javierre, M. Q., Dias da Silva, W. and Camara, D. S. (1974). *Experientia (Basel)*, 30, 945
Merluzzi, V. J., Badger, A. M., Kaiser, C. W. and Cooperband, S. R. (1975). *Clin. exp. Immunol.*, 22, 486
Olson, J. A., Nelms, D. C., Silverman, S. and Spitler, L. E. (1976). *Oral Surg. Med. Path.*, 41, 588
Pabst, H. F. and Crawford, J. (1975). *Clin. exp. Immunol.*, 21, 468
Pike, M. C. and Snyderman, R. (1976). *Nature*, 261, 136
Renoux, G. and Renoux, M. (1973). *Infect. Immun.*, 8, 544
Renoux, G. and Renoux, M. (1977). *J. exp. Med.*, 145, 466
Renoux, G., Kassel, R. L., Renoux, M., Fiore, N. G., Guillaumin, J. M. and Palat, A. (1974) *Proc. 3rd. Con. Modulation of Host Immune Resistance in the Prevention of Treatment of Induced Neoplasias*, Bethesda, MD
Renoux, G., Renoux, M., Teller, M. N., McMahon, N. and Guillaumin, J. M. (1976). *Clin. exp. Immunol.*, 25, 288

Rogers, R. S., Sams, W. M. and Shorter, R. G. (1974). *Archs. Derm.*, 109, 361
Sampson, D. and Lui, A. (1976). *Cancer Res.*, 36, 952
Schultz, R. M., Papamathiallis, J. D., Luetzler, J. and Chirigos, M. A. (1977). *Cancer Res.*, 37, 3338
Symoens, J. and Rosenthal, M. (1977). *J. reticuloendothel. Soc.*, 21, 175
Tripodi, D., Parks, L. C. and Brugmans, J. (1973). *New Eng. J. Med.*, 289, 354
Verhaegen, H., De Cree, J. and Brugmans, J. (1973). *Lancet*, ii, 842

8
New developments in drugs enhancing the immune response: activation of lymphocytes and accessory cells by muramyl-dipeptides

R. H. Gisler, F. M. Dietrich, G. Baschang, A. Brownbill, G. Schumann, F. G. Staber, L. Tarcsay, E. D. Wachsmuth and P. Dukor (Research Department, Pharmaceuticals Division, CIBA-GEIGY Limited, Basel, Switzerland)

ADJUVANT EFFECTS AND SYSTEMIC IMMUNOSTIMULATION

Recently, stimulation of host defence mechanisms has become a major goal of pharmacotherapeutic research. Immunopotentiating compounds exert their effects in different ways. On the one hand, they may enhance non-specific effector mechanisms operative in the resistance of infectious agents and to neoplastic cells. On the other hand, they may non-specifically increase specific immune responses elicited by the recognition of antigenic determinants. Of course, the two mechanisms operative in the resistance to infectious agents and to neoplastic cells. On may be mediated by the pharmacological activation of common target cells, that is macrophages and other accessory cells, such as polymorphonuclear leucocytes.

In principle, immunopotentiating agents can be used either as adjuvants *sensu strictiori* or as systemic immunostimulants (figure 8.1). In the first case, they are admixed to poorly immunogenic antigens to increase their immunogenicity. In the second case, they are administered by themselves to increase the immunological responsiveness of the recipient to either extrinsic or intrinsic antigens. Some immunostimulants may act as polyclonal activators (Coutinho and Möller, 1975), triggering non-specifically — in the absence of any known antigenic stimulation — the proliferation of multiple lymphocyte clones that will then express their genetically predetermined immunological potential. Although this mechanism could play an important role in the induction of non-specific resistance, it might also carry considerable risks such as activation of 'forbidden' autoreactive cell populations. Accordingly, several types of potential use of immuno-stimulating agents can be distinguished (table 8.1). New and better adjuvants are urgently required to facilitate the development of novel vaccines and of improved vaccination pro-

133

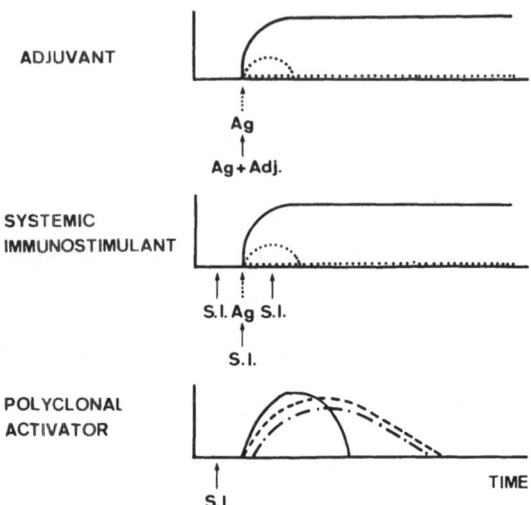

Figure 8.1   Schematic representation of different types of immunopotentiation
Immune response (ordinate) over time (abscissa) with (—, – – – –, · – · –) and without
(· · · ·) administration of an immunopotentiating agent. —, – – – –, · – · –, denote different
specificities. Ag, Antigen; Adj., adjuvant; S.I., systemic immunostimulant.

cedures. This is particularly important for conditions that are mainly controlled
by cell-mediated rather than humoral immunity, as appears to be the case in many
intracellular infections and in parasitic diseases.

Systemic immunostimulants have found wide-spread application in trials of
tumour immunotherapy and may prove valuable in combination chemotherapy
and prophylaxis of infectious diseases. Moreover, they may be used for the
correction of generalised immunodeficiencies, particularly those resulting from
immunosuppressive regimens, and in some disorders that may be associated with
genetically determined selective immunological defects.

MUREIN, AND SYNTHETIC MURAMYL-DIPEPTIDES WITH IMMUNO-STIMULANT ACTIVITY

With the exception of levamisole (Symoens and Rosenthal, 1977), most clinical
and also preclinical experience with immunostimulants has been restricted to
bacterial vaccines, crude bacterial extracts and complex macromolecular preparations. It is in the field of bacterial cell-wall biochemistry, however, that particularly promising advances have been made over the past few years. Many bacteria,
notably gram-negative micro-organisms, contain a whole range of structurally
distinct constituents with marked immunopotentiating properties: murein (the
cell-wall peptidoglycan skeleton), phospholipids, lipopolysaccharides and other
glycolipids (including cord factors), lipoprotein, teichoic acids, etc.

Since phylogenetically the vertebrates have co-evolved with pathogenic micro-
organisms, it is tempting to speculate that the immune system became adapted to

Table 8.1   Potential uses of immunostimulants

A. Improvement of vaccines (adjuvanticity)

    (a)   Novel vaccines
    (b)   Simplified vaccination procedures
    (c)   Replacement of attenuated live vaccines
          by killed vaccines (subunit vaccines)

B. Enhancement of resistance to tumours*

    (a)   Induction of remissions
    (b)   Prevention of relapses

C. Enhancement of resistance to infections†

    (a)   Prevention and therapy of acute infections
    (b)   Prevention and therapy of chronic infections

D. Treatment of generalised immune deficiencies

    (a)   Congenital
    (b)   Acquired

E. Treatment of selective immunological defects

    (a)   Rheumatoid arthritis
    (b)   Multiple sclerosis
    (c)   Autoimmune disorders

---

*In combination with surgery, radiotherapy and chemotherapy.

†In combination with antibiotics and chemotherapeutic agents.

recognise some of the widely represented bacterial components as signals for the enhancement or modulation of immune responses irrespective of their antigenic specificity (Melchers *et al.*, 1975).

Many laboratories have been engaged in the isolation and fractionation of such constituents to define the smallest biologically effective fragments. This approach is exemplified by the characterisation of the active principle of the mycobacterial component in complete Freund's adjuvant (CFA; Freund, 1947). CFA is prepared as a water-in-oil emulsion containing antigen in the aqueous phase and killed mycobacteria in the oil phase, which is made up of mineral oil and an emulsifying agent. The mycobacteria further enhance the antibody response already stimulated by the paraffin oil (Freund *et al.*, 1937), but more strikingly they also allow for the development of persistent delayed hypersensitivity (Freund and McDermott, 1942). Three different groups independently demonstrated that water-soluble peptidoglycan fractions could effectively substitute for whole mycobacteria in inducing manifestations of cell-mediated immunity (Adam *et al.*, 1972; Migliore-Samour and Jollès, 1972; Hiu, 1972). More recently, Lederer and his associates were able

Drugs and Immune Responsiveness

to identify the muramyl-dipeptide moiety (*N*-acetyl-muramyl-L-alanyl-D-isogluta-mine, MDP) as the minimum structure still carrying much of the immunopharm-acological activity of the parent molecule (Ellouz *et al.*, 1974).

MDP was first synthesised by Merser *et al.* (1975) and by Kotani *et al.* (1975) and in the meantime a large number of modified analogues of this prototype mole-

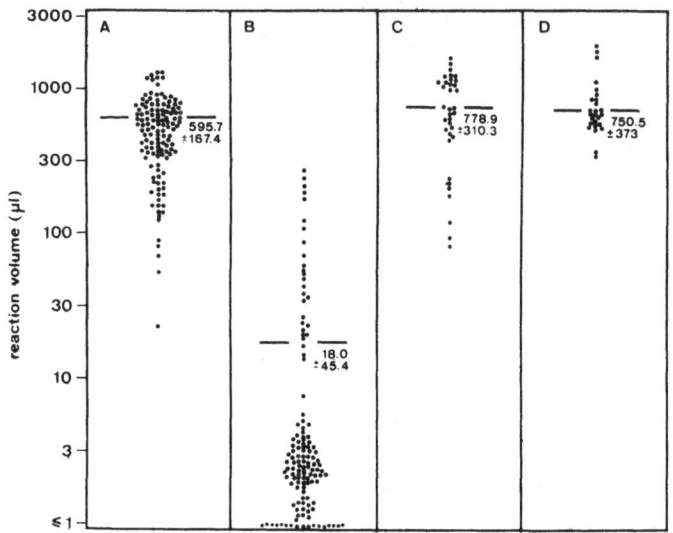

Figure 8.2 MDP-mediated induction of delayed hypersensitivity to BSA in guinea pigs
Female Pirbright guinea pigs (250–300g) immunised on day 0 by s.c. (subcutaneous) injection into both hind foot pads of 2 × 0.1 ml of a standardised water-in-oil emulsion containing one part PBS (phosphate-buffered saline) supplemented with BSA (total dose 1 mg per recipient) and MDP, and one part oil phase (8.5 parts of Bayol F and 1.5 parts of Arlacel A). Challenge on day 21 was by i.c. (intracutaneous) injection of 100 μg of BSA in 0.1 ml of PBS into the shaved skin of the flank using a Panjet injector (Schuco). At 24 h later, the area of redness and skin thickness at the antigen-injection site were determined by measuring two diameters, and compared with an adjacent site injected with PBS alone, by using a skin-fold caliper fitted with a constant-pressure device. Calculation of reaction volume (μl) = increase in skin thickness (mm) × area of redness (mm)^2 as described by Maurer *et al.* (1975). For each group, values of individual animals and arithmetic means ± s.d. are indicated. Immunisation vehicles: A, CFA (Difco); B, IFA (Difco); C, IFA supplemented with MDP (100 μg/recipient), D, IFA supplemented with Nor-MDP (100 μg/recipient). MDP and Nor-MDP were synthesised by Drs J. Stanek and A. Hartmann (CIBA-GEIGY Ltd, Basel).

cule have become available (Audibert *et al.*, 1977; Kotani *et al.*, 1977; Baschang *et al.*, 1977; Jones *et al.*, 1978). The structural requirements for the adjuvant act-ivity of MDPs are rather narrow and quite well-defined. A D-glucosamine con-figuration without stable substitution in C-1 or C-4 appears to be important for high activity. Reduction of the sugar moiety invariably is associated with inactiva-tion (Adam *et al.*, 1976). *N*-Benzoyl derivatives (Jones *et al.*, 1978; unpublished results) and 6-*O*-acyl derivatives (Kotani *et al.*, 1977) retain considerable immuno-

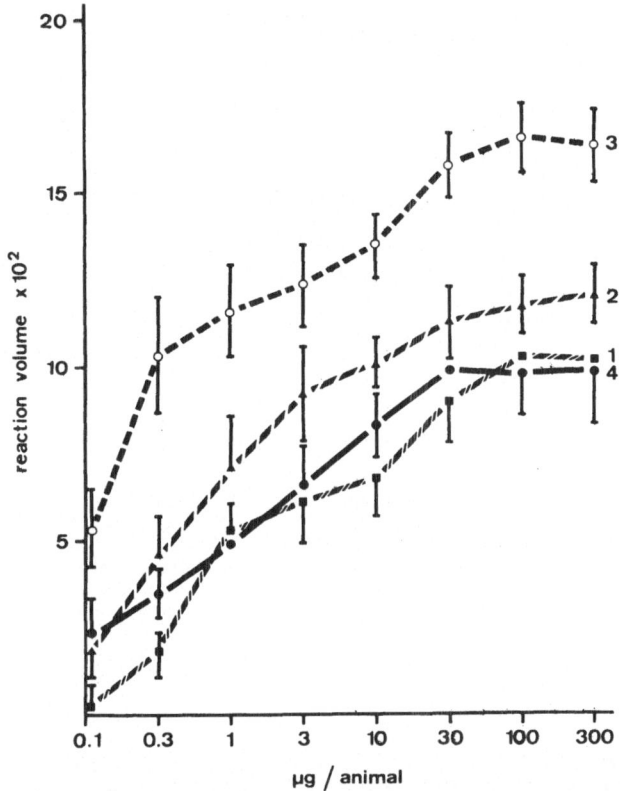

Figure 8.3 MDP-mediated induction of delayed hypersensitivity to BSA in guinea pigs: comparative activity of different MDP derivatives
Ordinate: reaction volumes (μl) 24 h after i.c. challenge with BSA on day 21 (arithmetic means of values obtained from six animals per group ± s.d.). Abscissa: μg of MDP per recipient in adjuvant mixture injected on day 0. 1, MDP (MurNac-L-Ala-D-isoGln): 2, Nor-MDP (Nor-MurNac-L-Ala-D-isoGln); 3, Nor-MurNac-L-Abu-D-isoGln; 4, Nor-MurNac-L-Ala-D-GluαN-Gly.NH$_2$.MDP derivatives were synthetised by J. Stanek and A. Hartmann. All groups were set up simultaneously. Otherwise immunisation and challenge as in figure 8.2.

stimulating properties in many assay systems. Substitution of the lactic acid moeity by glycolic acid (Nor-MDP derivatives) does not interfere with activity (figures 8.2 and 8.3; Jones *et al.*, 1978) but leads to a remarkable reduction in toxicity in non-rodents (Jones *et al.*, 1978). The amino acid composition of the dipeptide chain appears to be critical (table 8.2). Thus substitution of L-Ala in position 1 by D-Ala, or by L-Leu or Gly has been reported to be associated with considerable reduction of activity in some of the models used. However, after substitution by L-Ser, L-Tyr, L-Pro and L-Thr, effectiveness is maintained. Substitution by L-Val or L-Abu will even yield derivatives of increased biological efficacy and greater potency (see also figure 8.3). On the other hand, in position 2, the D-configuration and the presence of the α-carboxamide group of the isoglutamine residue appears to be crucial for retention of the full adjuvant activity.

Table 8.2 Adjuvant activity of synthetic MDP derivatives: effect of amino acid substitution

AA 1	Adjuvant activity	AA 2	Adjuvant activity
L-Ala	++	D-isoGln	++
D-Ala	−	L-isoGln	−
L-Leu	−	D-Gln	(+)
Gly*	(+)	L-Gln	−
L-Ser	++	D-Glu	+
L-Tyr	++	L-Glu	−
L-Pro	++	D-Glu (OCH$_3$)$_2$	+
L-Thr	++(+)	L-GluαN-Gly·NH$_2$	++
L-Val	+++		
L-Abu	+++		

Data are from Kotani *et al.* (1975), Adam *et al.* (1976), Chedid *et al.* (1976), Audibert *et al.* (1977), Jones *et al.* (1978) and Nagai *et al.* (1978*b*): AA 1 and AA 2 are the first and second amino acids (AA) of MDP (MurNac-AA1-AA2). Adjuvant activity was assessed by induction of delayed hypersensitivity to heterologous proteins in guinea pigs immunised with MDP-supplemented antigen–mineral oil emulsions.–, No activity; +, activity < MDP; ++, activity in the range of MDP; +++, activity > MDP.

*Full adjuvant activity was retained in induction of experimental allergic encephalo-myelitis in guinea pigs (Nagai *et al.*, 1978*b*)

INDUCTION OF DELAYED HYPERSENSITIVITY AND OTHER MANIFESTATIONS OF T-CELL-MEDIATED IMMUNITY BY MDP *IN VIVO*

The induction of delayed hypersensitivity to protein antigens in guinea pigs is the hallmark of the adjuvant activity of MDP and MDP derivatives. If administered together with the antigen in water-in-mineral-oil emulsions synthetic MDPs induced manifestations of cell-mediated immunity to ovalbumin (Ellouz *et al.*, 1974; Kotani *et al.*, 1975; Audibert *et al.*, 1976), bovine serum albumin (BSA) (figures 8.2 and 8.3; tables 8.3 and 8.4), azobenzene arsonate (ABA) *N*-acetyl-L-tyrosine (Audibert *et al.*, 1976; Azuma *et al.*, 1976*a*). Similarly, MDP derivatives effectively promoted the development of experimental allergic encephalomyelitis in guinea pigs immunised with encephalitogens (Nagai *et al.*, 1978*a,b*).

In the guinea pig BSA model (figure 8.2) both MDP and demethylated MDP (Nor-MDP) fully substitute for whole mycobacteria in CFA, whereas immunisation with BSA in incomplete Freund's adjuvant (IFA) fails to induce any delayed hyper-sensitivity to this heterologous protein. However, the time course of MDP-promoted delayed reactivity may differ markedly from that after sensitisation with CFA: whereas MDP-mediated induction of sensitivity occurs fast, but is maintained only for a few weeks, CFA-induced sensitivity is much slower to rise, but persists longer (unpublished results). Similar observations were recently reported when antibody responses to ovalbumin (OA) in guinea pigs were compared after immunisation with MDP in IFA and CFA respectively (Souvannavong *et al.*, 1978). On the other hand, as summarised above (table 8.2), the relative efficacy and potency of closely related

Table 8.3   MDP-mediated induction of delayed hypersensitivity to BSA in guinea pigs*: effect of separate administration of MDP and antigen

Foot-pad immunisation (day 0) with IFA containing		Systemic administration of MDP (day 0 to 4)	Reaction volume (challenge day 21)	
			4h	24h
BSA		−	56	9
BSA	+ MDP†	−	314	936
BSA		MDP‡	290	60
dBSA		−	8	7
dBSA	+ MDP†	−	5	74
dBSA	+ Nor-MDP†	−	7	133
dBSA		MDP∮	7	40
dBSA		Nor-MDP∮	4	62

*As in figure 8.2. Mean values of six animals per group.
Reaction volume (μl) after i.c. challenge with BSA given at a dose of 1 mg/animal. dBSA, heat-denatured BSA (100°C, 30 min) given at 1 mg/animal. MDP and Nor-MDP doses: †10 μg/animal; ‡5 × 300 mg/kg p.o.; ∮5 × 300 mg/kg s.c.

Table 8.4   MDP-mediated induction of delayed hypersensitivity to BSA* in preimmunised guinea pigs with established humoral immunity

1st immunisation (day 0)	Antibody titre (day 16)	2nd immunisation (day 16)	Reaction volume (challenge day 37)
None	0	1 mg of BSA in IFA + MDP	691 ± 188
None	0	1 mg of BSA in IFA	28 ± 12
0.1 mg of BSA in IFA	5.1 ± 0.6	1 mg of BSA in IFA + MDP	620 ± 138
1 mg of BSA in IFA	18.4 ± 3.1	1 mg of BSA in IFA + MDP	258 ± 63
10 mg of BSA in IFA	11.8 ± 1.7	1 mg of BSA in IFA + MDP	342 ± 102

*As in figure 8.1. Mean values ± s.d. of six animals per group.

Antibody titre was determined in individual sera by passive haemagglutination of glutaraldehyde-coupled BSA-SRBCs (Avrameas *et al.*, 1969) in microtitre plates. Titres expressed as $\log_2$ of reciprocal final agglutinating dilution. Reaction volume (μl) was determined 24 h after i.c. challenge with BSA. MDP dose was 50 μg/animal.

MDP derivatives may differ markedly in this system. Indeed, Nor-MurNac-L-Abu-D-isoGln (figure 8.3) and MurNac-L-Val-D-isoGln (unpublished results) induced stronger delayed-type reactions to BSA and were active at 10–100 times smaller doses than MDP. The induction of manifestations of cell-mediated immunity by

MDP — at least in non-cyclophosphamide-treated animals — critically depends on the immunisation scheme used and the vehicle in which antigen and adjuvant are injected. If water-soluble MDP is mixed with a protein antigen, it usually has to be incorporated into a mineral-oil emulsion to induce delayed-type hypersensitivity. Many other vehicles, including numerous metabolisable oils, have so far proved to be incorporated into a mineral-oil emulsion to induce delayed-type hyper-sensitivity. Many other vehicles, including numerous metabolisable oils, have so far proved to be ineffective in this respect. Unfortunately, this has practical implications, since the medical use of CFA in vaccination has been made impossible by its toxicity, which was documented in man (Chapel and August, 1976). Although clinical use (Hilleman, 1966). It is most encouraging in this context, that successful induction of delayed reactivity to ovalbumin has recently been reported using fully metabolisable liposomes into which the antigen was incorporated together with lipophilic 6-*O*-acyl derivatives of MDP (Kotani *et al.*, 1977). To induce cell-mediated immunity to heterologous proteins in guinea pigs, it is also mandatory that both MDP and antigen are injected together. If BSA is administered separately from the MDP-mineral-oil mixture, for example by the intraperitoneal (i.p.) route, no de-layed reactivity occurs. The same is true if the schedule is reversed. As shown in table 8.3, systemic administration of MDP to guinea pigs simultaneously immunis-ed with BSA in IFA, stimulates only immediate-type skin reactivity, reflecting en-hanced formation of circulating antibodies to BSA. However, a rather different result is obtained if heat-denatured BSA, which is incapable of inducing humoral antibody formation, is used for immunisation instead of BSA. Although denatured BSA in IFA fails to induce any response at all, admixture of MDP or Nor-MDP to the antigen–IFA emulsion stimulates a small, but definite, pure delayed reaction. Separate application of MDP or Nor-MDP by the systemic route (s.c.) has the same effect. It must be concluded, that systemically administered MDP in aqueous sol-ution is perfectly capable of stimulating cell-mediated immunity, provided its enhancing effect on antibody formation does not depress the T-cell-mediated response. Clearly, the latter is the case with the many antigens that elicit both cell-mediated and humoral immunity.

These experiments are compatible with a simple model for the induction of persistent cell-mediated immunity by adjuvants and systemic immunostimulants. (1) Cell-mediated immunity is established by simultaneous activation of target cells by both antigen and adjuvant in a T-cell compartment. (2) Cell-mediated immunity can only persist in the absence of significant B-cell activation resulting from the simultaneous interaction of antigen and adjuvant with target cells in a B-cell com-partment. According to this model, the establishment of cell-mediated immunity depends on the selective localisation of antigen and/or adjuvant in an area accessible predominantly to T lymphocytes, but not to B lymphocytes. Moreover, in the con-text of this hypothesis the experimental data suggest that IFA and appropriately constituted liposomes favour the distribution of s.c. injected BSA and MDP into T-cell compartments. Indeed, mineral oil is known to be retained selectively in thymus-dependent areas (Boitnott and Margolis, 1966). Also, lipophilically sub-stituted protein antigens induced delayed-type hypersensitivity and were localised exclusively in the paracortical areas of draining lymph nodes (Coon and Hunter, 1973). In view of the well-documented B-cell suppression of T-cell-mediated immunity (see Turk and Parker, chapter 5, and Polak, chapter 11 of this book) it

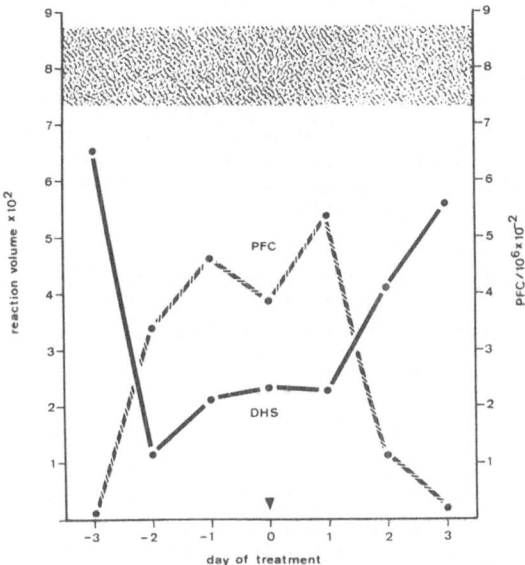

Figure 8.4   Effect of systemic administration of MDP on delayed hypersensitivity and antibody formation to SRBCs in mice.
Male (C57BL/6 $\times$ DBA2) F_1 mice immunised on day 0 by i.v. injection of 3 $\times$ 10^5 SRBCs and treated with 300 mg of MDP/kg i.v. at various times relative to the day of immunisation as indicated on the abscissa. On day 4 each group was divided into two subgroups: (a) challenged with 10^8 SRBCs in 20 μl of PBS injected into a hind paw and increases in paw volume (μl) (compared with PBS-injected contralateral paw) were determined volumetrically 24 h later; (b) killed for enumeration of direct anti-SRBCs plaque-forming cells (PFCs) in the spleen by the Cunningham technique. Mean values of six mice per point. Shaded area indicates paw reaction volumes of mice immunised but not treated with MDP.

appeared interesting to see whether, in preimmunised hosts with established humoral immunity, MDP could still induce delayed hypersensitivity. As table 8.4 shows, this is in fact the case. Nevertheless, a marked reduction of the 24 h skin reactions was apparent in guinea pigs presensitised with high doses of BSA in IFA before injection of BSA in MDP-supplemented I FA.

Since systemic administration of MDP in aqueous solution has been shown to favour humoral antibody formation, it would be expected that — with an appropriate antigen — it should at the same time also suppress manifestations of T-cell-mediated immunity. This was in fact demonstrated by the experiment in figure 8.4. Intravenous (i.v.) injection into mice of small numbers of sheep erythrocytes (SRBCs) induces pure delayed hypersensitivity without attendant antibody formation. However, i.v. administration of MDP shortly before, together with, or after immunisation with SRBCs is associated with a measurable anti-SRBCs plaque response in the spleen and a parallel suppression of the delayed foot-pad reaction that can be elicited in non-MDP-treated mice.

In several other systems, failure to induce cell-mediated immunity by systemic administration of MDP and MDP derivative in aqueous solution has also been reported. Thus MDP and 6-*O*-steaoryl-MDP in PBS (phosphate-buffered saline) did not enhance the generation of cytotoxic lymphocytes in mice immunised with allogeneic mastocytoma cells (Azuma *et al.*, 1976*b*). Also, the growth of an immunogenic transplantable murine tumour was not inhibited by these compounds (Yamamura *et al.*, 1977). However, the highly lipophilic 6-*O*-mycoloyl-MDP (suspended in PBS or dissolved in oil) markedly enhanced the cytotoxic response to allogeneic tumour cells in mice *in vivo* (Yamamura *et al.*, 1976) and displayed a potent anti-tumour activity against a mouse hepatoma (Yamamura *et al.*, 1977). Taken together, the presently available data suggest therefore that the MDP moiety by itself can augment T-cell-mediated immunity *in vivo*, provided that it is either used together with antigens that do not induce humoral antibody formation, or that it is administered in suitable lipid vehicles and/or substituted with appropriate side-chains, both of which may alter its localisation in strategic tissue compartments.

STIMULATION OF HUMORAL ANTIBODY FORMATION BY MDPs *IN VIVO*

In parallel with their adjuvant effect on delayed hypersensitivity, MDP and MDP-derivatives administered to guinea pigs, together with ovalbumin in IFA or liposomes, also enhanced humoral antibody formation (Ellouz *et al.*, 1974; Kotani *et al.*, 1975; Audibert *et al.*, 1976; Kotani *et al.*, 1977; Souvannavong *et al.*, 1978; Jones *et al.*, 1978). Under comparable conditions, antibody titres to bacterial α-amylase (Azuma *et al.*, 1976*a*) or to BSA (unpublished work) are only marginally increased. With these two antigens, IFA by itself appears to exert an already

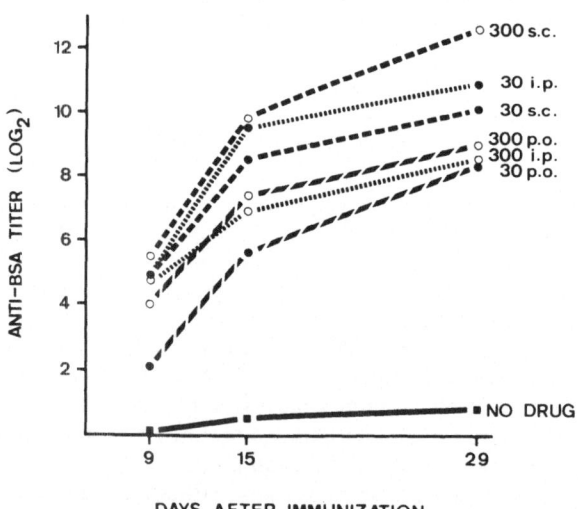

Figure 8.5 Potentiation by MDP of antibody formation to a subimmunogenic dose of BSA in mice
Male Tif: MAGf(SPF) mice (7–8 weeks old) immunised with 10 μg of BSA in PBS i.p. on day 0 and treated daily with MDP (300 or 30 mg/kg per day) for five consecutive days, starting on day 0, by different routes of administration. Serum sampling on days 9, 15 and 29. Antibody determination was as indicated in table 8.4. Mean values of 10 mice per group.

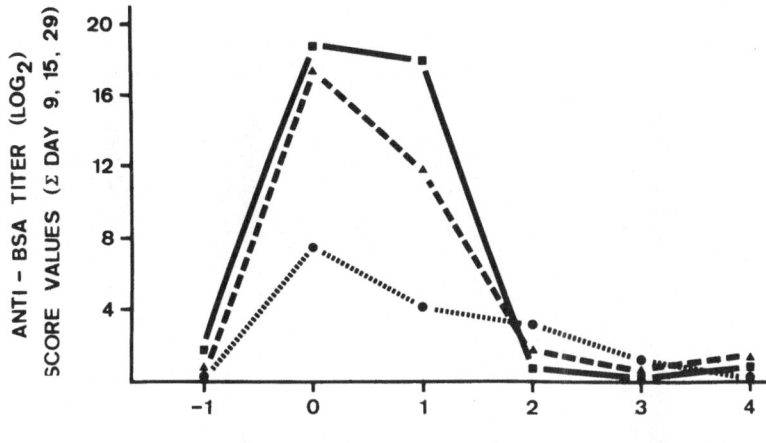

DAY OF DRUG TREATMENT (IMMUNIZATION ON DAY 0)

Figure 8.6   Potentiation by MDP of antibody formation to a subimmunogenic dose of BSA in mice: effect of timing of MDP administration
MDP administered in a single s.c. dose before, simultaneously with or after antigen injection as indicated on the abscissa (■–■, 30 mg/kg, ▲–▲, 3 mg/kg, ●–●, 0.3 mg/kg). Antibody response expressed as sum of differences between mean titres of MDP-treated and untreated groups on days 9, 15 and 29 (=score value). Mean values of 10 animals per group. Otherwise, mice, immunisation and antibody determination were as in figure 8.5.

optimal stimulatory effect with respect to humoral, though not to T-cell-mediated immunity.

In contrast to delayed hypersensitivity, MDP-mediated protentiation of antibody synthesis does not depend on the use of a lipid vehicle. Thus MDP and MDP derivatives administered in saline or PBS together with antigen to mice were shown specifically to stimulate humoral immunity to BSA (Audibert *et al.*, 1976; Chedid *et al.*, 1976; see also figures 8.5, 8.6 and 8.7), ovalbumin (Kotani *et al.*, 1976; Ohkuni *et al.*, 1977), human gamma-globulin (unpublished results), bacterial α-amylase (Azuma *et al.*, 1976*b*), TNP (trintrophenol)-ovalbumin and TNP-keyhole limpet haemocyanin (Sugimoto *et al.*, 1978), SRBCs (Löwy *et al.*, 1977; see also figure 8.4) and – if only slightly – to the T-independent antigen DNP (dinitrophenol)-Ficoll (Azuma *et al.*, 1976*b*). Similarly, enhancement of antibody responses by MDP in aqueous solution was also observed after immunisation with ovalbumin in rats (Ohkuni *et al.*, 1977) and with influenza virus subunit vaccines in hamsters (Webster *et al.*, 1977).

Clearly, formation of IgM, IgG (Sugimoto *et al.*, 1978) and IgE antibodies (Ohkuni *et al.*, 1977) can all be increased by MDP. It remains to be shown, however, whether, under selected conditions of immunisation, stimulation with MDP would not shift immunoglobulin production from one class to another. It is also evident that adjuvation of antigen during priming not only leads to an increased primary response, but also to greatly enhanced secondary responses, even if the challenge is carried out in the absence of MDP (Audibert *et al.*, 1976; Sugimoto *et al.*, 1978). By using adoptive transfer systems it was convincingly demonstrated that MDP promotes the priming of helper T cells by carrier moieties (Löwy *et al.*, 1977; Webste *et al.*, 1977).

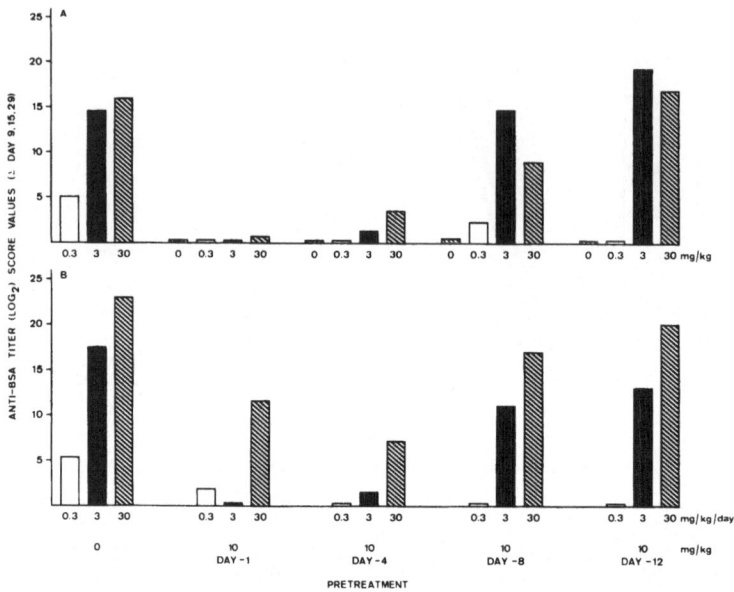

Figure 8.7 Inhibition of the potentiating effect of MDP on antibody formation to BSA in
mice by a single injection of MDP before immunisation and drug treatment
Immunisation with BSA (day 0) and treatment with graded doses of MDP (0.3, 3 or 30 mg/kg
s.c. as indicated on the abscissa) either once on day 0 (A) or daily for 4 consecutive days
(days 0 to 3) (B). In either case, animals were pretreated with a single injection of MDP (10 mg/
kg s.c.) on days −1, −4, −8, or −12, as indicated at the bottom of the figure. Mean values of
10 animals per group. Otherwise, mice, immunisation and antibody determination were as in
figure 8.5, score values as in figure 8.6.

This does not imply, however, that carrier-responsive helper lymphocytes represent a primary target of MDP action.

In the BSA and in the OA model in mice, MDP retains its activity even when
given separately from the antigens (Chedid *et al.*, 1976; Kotani *et al.*, 1976). I.p.
injection of 10 μg of BSA into mice is subimmunogenic and does not induce significant production of humoral antibodies (figure 8.5). Separate administration of
MDP by the i.p., s.c. or even oral route is associated with a marked potentiation
of the antibody response.

On the other hand, the timing of the MDP application relative to the immunisation is critical. Figure 8.6 shows the MDP-mediated increase in anti-BSA titres
as a function of the day of drug treatment, day 0 representing the day of immunisation with BSA. It is obvious that MDP is only active in this system, if given at
about the same time as or, at most, 24 h after the antigen.

During investigation of the effect of repeated administration of MDP, a phenomenon resembling tachyphylaxis became apparent. In fact, as shown in figure 8.7,
the immunostimulatory effect of MDP can be inhibited by a single injection of the
same compound before immunisation and MDP treatment. If 10 mg of MDP/kg
was given 1 or 4 days before adjuvant-promoted immunisation, antibody forma-

tion was no longer induced or was greatly diminished, i.e. there was a temporary unresponsiveness to the immunostimulatory effect of MDP. Pretreatment 8 or 12 days before was no longer inhibitory. This effect appears to be adjuvant-type specific, since pretreatment with IFA, LPS or lipoprotein failed to abrogate immunopotentiation by MDP (unpublished results). The nature of this refractory state has not been elucidated. It is not clear whether there is depletion or blockade of an MDP receptor, exhaustion of a cellular or subcellular compartment selectively involved in antigen-specific immunopotentiation by MDP, and also whether there is cross-tolerance to other MDP derivatives.

INDUCTION BY MDPs OF NON-SPECIFIC RESISTANCE TO INFECTIONS

As was first discovered by Chedid *et al.* (1977*a,b*) MDP and several of its derivatives are capable of enhancing non-specific resistance to *Klebsiella pneumoniae* infections in mice. Again, administration by various routes, including oral application, proved to be effective. Apparently, protection is not immediately linked to the intrinsic adjuvanticity of MDP, since several adjuvant-active analogues were shown to lack protective properties (Chedid *et al.*, 1977*b*). Figure 8.8 demonstrates the effect of different treatment schedules. Evidently, daily administration of 30 mg of MDP/kg s.c. for 3 days starting 24 h before a lethal infection conferred almost complete protection and proved superior to earlier, later or shorter regimens. The spectrum of pathogenic micro-organisms against which MDP derivatives may actually protect is presently under active investigation in many laboratories.

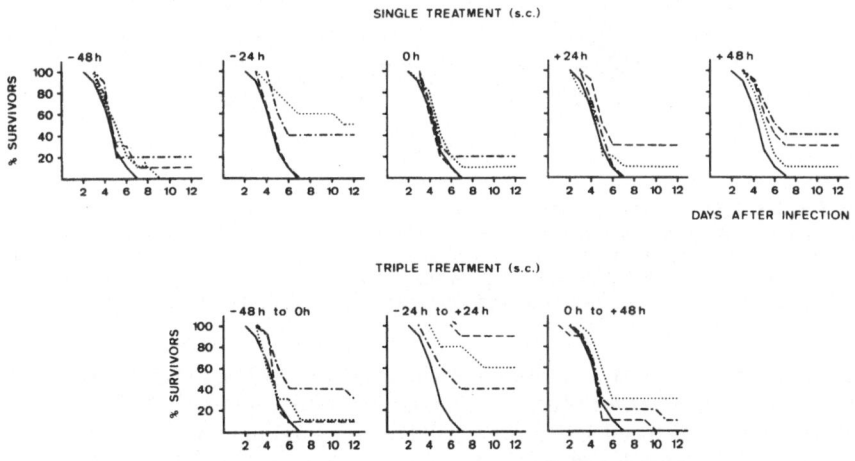

Figure 8.8   Effect of MDP on resistance to infection with *K. pneumoniae* in mice
I.p. infection of Tif:MF2f(SPF) mice with 2.1 × 10³ *K. pneumoniac* 329. Administration of MDP s.c. either once (upper panels) or daily on 3 consecutive days (lower panels) at different time intervals relative to the day of infection, as indicated in the figure; 10 animals per group. Treatment: ——, no drug; · · · · ·, 5; —·—, 10; — — — —, 30 mg/kg/per day. Curves show cumulative mortality in simultaneously infected groups treated with different regimens. Data kindly provided by Dr H. Hariharan (CIBA-GEIGY Ltd, Goregaon, India).

It remains to be shown whether MDP-mediated enhancement of non-specific resistance is of potential clinical interest.

B cell mitogenicity of MDPs
To define the possible mode of action of MDPs, their immunostimulatory effects were investigated in various tissue-culture systems. As shown in figure 8.9, MDP is a selective B-cell mitogen. Thus thymidine incorporation appears to be triggered in cultures of mouse B lymphocytes (spleen cells from congenitally athymic nude mice), but not of T lymphocytes (cortisone-resistant thymus cells). However, the experiment represented in figure 8.10 puts this observation in perspective. Compared with other bacterial immunostimulants such as lipid A (Andersson *et al.*,

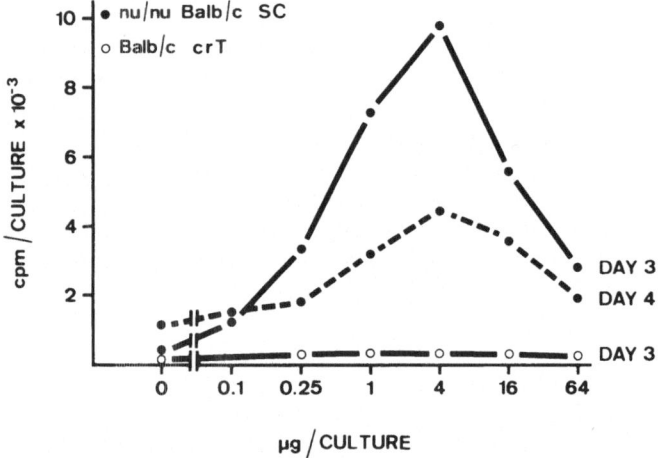

Figure 8.9 B-cell mitogenicity of MDP
[^{3}H] Thymidine incorporation in serum-free 2 ml cultures of BALB/c nu/nu spleen cells (SCs) or BALB/c cortisone-resistant thymus cells (crTs; 5 × 10^5 cells/well) set up in the presence of graded concentrations of MDP, as indicated on the abscissa. Mean values of triplicate experiments. For details of culture conditions and assay technique see Staber *et al.* (1978*a*).

1973; Chiller *et al.*, 1973), lipoprotein (Melchers *et al.*, 1975), low-molecular-weight lipopeptides (Bessler *et al.*, 1976) and murein (Staber *et al.*, 1978*a*), which are all very powerful B-cell activators, MDP is a comparatively weak mitogen for mouse B lymphocytes. Nevertheless, the effect is consistent and readily demonstrable in serum-free cultures of low cell density.

For some time, the published data on the B-cell mitogenicity of murein, MDP and MDP derivatives have been somewhat controversial. Thus a water-soluble peptidoglycan preparation (Bona *et al.*, 1974) as well as synthetic MDP (Damais *et al.*, 1975; Rook and Stewart-Tull, 1976; Azuma *et al.*, 1976*b*; Specter *et al.*, 1977) were reported to be devoid of mitogenicity. More recent evidence based on the use of more sensitive culture conditions indicates that water-soluble peptidoglycan and MDP exhibit a definite mitogenic effect on lymphocytes from mice (Damais *et al.*,

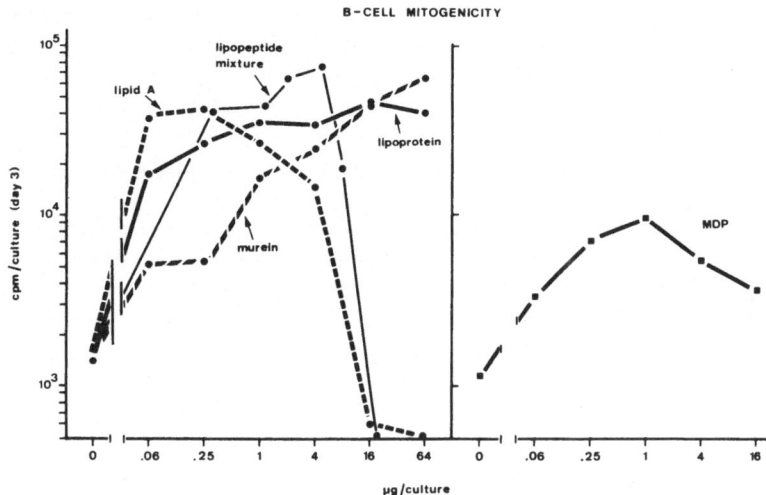

Figure 8.10 Comparative B-cell mitogenicity of MDP and some purified bacterial cell-wall components
[³H] Thymidine incorporation in 3 -day cultures of BALB/c nu/nu spleen cells exposed to graded concentrations of MDP (right-hand panel) and several other bacterial immunostimulants (left-hand panel). Purified murein from *Escherichia coli* B (Staber *et al.*, 1978*a*), lipid A isolated from *Salmonella minnesota* R595 (according to Galanos *et al.*, 1969) purified lipo-protein from *E. coli* B (as described by Braun and Rehn, 1969 and by Braun and Sieglin, 1970) and low-molecular-weight lipopeptides containing 1–4 amino acids bound to *N*-acyl-*S*-diacyloxypropylcysteine from *E. coli* B (Hantke and Braun, 1973 and Staber *et al.*, 1978*a*). Otherwise details are as in the legend to figure 8.9.

1977). Interestingly, there are considerable differences in the susceptibility of spleen cells from different mouse strains to the mitogenic action of MDP (DBA/2; BALB/c, CBA > AKR >> C57BL/6 and C3H/HeJ; Damais *et al.*, 1978). Mitogenic activity of MDP was also demonstrated in spleen lymphocyte cultures from guinea pigs (Takeda *et al.*, 1977.)

By comparing different MDP derivatives, a correlation between mitogenicity and adjuvant activity in aqueous solution has been tentatively established (Damais *et al.*, 1978). It is doubtful, however, whether this reflects a direct link between the two properties, since C57BL/6 mice (reported to be resistant to the mitogenic effect of MDP) are just as responsive to the adjuvant action of MDPs as BALB/c recipients (unpublished results).

Although spleen cell cultures from athymic mice predominantly contain B lymphocytes, B cells are not necessarily the target of the MDP effect. It has been suggested that MDP might stimulate the division of immature precursor T cells (Damais *et al.*, 1977) which are present in the spleen lymphocyte pool of nu/nu mice (Loer and Roelants, 1974). Alternatively, the action of MDP could be mediated by accessory cells. Other immunostimulating B-cell activators, such as LPSs (lipopolysaccharides), stimulate not only B cells, but also macrophages (Spitznagel and Allison, 1970; Edelson *et al.*, 1975). Activated macrophages secrete factors that directly influence T-cell proliferation and antigen recognition (Gery and Waksman,

1972; Gery *et al.*, 1972; Rosenwasser and Rosenthal, 1978) as well as B-lymphocyte functions (Calderon *et al.*, 1975). Hence it is appropriate to examine the
effect of MDP on the immunological triggering of both T and B lymphocytes in
the context of this possibility.

Potentiation by MDP of T-cell reactivity and generation of killer cells in mixed lymphocyte cultures

Although MDP fails to trigger the division of T cells by itself, it greatly facilitates
the proliferation of T lymphocytes in mouse mixed lymphocyte cultures set up with
suboptimal numbers of allogeneic stimulator cells. A representative experiment is
shown in figure 8.11. Although cortisone-resistant thymus cells are stimulated to
divide by concanavalin A (Con A), but not by LPS or MDP, the addition of MDP
greatly enhances the response to irradiated histo-incompatible lymphocytes. In

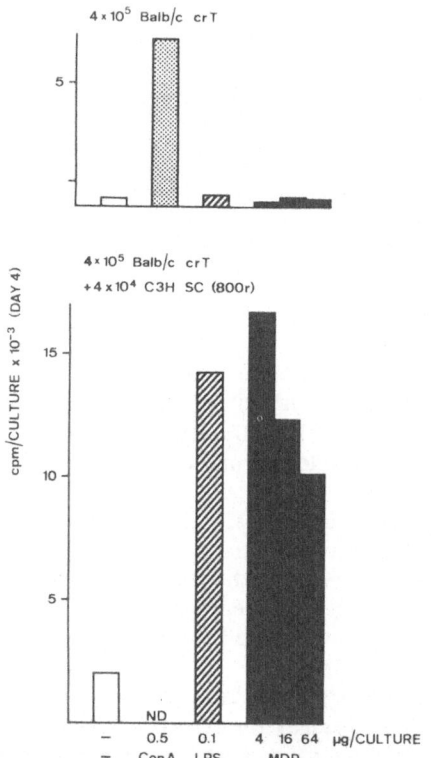

Figure 8.11   Potentiation by MDP and LPS of T-cell reactivity in mixed lymphocyte cultures
set up with suboptimal numbers of stimulator cells
[³H] Thymidine incorporation in 4-day cultures (0.2 ml) of 4 × 10⁵ BALB/c cortisone-
resistant thymus cells (crTs) sert up alone (upper panel) or with 4 × 10⁴ 800 r-irradiated C3H
spleen cells (SCs) (lower panel) in the presence of optimal concentrations of Con A, LPS
S. minnesota R345 (Galanos *et al.*, 1969) or graded concentrations of MDP. Culture conditions and assay were as in figure 8.9. ND, not determined.

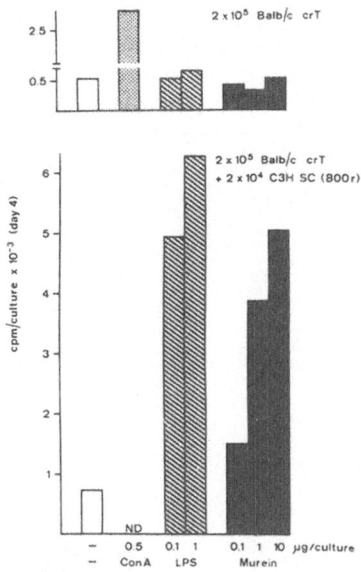

Figure 8.12   Potentiation by murein and LPS of T-cell reactivity in mixed lymphocyte cultures set up with suboptimal numbers of stimulator cells
[^{3}H] Thymidine incorporation in 4-day cultures (0.2 ml) of 2×10^5 BALB/c cortisone-resistant thymus cells (crTs) set up alone (upper panel) or with 2×10^4 800 r-irradiated C3H spleen cells (SCs) (lower panel) in the presence of optimal concentrations of Con A, LPS *S. minnesota* R345 (Galanos *et al.*, 1969) or graded concentrations of murein (see figure 8.10). Culture conditions and assay were as in figure 8.9. ND, not determined.

this respect, it mimics the effect of other B-cell activating bacterial cell-wall components with immunopotentiating properties. Murein (figure 8.12), LPS (figures 8.11, 8.12 and 8.13), lipoprotein and low-molecular-weight lipopeptides (figure 8.13) all enhance the alloantigen-induced proliferation of T lymphocytes. Moreover, in similar culture systems, MDP and MDP derivatives are also capable of potentiating the generation of cytotoxic T lymphocytes. This does not occur only in allogeneic mixed lymphocyte cultures, but also in syngeneic mixed lymphocyte tumour-cell cultures. In the experiment shown in figure 8.14, C57BL/6 responder cells were cultured in the presence of irradiated syngeneic El 4 lymphoma cells, which exhibit only minor antigenic differences, and the resulting specific cytotoxicity was determined by an isotope release assay. In contrast to the strong cytotoxicity developing in allogeneic combinations, only minimal cytotoxicity was generated against the syngeneic tumour cells. However, addition of graded doses of Nor-MDP, at the onset of the culture, clearly enhanced the formation or the efficacy of the cytotoxic T-effector cells. Comparable effects can be obtained with MDP and other MDP analogues, as well as by addition of purified immunostimulatory bacterial cell-wall components (unpublished results).

Similar data have recently been reported by others. MDP and 6-*O*-steaoryl-MDP augmented cell-mediated lymphocytolysis in allogeneic mouse mixed lymphocyte cultures (Azuma *et al.*, 1976*b*). In another model, mice were immunised *in vivo* against mitomycin-treated syngeneic mastocytoma cells. *In vitro*, secondary stimulation of spleen cells from the primed donors in the presence of MDP or 6-*O*-mycoloyl-MDP yielded greatly increased cytotoxic activity (Igarashi *et al.*, 1977).

The proliferation of lymphocytes in mixed lymphocyte cultures and the attendant development of killer cells requires the presence of a critical number of macrophages (Alter and Bach, 1970; Bach *et al.*, 1970; Wagner *et al.*, 1972). Earlier

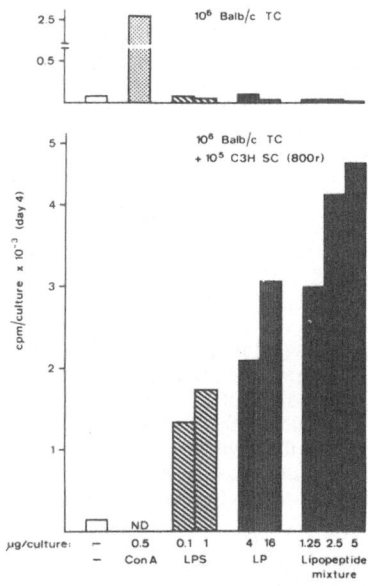

Figure 8.13   Potentiation by lipoprotein, lipopeptides and LPS of T-cell reactivity in mixed lymphocyte cultures set up with suboptimal number of stimulator cells
[³H] Thymidine incorporation in 4-day cultures (0.2 ml) of 10⁶ BALB/c thymus cells (TCs) set up alone (upper panel) or with 10⁵ 800 r-irradiated C3H spleen cells (SCs) (lower panel) in the presence of optimal concentrations of Con A, LPS *S. minnesota* R345 (Galanos *et al.*, 1969) or graded concentrations of lipoprotein (LP) or lipopeptide mixture (see figure 8.10). Culture conditions and assay were as in figure 8.9. ND. not determined.

reports from our laboratory (Perren *et al.*, 1974; Dukor *et al.*, 1975), as well as from other workers (Ritter *et al.*, 1975), have indicated that LPS-mediated potentiation of cytotoxic sensitisation is strictly macrophage-dependent. Moreover, it was shown that LPS exerts other T-cell-activating properties through its effect on macrophages (Gery *et al.*, 1972; Gery and Waksman, 1972). Hence it is tempting to speculate that a similar mechanism accounts for MDP-induced stimulation of T-cell functions.

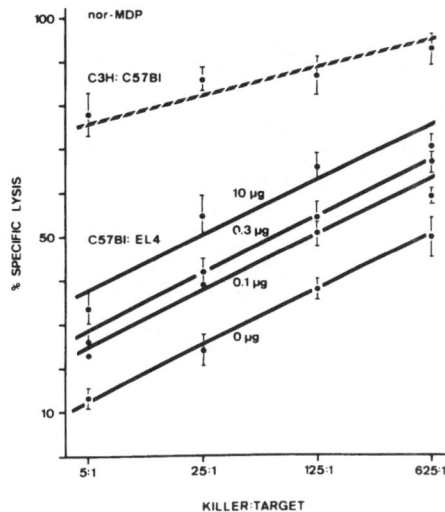

Figure 8.14   Potentiation by Nor-MDP of killer-cell generation in syngeneic mixed lymphocyte
tumour-cell cultures
C57BL/6 spleen cells (25×10^6) were cultured for 6 days with 5×10^6 6000 r-irradiated E1 4
lymphoma cells in the presence of 5 per cent foetal calf serum and different concentrations of
Nor-MDP (total volume 20 ml). Graded numbers of killer lymphocytes incubated for 4 h with
2×10^3 ^{51}Cr-labelled E1 4 target cells (150 μl of reaction mixtures in Dynatech microtitre
plates). Specific lysis of tumour cells was determined by isotope release into the supernatant.
— —, Specific lysis of E1 4 cells by syngeneic killer cells generated in the presence or absence
of Nor-MDP. - - - -, Specific lysis of E1 4 cells by allogeneic C3H killer cells generated by co-
cultivation with 800 r-irradiated C57BL/6 spleen cells in the absence of Nor-MDP under
otherwise identical conditions.

Operational T-cell substitution and potentiation of antibody formation by MDP *in vitro*

B-cell mitogens substitute operationally for T cell help in responses to T-dependent
antigens *in vitro* (Sjöberg *et al.*, 1972; Schrader, 1974). Therefore the ability of
MDPs to allow for a plaque response against SRBCs in cultures of spleen cells from
congenitally athymic nu/nu BALB/c mice was investigated. For comparison, other
bacterial immunopotentiating B-cell activators were examined in the same system.
As shown in figure 8.15, addition of appropriate concentrations of lipid A, lipoprotein, low-molecular-weight lipopeptides or murein led to a full restoration of
the antibody response to SRBCs in T-cell deficient cultures of spleen cells from
ALB/c nu/nu mice. Some restoration was achieved by supplementation of the
defective cultures with MDPs. Its effect, however, was much smaller than that of
the other bacterial B-cell activators. Other MDP-derivatives, including Nor-MDP,
gave similar results, whereas Nor-MurNac-D-Ala-D-isoGln was completely inactive
(unpublished). By comparing figure 8.9 and 8.10, it becomes apparent that the

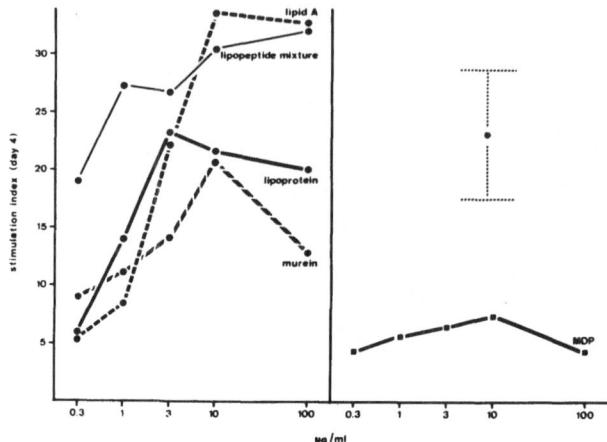

Figure 8.15 Operational T-cell substitution by MDP and some purified bacterial cell-wall components

Direct antibody-plaque formation to SRBCs in T-cell-deficient cultures containing BALB/c nu/nu spleen cells (8 × 10⁶/ml) stimulated with SRBCs in the presence of 5 per cent foetal calf serum and graded amounts of MDP, murein, lipid A, lipoprotein or low-molecular-weight lipopeptides (as in figure 8.10). Enumeration of PFCs on day 4 using the Cunningham technique. Responses expressed as stimulation indices (PFCs in experimental cultures/PFCs in simultaneously run control cultures without immunostimulant). Mean values of triplicate cultures. Point ± s.d. in the right panel indicates response in cultures supplemented with 2 × 10⁶ cortisone-resistant thymus cells in the absence of immunopotentiating agents. Otherwise culture technique and assay as described in Gisler and Fridman (1975).

dose–response curves for T-cell replacement differ from those for B-cell mitogenicity. Maximum T-cell substitution was obtained with doses that already inhibited B-cell proliferation, but these discrepancies may simply reflect methodological differences in the two culture systems.

The mechanism of operational T-cell replacement by B-cell mitogens is not fully understood. It is of course quite possible that the T-cell substituting effect of such agents is a direct consequence of their binding to B cells and of their mitogenicity (Sjöberg *et al.*, 1972). Alternatively, they might not be acting as mitogens (as suggested by Coutinho and Möller (1975) in the framework of their one-signal hypothesis of B-cell activation), but rather as completing an inductive stimulus to antigen-stimulated B lymphocytes (Watson *et al.*, 1973). Of course, both mechanisms may instead be mediated via a cooperating cell population. It is noteworthy that T-cell substitution in cultures of nu/nu spleen cells has also been achieved by the use of soluble factors from macrophages (Calderon *et al.*, 1975). Again, it would appear plausible that MDP and other bacterial immunostimulants initiate the release of such mediators from stimulated macrophages.

The effect of MDP and MDP derivatives on antibody formation in normal lymphocyte cultures may depend on a similar mechanism. It has been reported that MDP, 6-*O*-stearoyl-MDP and some other analogues augment the formation of plaque-forming cells (PFCs) in mouse spleen-cell cultures stimulated with suboptimal numbers of SRBCs (Azuma *et al.*, 1976*b*; Specter *et al.*, 1978; Leclerc *et al.*,

1978). Further, even in the absence of SRBCs, a significant increase of background-PFCs was induced by these compounds. This is compatible with the notion that MDP acts as a polyclonal activator, but alternatively, it might simply reflect potentiation, by MDP, of responsiveness to culture constituents such as foetal calf serum which is known to cross-react with SRBCs.

ACTIVATION OF ACCESSORY CELLS BY MDPs

In a more direct approach, the release of a lymphocyte-activating factor from MDP-stimulated macrophages could be demonstrated as follows. As we have shown before, mouse lymph-node cells barely respond with antibody formation if they are cultured in the presence of SRBCs.This unresponsiveness can be overcome by supplementation of the lymph-node cells with appropriate numbers of macrophages (Gisler and Dukor, 1972). Instead, in the experiment represented in figure 8.16, the antibody forming potential of such cultures was successfully restored by supernatants from MDP-stimulated purified mouse macrophages. Addition of supernatants from unstimulated macrophage cultures suppressed rather than restored responsiveness, whereas direct addition of MDP to the lymph-node cells was

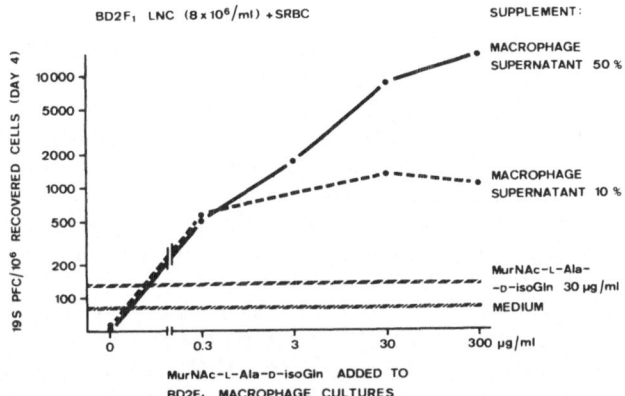

Figure 8.16 Reconstitution of macrophage-deficient lymph-node cell cultures by supernatants from MDP-treated macrophages
Preparation of supernatants. Peritoneal washout cells from (C57BL/6 × DBA/2)F$_1$ mice were preincubated for 5 h in the presence of serum-free medium and freed of non-adherent cells by vigorous washing. Adherent cells were exposed to graded concentrations of MDP in the presence of fresh medium RPMI 1640 for 24 h in the absence of serum. Cell-free supernatants were harvested and assayed for lymphocyte-activating capacity. Activation of lymph-node cell (LNC) cultures. Mesenteric (C57BL/6 × DBA/2)F$_1$ lymph-node cells (8 × 10⁶/ml) stimulated with SRBCs, cultured and assayed as in figure 8.15.╼╼╼╼, LNC control cultures; ╼╼╼╼,LNC cultures set up with MDP (30 µg/ml);╌╌╌╌LNC cultures supplemented with 10 per cent supernatant from macrophages exposed to MDP as indicated on the abscissa; ━━━ , LNC cultures supplemented with 50 per cent supernatant. Antibody responses on day 4 are expressed as direct PFCs/10⁶ recovered cells, mean values from triplicate cultures.

barely effective. It is concluded that MDP stimulates mouse macrophages to release T-and/or B-lymphocyte-activating factors which allow lymph-node cells to respond to antigen. This finding agrees with observations of Modolell *et al.* (1974), who reported that the immunostimulatory effect on antibody synthesis *in vitro* of water-soluble adjuvant from mycobacteria was also mediated by macrophages.

Moreover, as Staber *et al.* (1978*a*) showed, several natural and synthetic bact-erial cell-wall components, with immunopotentiating properties, share the capacity of inducing the release of colony-stimulating activity (CSA, the factor responsible for proliferation and differentiation of committed myeloid precursor cells (Metcalf, 1971)) from cultures of purified macrophages. A representative experiment is summarised in table 8.5. It can be seen that MDP, murein, lipid A, lipoprotein and low-molecular-weight lipopeptides all proved to be very effective in this respect. Although lipid A and lipoprotein were much more potent than MDP, the peak levels of CSA induced by the synthetic compound were as high as those in lipo-protein-treated cultures. Supernatants from untreated macrophages to which the inducing agent was added only before testing for CSA ('reconstituted superna-tants') showed only very low levels of activity. Treatment of the cultures with appropriate antisera and complement made it highly unlikely that contaminating cells other than macrophages were responsible for the observed release of CSA (Staber *et al.*, 1978*a*).

Likewise, induction and release of CSA by immunopotentiating bacterial cell-wall components could be demonstrated *in vivo* (Staber *et al.*, 1978*b*). In unpub-lished experiments, synthetic MDP also proved effective in this respect. Moreover, lipid A and lipoprotein triggered noncommitted haemopoietic stem cells (CFU-S) into cell cycle, to increase the pool size of committed precursors of myeloid cells (CFU-C) in the spleen (Staber *et al.*, 1978*b*) and to stimulate the differentiation of cultured immature marrow-derived monocytes to functional mature macrophages with accessory-cell activity (unpublished results). It will be interesting to see whether MDP derivatives show similarities with lipid A and lipoprotein also in these respects. Nevertheless, present data are sufficient to suggest that MDP may have profound effects on the differentiation of monocytes, macrophages and polymorphs from the committed stem-cell pool.

Several other observations implicate macrophages as target cells of MDP. *In vitro*, macrophages are activated by MDP to inhibit the growth of mastocytoma cells (Juy and Chedid, 1975). On the other hand, MDP, but not an adjuvant-inactive stereoisomer, was reported to inhibit the migration of normal guinea pig macrophages (Yamamoto *et al.*, 1978). Finally, it was claimed that the carbon-clearance rate of mice could be significantly enhanced by MDP, although a stereoisomer was again ineffective (Tanaka *et al.*, 1977).

Macrophages may not be the only accessory cells to be involved in the mediation of effects of MDP. Indeed, a possible role of polymorphonuclear leucocytes was suggested by a recent histological study of the local cellular reaction to Nor-MDP (Wachsmuth, 1978). In these experiments, Nor-MDP in PBS, Nor-MDP in IFA, IFA or CFA were injected i.c. into guinea pigs. Figure 8.17 demonstrates the out-ward appearance of the inflammatory lesions at the injection sites. Although the reaction to Nor-MDP was minimal, IFA caused considerable erythema and indur-ation, whereas CFA led to a still stronger inflammatory reaction with central necrosis. The same reaction was observed when Nor-MDP, instead of mycobacteria,

Table 8.5 CSA in supernatants from cultured C57BL/6 adherent peritoneal cells (aPC) stimulated with MDP and other immunopotentiating agents

Supernatants from	Number of colonies per 10^5 C57BL/6 bone-marrow cells at the given concentration of immunostimulant (mg/ml)								
	10^{-9}	10^{-8}	10^{-7}	10^{-6}	10^{-5}	10^{-4}	10^{-3}	10^{-2}	10^{-1}
MDP-treated aPC	8	26	47	48	71	80	82	202	173
Untreated aPC, reconstituted with MDP	0	12	16	11	10	9	15	16	7
Murein-treated aPC	0	0	0	8	44	108	142	131	n.d.
Untreated aPC, reconstituted with murein	0	0	0	0	0	0	0	0	n.d.
Lipid-A-treated aPC	121	n.d.	128	125	131	111	26	0	n.d.
Untreated aPC, reconstituted with lipid A	13	n.d.	46	37	14	11	10	n.d.	n.d.
Lipoprotein-treated aPC	26	48	61	138	193	140	129	80	n.d.
Untreated aPC, reconstituted with lipoprotein	0	0	0	0	3	4	3	4	n.d.
Lipopeptide mixture-treated aPC	22	25	30	39	45	81	96	85	n.d.
Untreated aPC, reconstituted with lipopeptide mixture	18	16	15	15	13	14	10	8	n.d.

For culture conditions and details of CSA assay see Staber et al. (1978a). Values are means of duplicate assays with pooled culture supernatants at a final dilution of 1:5. Murein, lipid A, lipoprotein and lipopeptides were prepared as in figure 8.10. n.d., Not determined.

was added to IFA. Histologically, injection of Nor-MDP led to a temporary accumulation of granulocytes and mononuclear cells which vanished rapidly. Addition of Nor-MDP to IFA augmented granulocyte infiltration (and, to a lesser degree, mononuclear cell and lymphocyte invasion as well as epitheloid-cell development) and led to a prolonged reaction similar to that elicited by CFA (figure 8.18). It was

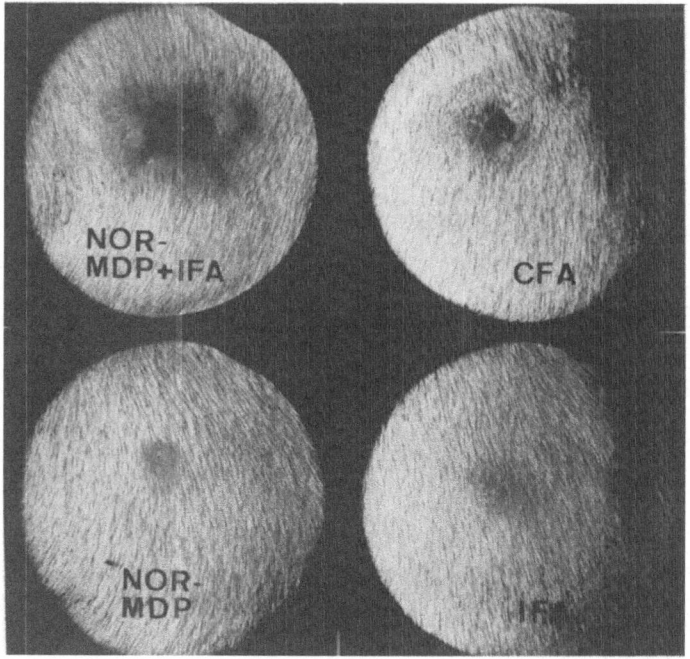

Figure 8.17   Inflammatory reactions to Nor-MDP and Freund's adjuvant in guinea pigs
Outward appearance of injection sites in Pirbright guinea pigs 14 days after i.c. administration
of 0.05 ml of Nor-MDP (5 mg in PBS), IFA, Nor-MDP + IFA or CFA.

concluded that granulocytes might play a more important role during the induction of immunity than has hitherto been believed. Moreover, persisting local inflammatory reactions and granulocyte infiltration might be prerequisites to the development of cell-mediated immunity.

Figure 8.18   Inflammatory reactions to Nor-MDP and Freund's adjuvant in guinea pigs
Histology of injection sites in Pirbright guinea pigs 14 days after i.c. administration of 0.05 ml
of Nor-MDP (5 mg in PBS), IFA, Nor-MDP + IFA or CFA. Muscularis at the bottom of each
picture. Note epitheloid cell development in the case of IFA, Nor-MDP + IFA, and CFA.
Marked granulocyte infiltration only in the case of Nor-MDP + IFA and CFA. Bar = 200μm.

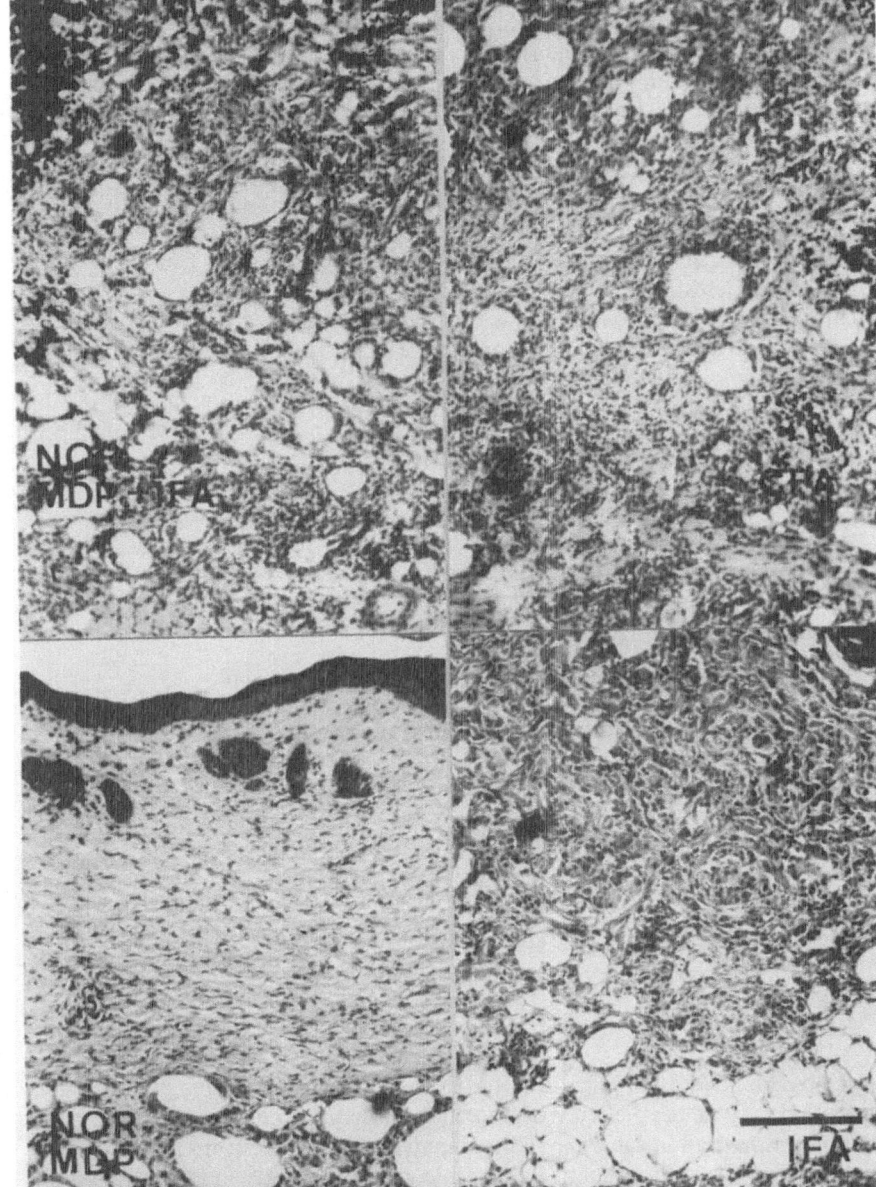

CONCLUSIONS

MDPs represent a new class of synthetic compounds that can be used as immuno-adjuvants and as systemic stimulants of both immunity and non-specific resistance. Induction of cell-mediated rather than humoral immunity by MDPs and their derivatives appears to be critically determined by the vehicles used for their administration. Also, lipophilic substitution may have the same effect. *In vitro*, MDPs appear to be selectively mitogenic for B cells, but were shown to potentiate both T- and B-lymphocyte functions in a variety of systems. These actions may be indirect, since MDPs were also found to have marked effects on accessory cells. Thus MDPs are capable of eliciting the release of lymphocyte-activating factors and of colony-stimulating activity from macrophages. The release of these mediators may facilitate the generation of still more macrophages in a positive feed-back loop and enhance the immunological responsiveness of both T lymphocytes and B lymphocytes. In parallel, the formation and recruitment of polymorphs would also occur. These mechanisms could account for the simultaneous potentiation by some MDPs of non-specific resistance to infections, non-specific cytotoxicity against tumour cells and of specific cell-mediated and humoral immunity.

Table 8.6   Potential risks of therapy with immunostimulants

(1)	Sensitisation to immunostimulant itself
(2)	Sensitisation to common extrinsic antigens
(3)	Sensitisation to autoantigens
(4)	Increased formation of blocking antibodies
(5)	Increased formation of suppressor cells
(6)	Toxicity for myelolymphoid cells
(7)	Neoplastic transformation of myelolymphoid cells

The possible medical application of MDPs is subject to the same potential hazards that may be connected with the clinical use of immunostimulants in general. They are summarised in table 8.6. Unfortunately, very little firm knowledge is available about the risks inherent in systemic and particularly in long-term administration of immunopotentiating agents. Certainly, sensitisation to the immunostimulant itself and to common environmental antigens, autoimmunisation, unwanted effects owing to the formation of blocking antibodies or immune complexes, or to the production of suppressor cells and finally direct toxicity for myeloid and lymphoid cells including the neoplastic transformation of these target cells have all to be reckoned with.

REFERENCES

Adam, A., Ciorbaru, R., Petit, J. F. and Lederer, E. (1972). *Proc. natn. Acad. Sci. U.S.A.*, **39**, 851

Adam, A., Devys, M., Souvannavong, V., Lefrancier, P., Choay, J. and Lederer, E. (1976). *Biochem. Biophys. Res. Commun.*, **72**, 339

Alter, B. J. and Bach, F. H. (1970). *Cell. Immun.*, **1**, 207

Andersson, J., Melchers, F., Galanos, C. and Lüderitz, O. (1973). *J. exp. Med.*, **137**, 943

Audibert, F., Chedid, L., Lefrancier, P. and Choay, J. (1976). *Cell. Immun.*, **21**, 243

Audibert, F., Chedid, L., Lefrancier, P., Choay, J. and Lederer, E. (1977). *Ann. Immun.*, **128C**, 653

Avrameas, S., Taudou, B. and Chuilon, S. (1969). *Immunochemistry*, **6**, 67

Azuma, I., Sugimura, K., Yamamura, Y., Kusumoto, S., Tarumi, Y. and Shiba, T. (1976a). *Jap. J. Microbiol.*, **20**, 63

Azuma, I., Sugimura, K., Taniyama, T., Yamawaki, M., Yamamura, Y., Kusumoto, S., Okada, S. and Shiba, T. (1976b). *Infect. Immun.*, **14**, 18

Bach, F. H., Alter, B. J., Jolliday, S., Zoschke, D. C. and Janis, M. (1970). *Cell. Immun.*, **1**, 219

Baschang, G., Stanek, J., Hartmann, A. and Sele, A. (1977). BE Patent No. 849.214 (Ciba-Geigy AG 10.12.1975).

Bessler, W., Hantke, K. and Resch, K. (1976). *Zeitschr. Immunitätsforsch.*, **152**, 75

Boitnott, J. and Margolis, S. (1966). *Bull. Johns Hopkins Hosp.*, **118**, 414

Braun, V. and Rehn, K. (1969). *Eur. J. Biochem.* **10**, 426

Braun, V. and Sieglin, U. (1970). *Eur. J. Biochem.*, **13**, 336

Calderon, J., Kiely, J. M., Lefko, J. L. and Unanue, E. R. (1975). *J. exp. Med.*, **142**, 151

Chapel, H. M. and August, P. J. (1976). *Clin. exp. Immun.*, **24**, 538

Chedid, L., Audibert, F., Lefrancier, P., Choay, J. and Lederer, E. (1976). *Proc. natn. Acad. Sci. U.S.A.*, **73**, 2472

Chedid, L., Parant, M. and Parant, F. (1977a) *C. R. Acad. Sci. Paris*, **284D**, 405

Chedid, L., Parant, M., Parant, F., Lefrancier, P., Choay, J. and Lederer, E. (1977b). *Proc. natn. Acad. Sci. U.S.A.* **74**, 2089

Chiller, J. M., Skidmore, B. J., Morrison, D. C. and Weigle, W. O. (1973). *Proc. natn. Acad. Sci. U.S.A.*, **70**, 2129

Coon, J. and Hunter, R. (1973). *J. Immun.*, **110**, 183

Coutinho, A. and Möller, G. (1975). *Adv. Immun.*, **21**, 113

Damais, C., Bona, C., Chedid. L., Fleck, J., Nauciel, C. and Martin, J. P. (1975). *J. Immun.*, **115**, 268

Damais, C., Parant, M. and Chedid, L. (1977). *Cell. Immun.*, **34**, 49

Damais, C., Parant, M., Chedid, L., Lefrancier, P. and Choay, J. (1978). *Cell. Immun.*, **35**, 173

Dukor, P., Vasella, S. Schläfli, E., Perren, B., Gisler, R. H., Dietrich. F. M. and Bitter-Suermann, D. (1975). In *Host Defense against Cancer and Its Potentiation*, (eds. D. Mizuno *et al.*) University Park Press, Baltimore, p.97

Edelson, P. J., Zwiebel, R. and Cohn, Z. A. (1975). *J. exp. Med.* **142**, 1150

Ellouz, F., Adam, A., Ciorbaru, R. and Lederer, E. (1974). *Biochem. Biophys Res. Commun.*, **59**, 1317

Freund, J. (1947). *A. Rev. Microbiol.*, **1**, 291

Freund, J. and McDermott, K. (1942). *Proc. Soc. exp. Biol. Med.*, **49**, 548

Freund, J., Casals, J. and Hosmer, E. P. (1937). *Proc. Soc. exp. Biol. Med.*, **37**, 509

Galanos, C., Lüderitz, O. and Westphal, O. (1969). *Eur. J. Biochem.*, **9**, 245

Gery, I. and Waksman, B. H. (1972). *J. exp. Med.*, **136**, 143

Gery, I., Gershon, R. K. and Waksman, B. H. (1972). *J. exp. Med.*, **136**, 128

Gisler, R. H. and Dukor, P. (1972). *Cell. Immun.*, **4**, 341

Gisler, R. H. and Fridman, W. (1975). *J. exp. Med.*, **142**, 507

Hantke, K. and Braun, V. (1973). *Eur. J. Biochem.*, **34**, 284

Hilleman, M. R. (1966). *Progr. Virol. méd.*, **8**, 131

Hiu, I. J. (1972). *Nature New Biol.*, 238, 241
Igarashi, T., Okada, M., Azuma, I. and Yamamura, Y. (1977). *Cell. Immun.*, 34, 270
Jones, G. H., Moffatt, J. G. and Nestor, J. J., Jr. (1978) US Patent 4.082.736
Juy, D. and Chedid, L. (1975). *Proc. natn. Acad. Sci. U.S.A.*, 72, 4105
Kotani, S., Watanabe, Y., Kinoshita, F., Shimono, T., Morisaki, I., Shiba, T., Kusumoto, S., Tarumi, Y. and Ikenaka, K. (1975). *Biken J.*, 18, 105
Kotani, S., Kinoshita, F., Morisaki, I., Shimono, T., Watanabe, Y., Takada, H., Kato, K., Shiba, T., Kusumoto, S., Okada, S. and Tamura, T. (1976). *Proc. Jap. Soc. Immun.* 6, 156
Kotani, S., Kinoshita, F., Morisaki, I., Shimono, T., Okunaga, T., Takada, H., Tsujimoto, M., Watanabe, Y. and Kato, K. (1977). *Biken J.*, 20, 95
Leclerc, C., Löwy, I. and Chedid, L. (1978). *Cell. Immun.*, 38, 286
Löwy, I., Bona, C. and Chedid, L. (1977). *Cell. Immun.*, 29, 195
Maurer, Th., Thomann, P., Weirich, E. G. and Hess, R. (1975). *Agents and Actions*, 5, 174
Melchers, F., Braun, V. and Galanos, C. (1975). *J. exp. Med.*, 142, 473
Merser, C., Sinay, P. and Adam, A. (1975). *Biochem. Biophys. Res. Commun.*, 66, 1316
Metcalf, D. (1971). *Immunology*, 21, 427
Migliore-Samour, D. and Jollès, P. (1972). *FEBS Letters*, 25, 301
Modolell, M., Luckenbach, G. A., Parant, M. and Munder, P. G. (1974). *J. Immun.*, 113, 395
Nagai, Y., Akiyama, K., Suzuki, K., Kotani, S., Watanabe, Y., Shimono, T., Shiba, T., Kusumoto, S., Ikuta, F. and Takeda, S. (1978a). *Cell. Immun.*, 35, 158
Nagai, Y., Akiyama, K., Kotani, S., Watanabe, Y., Shimono, T., Shiba, T. and Kusumoto, S. (1978b). *Cell. Immun.*, 35, 168
Ohkuni, H., Norose, Y., Hayama, M., Kimura, Y., Kotani, S., Shiba, T., Kusumoto, S., Yokogawa, K. and Kawata, S. (1977). *Biken J.*, 20, 131
Perren, B., Schläfli, E., Schumann, G. and Dukor, P. (1974) In *Contact Hypersensitivity in Experimental Animals, Monogr. Allergy*, (eds. D. L. Parker and J. L. Turk), Vol. 8., Karger, Basel, p. 125
Rook, G. A. W. and Stewart-Tull, D. E. S. (1976). *Immunology*, 31, 389
Ritter, J., Lohmann-Matthes, M. L., Sonntag, H. G. and Fischer, H. (1975). *Cell. Immun.*, 16, 153
Rosenwasser, L. J. and Rosenthal, A. S. (1978). *J. Immun.*, 120, 1991
Schrader, J. W. (1974). *Eur. J. Immun.*, 4, 20
Sjöberg, O., Andersson, J. and Möller, G. (1972). *Eur. J. Immun.*, 2, 326
Souvannavong, V., Adam, A. and Lederer, E. (1978). *Infect. Immun.*, 19, 966
Specter, S., Friedman, H. and Chedid, L. (1977). *Proc. Soc. exp. Biol. Med.*, 155, 349
Specter, S., Cimprich, R., Friedman, H. and Chedid, L. (1978). *J. Immun.* 120, 487
Spitznagel, K. J. and Allison, A. C. (1970). *J. Immun.*, 104, 128
Staber, F. G., Gisler, R. H., Schumann, G., Tarcsay, L., Schläfli, E. and Dukor, P. (1978a). *Cell. Immun.*, 37, 174
Staber, F. G., Tarcsay, L. and Dukor, P. (1978b). *Infect. Immun.*, 20, 40
Sugimoto, M., Germain, R. N., Chedid, L. and Benacerraf, B. (1978). *J. Immun.*, 120, 980
Symoens, J. and Rosenthal, M. (1977). *J. Reticuloendothel. Soc.* 21, 175
Tanaka, A., Nagao, S., Saito, R., Kotani, S. Kusumoto, S. and Shiba, T. (1977). *Biochem. Biophys. Res. Commun.*, 77, 621
Wachsmuth, E. D. (1978). *Proceedings of the VIth International Conference on Lymphatic Tissue and Germinal Centers in Immune Reactions*, (in press)
Wagner, H., Feldmann, M., Boyle, W. and Schrader, J. W. (1972). *J. exp. Med.*, 136, 331
Watson, J., Trenkner, E. and Cohn, M. (1973). *J. exp. Med.*, 138, 699
Webster, R. G., Glezen, W. P., Hannoun, C. and Laver, W. G. (1977). *J. Immun.*, 119, 2073
Yamamoto, Y., Nagao, S., Tanaka, A., Koga, T. and Onoue, K. (1978). *Biochem. Biophys. Res. Commun.*, 80, 923
Yamamura, Y., Azuma, I., Sugimura, K., Yamawaki, M., Kusumoto, S., Okada, S. and Shiba, T. (1976). *Gann*, 67, 867
Yamamura, Y., Azuma, I., Sugimura, K., Yamawaki, M., Uemiya, M., Kusumoto, S., Okada, S. and Shiba, T. (1977). *Proc. Jap. Acad.*, 53, 63

9

Drugs as haptens

Janet M. Dewdney (Beecham Pharmaceuticals, Brockham Park, Betchworth, Surrey RH3 7AJ, U.K.)

The clinical importance of the ability of some drugs to act as haptens and to participate in immunological reactions relates to the development of allergic drug-induced reactions either during therapy or in circumstances of occupational exposure to the drug. The majority of adverse reactions to drugs are not immunologically mediated but can be understood on the basis of direct toxicity owing to overdosage, to side effects and to secondary effects dependent on the primary beneficial action of the drug and in some instances to an unexplained pattern of drug handling on the part of the patient. It is these idiosyncratic adverse reactions that cause the main problems in differential diagnosis of allergic drug reactions. However, only the unambiguous demonstration of the immunochemical properties of the drug, or of a drug-derived product allows a firm diagnosis of drug allergy.

It has been well recognised since the work of Landsteiner (1933) and Eisen *et al.* (1952) that the ability of low-molecular-weight chemical compounds to stimulate a specific immune response is a direct function of reactivity with protein amino groups or other nucleophiles. In these studies, it was demonstrated that the ability of the chemical to form covalent bonds with carrier macromolecules correlated with their ability to induce contact hypersensitisation in guinea pigs, an essentially cell-mediated form of sensitisation.

The question then is whether this concept of obligatory covalent reaction with nucleophiles in proteins as the first step in the immunogenicity of chemical substances can be held to explain the undoubted ability of some drugs to stimulate immune responses and to explain, in general terms, allergic reactions to drugs.

The answer is that it cannot without some difficulty. The majority of drugs do not possess an adequate degree of reactivity and this is to be expected, in that drugs highly reactive with mammalian macromolecular structures are likely to reveal themselves in preclinical safety testing as toxic, possibly as mutagens or carcinogens. The situation is different for chemical substances used as intermediates in synthetic processes. These compounds may possess a high degree of reactivity and would be expected to induce immunological reactions as a consequence of covalent binding to proteins. Allergic responses induced therefore by compounds acting as haptens are more a problem in the context of occupational experience than a hazard of drug therapy, and the available data on, for example,

161

the causative agents of contact hypersensitivity in man supports this view (Adams, 1969; Fisher, 1973).

A consideration of drug immunogenicity involves a detailed evaluation of the possible sources of potentially haptenic groupings and of the conditions under which facilitated interactions with macromolecular structures might occur.

Table 9.1 summarises the possible routes to drug immunogenicity. The role of macromolecular products as impurities, as additives or as metabolic products is not discussed further here as it is beyond the scope of this paper, which is directed towards consideration of the evidence for the haptenic properties of low-molecular-weight drugs.

Table 9.1   Immunochemical factors determining drug immunogenicity

---

(1) Covalent binding of drug to macromolecule.
(2) Covalent binding of drug metabolite(s) to macromolecule.
(3) Covalent binding of reactive product impurity to macromolecule *in vivo* or *in vitro*.
(4) Presence of macromolecular impurity: (a) drug related specificity;
                                                          (b) non-drug related specificity.
(5) Macromolecular rearrangement products formed *in vivo* or *in vitro*.

The classic example of the ability of drugs to react to form covalent bonds with protein amino groups is that of the β-lactam antibiotics. The antigenic determinant, the penicilloyl group, is formed by direct acylation of protein amino groups by the β-lactam carbonyl group, a reaction facilitated by high pH but which has been shown to proceed at physiological pH also (Batchelor *et al.*, 1965; Schneider and de Weck, 1965).

More recently we have studied the ability of the drug penicillamine to act as a hapten. Adverse reactions have occurred with penicillamine in the treatment of rheumatoid arthritis and there is some evidence, reviewed by Dewdney (1977*a*), that it can be rendered immunogenic. Rabbits were immunised with D-penicillamine emulsified in Freund's complete adjuvant, each receiving 50 mg by the intradermal route and booster injections subcutaneously in saline of 10 mg at weeks 3, 5, 7 and 9. The production of IgG antibody was assessed in a radioimmunoassay under development in our laboratory. Penicillamine was coupled to an activated Sepharose under non-oxidative conditions. The Sepharose used was activated thiol-Sepharose 4B (Pharmacia Fine Chemicals Ltd.) and comprised cyanogen bromide-activated Sepharose 4B coupled to a mixed disulphide formed between 2–2'-dipyridyl disulphide and glutathione. Penicillamine coupling to this support is accomplished under mild conditions with the release of 2'-thiopyridone and the formation of a mixed disulphide between the drug and the support (figure 9.1). The use of this support in a radioimmunoassay, developed using goat anti-rabbit IgG antibody, has provided evidence for the immunogenicity of penicillamine in the rabbit and the specificity of the reaction has been confirmed by inhibition data (figure 9.2). The assay requires further development, but it has provided two critical pieces of information. One, that penicillamine will form mixed disulphides with appropriate thiols under mild conditions and two, that the potential haptenic determinant so formed is that formed *in vivo* and responsible at least in part for the immune response to this drug.

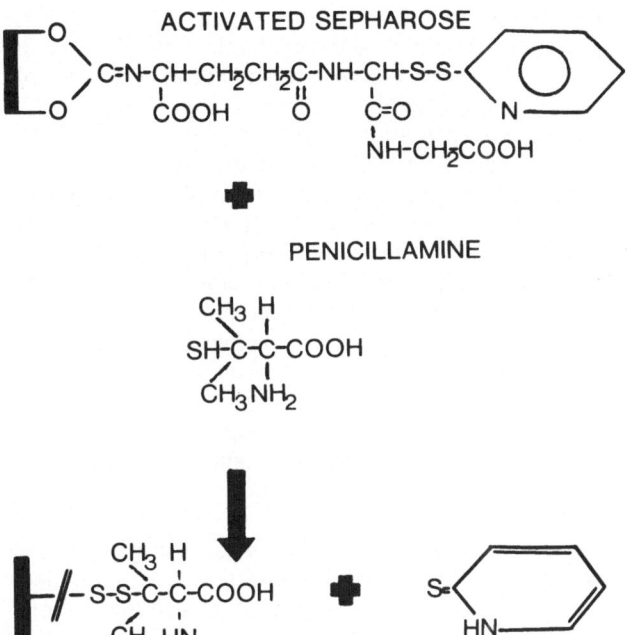

Figure 9.1 The formation of mixed disulphides between D-penicillamine and activated thiol-Sepharose

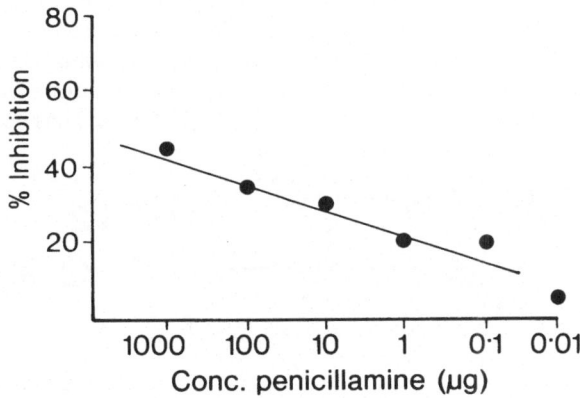

Figure 9.2 Inhibition by D-penicillamine of reaction between activated thiol-Sepharose–D-penicillamine and rabbit IgG antibody. Radioimmunoassay was performed in plastic tubes in PBS (phosphate-buffered saline), bovine serum albumin and Tween buffer. Sepharose–penicillamine was incubated with rabbit antiserum at RT, then washed and goat anti-rabbit IgG ^{125}I-labelled serum was added and the mixture was incubated, then washed and counted for radioactivity (Spackman, D., personal communication)

For the vast majority of drugs, this type of immunochemical evidence is lacking and for many, where clinical experience suggests that allergic mechanisms are involved in adverse reactions, there are postulated pathways to the biotransformation of drugs to protein-reactive metabolites. Remmer and Schüppel (1972) have reviewed this topic, drawing attention to the fact that many products of drug hydroxylation can conjugate to proteins covalently, as for example, the formation of hydroxylated amines from imipramine and from phenothiazine, the formation of sulphoxides from chlorpromazine and of aldehydes from phenothiazines.

It should be noted that these are theoretical pathways to the formation of haptens from drugs. Amos *et al.* (1977) have developed an interesting method by which it may be possible to demonstrate the relevance of some of these pathways. These workers were able to generate reactive metabolic products from the β-blocker drug practolol using, *in vitro*, a rat liver mixed-function oxidase complex and allowing spontaneous coupling of the reactive products to a non-agglutinating rabbit anti-human erythrocyte serum. The antibody reagent was then used to sensitise human erythrocytes to provide an indicator system in an antibody assay. This approach may form the basis of important further studies related to drug immunogenicity.

It has been clearly demonstrated that impurities in drug preparations may be responsible for the introduction of haptenic groups into macromolecules. Benzyl penicillenic acid may be important in this respect, as a source of both penicilloyl and penicillenate antigenic determinants (Dewdney, 1977*b*), and de Weck (1971) has shown unequivocally that the presence of an impurity, aspirin anhydride, in aspirin samples is responsible for the formation of *N*-aspiryl-substituted proteins and immunogenicity.

A number of factors will influence the ability of drugs, or metabolites, or reactive impurities to form hapten–protein conjugates *in vivo*. Bundgaard (1976) has drawn attention to potential immunological implications of the administration of drug in pro-drug form. A recent development in antibacterial chemotherapy has been the introduction of thiazolidine C-3 esters of ampicillin which in man give rise to early and high peak concentrations of the parent antibiotic in serum. A similar thiazolidine C-3 ester of benzyl penicillin (figure 9.3) has been shown

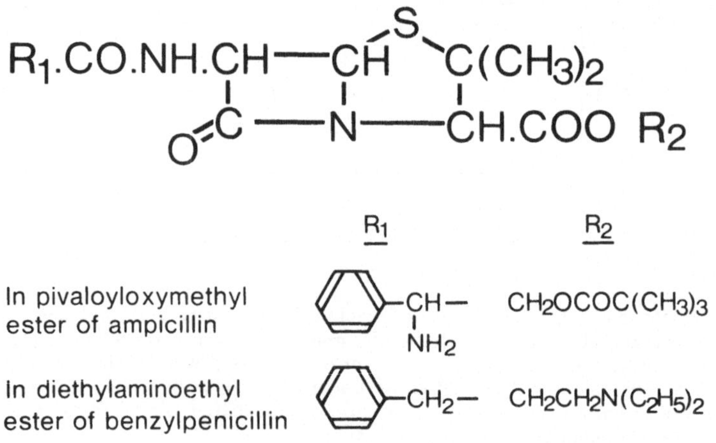

$$R_1.CO.NH.CH—CH \overset{S}{\diagdown} C(CH_3)_2$$
$$O \overset{\diagup}{=} C —N—CH.COO \ R_2$$

	R_1	R_2
In pivaloyloxymethyl ester of ampicillin	⬡–CH– NH$_2$	CH$_2$OCOC(CH$_3$)$_3$
In diethylaminoethyl ester of benzylpenicillin	⬡–CH$_2$–	CH$_2$CH$_2$N(C$_2$H$_5$)$_2$

Figure 9.3 Structures of some thiazolidine C-3 esters of penicillins

in clinical practice to produce contact hypersensitivity (Hjorth, 1967) and, in our laboratories, A. C. Munro and D. Moran (personal communication) demonstrated the sensitising capacity of esters of benzyl penicillin and ampicillin compared with the parent penicillin in an experimental model in the guinea pig. Figure 9.4 shows

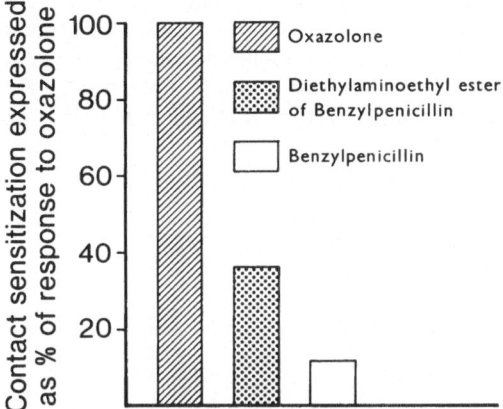

Figure 9.4   Contact sensitisation to benzyl penicillin and diethylaminoethyl ester of benzyl penicillin in the guinea pig. Sensitisation was with 6 × 0.05 ml samples (0.03M concentrations) of the ester and penicillin, and 6 × 0.05 ml of 3 per cent oxazolone (Levine, 1960). Challenge was on day 28, with 0.05 ml of 0.1 M and 0.01 M solutions (A. C. Munro and D. M. Moran, personal communication)

results obtained with benzyl penicillin in which sensitisation is expressed as a proportion of that achieved by oxazolone. In a further series of experiments, they showed that there was cross-sensitisation in this system between the esters but not between ester and parent penicillin. The conclusion reached was that the application of ester to guinea pig skin resulted in the introduction of the penicillanyl determinant (figure 9.5), a chemical grouping shown by Feinberg (1970) to be non cross-reactive with the penicilloyl group introduced on to proteins by parent antibiotics. These results are not of clinical importance when esters are administered orally and in fact Iwata and Serizawa (1974) have shown that the pivaloyloxymethyl ester of ampicillin was only poorly immunogenic compared with ampicillin itself. However, the results indicate a general principle in relation to the ability of drugs to act as haptens and it is clear that pro-drugs may have a spectrum of immunological reactivity quantitatively and qualitatively different from that of their parent antibiotics.

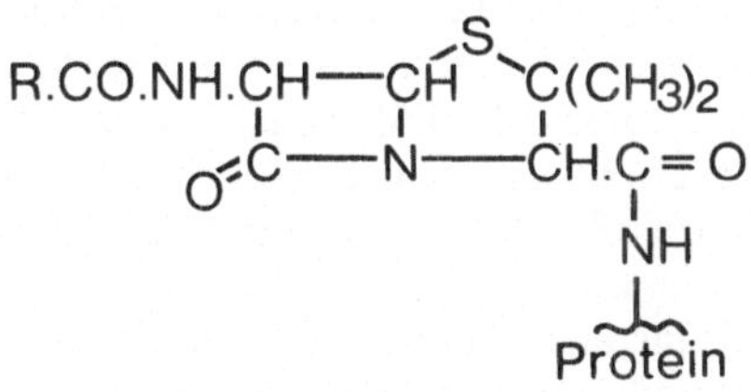

The penicillanyl determinant.

Figure 9.5   Structure of the penicillanyl determinant

Experimental work in our laboratories has indicated that although the contact-sensitisation model in the guinea pig is of value in the assessment of drug immunogenicity, only a low level of sensitisation is achieved compared with the classic sensitisers, oxazolone or the dinitrophenyl analogues. Use is being made of the observations of Turk *et al.* (1972) that pretreatment of guinea pigs with the drug cyclophosphamide will, by elimination of a population of suppressor lymphocytes, enhance contact-sensitisation reactions. Figure 9.6 shows data using benzyl penicillin and a semi-synthetic penicillin in this model. Clear enhancement was achieved and this may be a useful model for further study of drug immunogenicity.

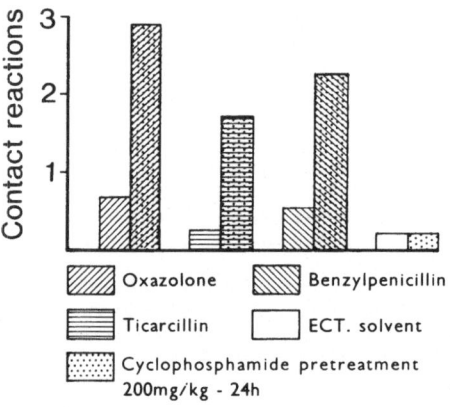

Figure 9.6 Cyclophosphamide enhancement of contact sensitisation in the guinea pig. Sensitisation was achieved with 5 × 0.1 ml samples of penicillins (0.1 M concentrations), or 3 per cent oxazolone. Challenge was made on day 28 with 0.1 M solutions. Cyclophosphamide (200 mg/kg i.p.)was given 24 h before sensitisation

Some years ago (Batchelor *et al.*, 1965), we showed that there was a striking correlation between the ability of a range of penicillins to introduce penicilloyl groups on to proteins and their capacity to bind reversibly to serum proteins. The implication of this work was that a high local concentration of drug, achieved through hydrophobic, reversible binding, at a site of potential covalent linkage, would facilitate antigenic substitution. This might be of even greater significance in relation to the cell membrane. Several observations suggest that the cell membrane is involved as a carrier of haptenic groups in drug allergy. It is known, for example, that the administration of high intravenous doses of benzyl penicillin, as required for the treatment of bacterial endocarditis, will result in a demonstrable penicilloylation of erythrocytes, and that this is by no means an isolated example is indicated by the fact that whereas blood dyscrasia, either haemolytic anaemia or thrombocytopenia, are exceedingly rare complications of the administration of therapeutic substances that are of a macromolecular nature, they are relatively common complications of drug allergy. The mechanism by which cell destruction is mediated is not clear in all instances, but in many it is due to the interaction of IgM or IgG antibody directed against drug haptenic determinants on the cell surface. Specific lymphocyte activation also seems to be more effectively achieved in some instances by drug presented on a cell membrane (de Weck *et al.*, 1974) and Thomas *et al.* (1977) have data that can be interpreted to suggest that the cell membrane of the macrophage may be a major site for haptenic interaction in the development of contact sensitisation in the guinea pig. Hydrophobic bonding capacity, in facilitating irreversible blinding to lipid membranes, might be as important as binding to proteins, and the study of Padfield and Kellaway (1973), which demonstrated the differential binding of two penicillins to a range of phospholipids, is of interest from this point of view.

The capability of drugs or chemical substances to act as haptens could be important also in the pathogenesis of some industrial lung diseases and in occupational asthma. Although immunological pathways are clearly involved in asthma resulting from the inhalation of dusts containing organic matter, as for example, in the case of the enzyme derived from *Bacillus subtilis* (Pepys, 1973), the aetiology of respiratory disease related to low M.W. dusts is less clear. Although in many instances, the data are suggestive of allergic mechanisms, only rarely has it proved possible to demonstrate the specific immunological nature of the reaction. One exception may be the case of asthma induced by trimellitic anhydride (TMA), a chemical used in the plastics industry. Zeiss and colleagues (1977) have reported the direct involvement of IgE antibody in TMA-induced occupational asthma and rhinitis and IgG antibody in a TMA-induced dyspnoea. The haptenic properties of this chemical were clearly demonstrated.

The apparent aetiological role of specific IgG antibody in this study is of interest and is similar to results reported by Shmunes *et al.* (1976) from an evaluation of occupational respiratory disease in an antibiotics factory in the U.S.A. A significant correlation was shown in this study between the development of symptoms in employees and dust levels in their work environment and between symptoms and the presence of benzyl penicilloyl-specific antibodies of the IgG class. Both studies demonstrate clearly the capability of organic chemical substances to stimulate specific immune responses in persons exposed to dusts in the environment, although the precise biological role of the IgG antibody remains unclear.

This paper has related only to the initiating step in the development of allergic drug reactions. Immunochemical properties, as described, are an essential and necessary pre-requisite of such a reaction but they do not determine in any way whether an allergic reaction will occur. The assessment of drug allergenicity is a much more complex topic and is not at the present time amenable to experimental investigation in the laboratory.

The efferent pathway of the pathogenesis of allergic drug reactions must take account of the genetic ability of the patient to respond immunologically to the drug, both from the point of view of recognition of the appropriate antigenic determinant group and of the ability to respond with appropriate antibody formation. Even in situations where, in immunological terms, the probability of an allergic reaction developing seems high, the actual experience of such a reaction will depend on multiple factors including concentrations of both drug and antibody, the availability of drug in appropriate form at critical sites, as for example, near tissue mast cells, the affinity of drug–antibody interactions and the affinity of interaction between tissue receptor sites and the mediators of allergic inflammation released from the initial drug–antibody interaction (Gero, 1972).

REFERENCES

Adams, R. M. (1969). *Occupational Contact Dermatitis*, J. B. Lippincott Co., Philadelphia
Amos, H. E., Lake, B. G. and Atkinson, H. A. C. (1977). *Clin. Allergy*, **7**, 423
Batchelor, F. R., Dewdney, J. M. and Gazzard, D. (1965). *Nature*, **206**, 362
Bundgaard, H. (1976). *Acta Pharm Suec*, **13**, *Suppl.*, 23
Dewdney, J. M. (1977a). In *The Antigens IV*, Academic Press, New York, p. 96
Dewdney, J. M. (1977b). In *The Antigens IV*, Academic Press, New York, p. 94
De Weck, A. L. (1971). *Int. Archs Allergy*, **41**, 393
De Weck, A. L., Spengler, H. L. and Geczy, A. F. (1974). *Monogr. Allergy*, **8**, 120
Eisen, H. N., Orris, L. and Belman, S. (1952). *J. exp. Med.*, **95**, 473
Feinberg, J. G. (1970). In *Penicillin Allergy. Clinical and Immunologic Aspects*, (eds. G. Stewart and J. P. McGovern), Thomas Springfield, Illinois, p. 90
Fisher, A. A. (1973). *Contact Dermatitis*, Lea and Febiger, Philadelphia
Gero, A. (1972). In *Hypersensitivity to Drugs*, vol. 1 (eds. M. Samter and C. W. Parker), Pergamon Press, Oxford, p. 11
Hjorth, N. (1967). *Berufs-Dermatosen*, **15**, 163
Iwata, M. and Serizawa, J. (1974). *Chemotherapy (Basel)*, **22**, 388
Landsteiner, K. (1933). In *The Specificity of Serological Reactions*, English Edition 1962, Dover Publications Inc., New York
Levine, B. B. (1960). *J. exp. Med.*, **112**, 1131
Padfield, J. M. and Kellaway, I. W. (1973). *J. Pharm. Pharmac.*, **25**, 285
Pepys, J. (1973). *Proc. R. Soc. Med.*, **66**, 930
Remmer, H. and Schüppel, R. (1972). In *Hypersensitivity to Drugs*, vol. 1, (eds. M. Samter and C. W. Parker), Pergamon Press, Oxford, p. 67
Schneider, C. H. and de Weck, A. L. (1965). *Nature*, **208**, 57
Shmunes, E., Taylor, J. S., Petz, L. D., Garratty, G. and Fudenberg, H. H. (1976). *Ann. Allergy*, **36**, 313
Thomas, D. W., Forni, G., Shevach, E. M. and Green, I. (1977). *J. Immun.*, **118**, 1677
Turk, J. L., Parker, D. and Poulter, L. W. (1972). *Immunology*, **23**, 493
Zeiss, C. R., Patterson, R., Pruzansky, J. J., Miller, M. M., Rosenberg, M. and Levitz, D. (1977). *J. All. Clin. Immun.*, **60**, 96

10
Allergic reactions to high-molecular-weight compounds

D. R. Stanworth (Department of Immunology, The Medical School,
University of Birmingham, U.K.)

INTRODUCTION

There is still much to be learnt about the nature of immediate-type allergic reactions
to high-molecular-weight, therapeutic compounds; particularly where these are
likely to associate or conjugate to carrier macromolecules *in vivo*. It would seem
worthwhile therefore first to outline current knowledge about the various factors
that are known to influence allergic responses to natural and experimental sensito-

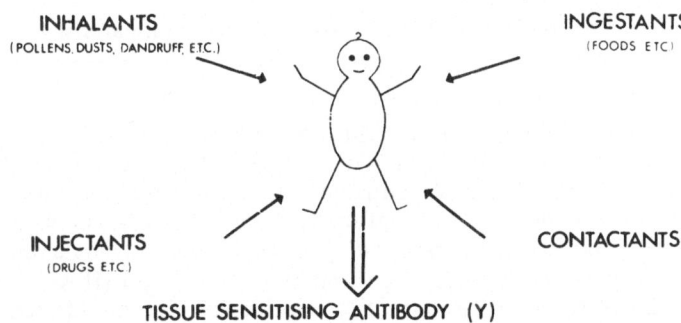

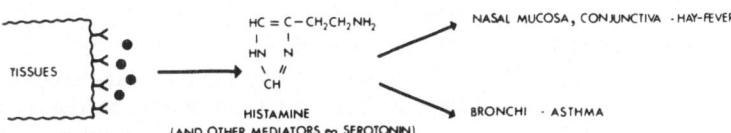

Figure 10.1 Schematic representation of immediate hypersensitivity system.

169

gens in general, before briefly considering structural characteristics of those allergens that have already been defined to any extent.

I propose then to discuss the manner in which interaction of allergen with antibody-sensitised mast cells (or basophils) could lead to the initiation of release of histamine and other mediators (figure 10.1). Finally, I shall draw attention to alternative immunological means of achieving the same end; a somewhat neglected aspect that could prove to be relevant to a greater understanding of allergic reactions to certain types of high-molecular-weight drugs.

FACTORS INFLUENCING IMMEDIATE-TYPE HYPERSENSITIVITY RESPONSE TO NATURAL AND EXPERIMENTAL SENSITOGENS

In considering the likelihood of a particular drug being capable of inducing, in the patient, an allergic response of the immediate type, it is worth considering first those factors (see table 10.1) that have been found to influence the sensitisation of mammals to common allergens, usually protein in nature.

Table 10.1   Factors influencing immediate-type hypersensitivity responses

(1)	Genetic status of host.
(2)	Immunological status of host – at both cellular and humoral levels.
(3)	Hormonal status of host
(4)	Mode of exposure to sensitising substance (sensitogen) – particle size, dose adjuvanicity, route of administration.
(5)	Nature of potential sensitogen.
(6)	Concomitant immunological stimuli – for example from parasite infections.

Foremost is a genetic predisposition, which has long been suggested from the case histories of patients with allergic conditions such as hay fever and extrinsic asthma, and which has now been substantiated from studies in atopic humans and animals. Thus it has become apparent that the total circulating IgE levels of humans are genetically determined (Hamburger *et al.*, 1973). Studies of allergic families have provided evidence that these are regulated by a single major HLA-linked gene (Marsh, 1976). Likewise, investigations into the influence of strain difference on IgE production in rats have suggested a genetic influence on both total and specific IgE antibody production (Pauwels *et al.*, 1978*a*); these parameters were also influenced by the age of the animals experimentally sensitised to ovalbumin using aluminium hydroxide $(Al(OH)_3)$ as adjuvant. A similar type of study on the influence of strain difference on IgE antibody production to proteins and hapten–protein conjugates in mice has prompted the conclusion that the genetic barrier to sensitisation exhibited by many individuals is not a reflection of an inability to develop immediate-type hypersensitivity response as such, but a manifestation of a genetic capability to inhibit synthesis of IgE antibody.

It is becoming increasingly apparent that this genetic control is expressed largely in terms of T-cell function. Much evidence is accumulating to indicate that it is the suppressor T cell that is primarily responsible for the control of IgE antibody production (as indicated, for example, by the studies of Tada (1975) in mice treated with antithymocyte serum to eliminate the dampening effect of suppresser T cells; and from the work of Ishizaka (1976) on IgE production in cultures of rabbit lymph nodes). In this context it is also worth mentioning the observations of Thomas *et al.* (1978) that mice painted with the contact-sensitising agent picryl chloride produce suppressor T cells concomitantly with both IgG and IgE circulating antibodies. These cells can inhibit responses of normal mice to picryl chloride as mediated by antibodies of the former but not the latter class.

At the humoral level, there is some evidence that circulating IgA can also influence the capacity of individuals to become primarily sensitised to common allergens. This evidence is based mainly on the observations (Taylor *et al.*, 1973) that there is a greater incidence of direct skin reactivity in infants (up to 1 year of age) with abnormally low serum IgA levels. However, the data obtained from comparable studies on adult atopic individuals (Stokes *et al.*, 1974) are not so convincing. Another immunological factor, which can obviously have a profound influence on IgE antibody production, is a concomitant helminth parasite infection. Thus it has been shown that the infection of rats with *Nippostrongylus brasiliensis* potentiates IgE antibody production to unrelated antigens like ovalbumin (Orr *et al.*, 1969). Subsequent studies have indicated that this effect is mediated by the release of a non-specific IgE-stimulating factor produced by parasite-specific T cells. This provides further confirmation of the important roles played by T cells in the control of immediate-type hypersensitivity responses.

Not surprisingly, the nature of the sensitising substance (i.e. sensitogen) and its form of presentation is also of some consequence in the induction of IgE-mediated hypersensitivity responses. For instance, it has been shown from experimental sensitisation studies in rats (Jarrett *et al.*, 1976) that presentation of very small amounts of protein antigen (1 μg intradermally or 10 μg orally) is capable of inducing an IgE antibody response provided that an adjuvant (for example Al(OH)$_3$) is used, although a booster response can be effected by subsequent presentation of antigen (1 μg intradermally or 1 μg orally) in the absence of adjuvant. In contrast, larger doses of antigen, irrespective of the route of presentation, are likely to produce only a transient IgE antibody response that cannot be boosted. The finding from this type of experimental animal study, that incomplete adjuvants, such as Al(OH)$_3$, appear to be more effective than complete ones in the induction of immediate hypersensitivity responses is interesting in view of the common practice of administering some drugs in a depot form, which might conceivably fulful this type of adjuvant requirement.

Despite the ability to achieve experimental sensitisation to a wide range of macromolecules (particularly proteins and hapten–protein conjugates) in this manner, there is still reason to suppose that native high-molecular-weight substances are not all equally sensitogenic. This aspect, particularly in relation to sensitivity to drugs, will be considered further in the next section.

THE NATURE OF ALLERGENIC SUBSTANCES

A primary requirement is, of coure, that the would-be sensitising material finds ready access to the respiratory or gastrointestinal tracts. This is not too surprising, as far as pollen grains are concerned, because their success in fulfilling their primary role of pollination depends very much on their capacity to readily pervade the atmosphere. Particles of other allergen materials such as animal danders and mite faeces, which are probably of similar size (20–60 μm diameter), can be expected likewise easily to find their way into the nasal passages of atopic individuals, and indeed human and animal epidermal particles have been identified in airborne matter by surface-fat analysis.

In view of the well-known chemical stability of the pollen membrane, it might seem surprising that a hypersensitivity response ensues with such speed. But, as the work of Knox *et al.* (1970) has suggested, after the pollen grains have become lodged in the aqueous medium within the nasal mucosae, the allergenic constituents (which have been shown to be located on sites within the intimae) diffuse out rapidly through the germinal pores. Yet, although a whole array of soluble protein constituents are leached out from the pollen grains in this manner, only certain of these appear to be allergenic. Similarly, my early work on the characterisation of horse dandruff allergen (Stanworth, 1957) showed that our group of horse-sensitive test subjects possessed skin reactivity to only one of the several major protein constituents of horse-dandruff extract distinguishable by immunological analyses (figure 10.2).

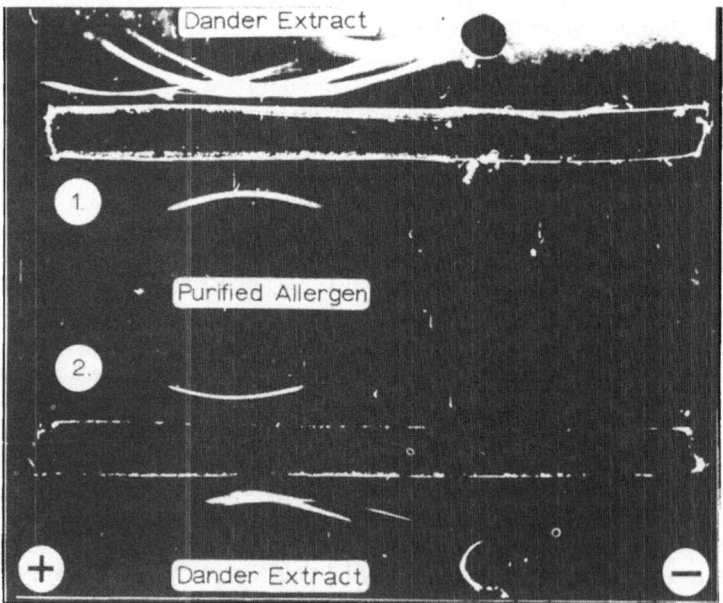

Figure 10.2 Immunoelectrophoretic pattern of purified horse dandruff allergen compared with that of horse dandruff extract; the antiserum used was rabbit anti-whole dander extract (reproduced from Stanworth, 1973).

This sort of observation inevitably raised the question whether there are certain structural features common to all native protein allergens. And, as I pointed out some time ago (Stanworth, 1973), many of the natural allergens (both inhalant and ingestant), which have been sufficiently well characterised, are predominantly protein in nature, of relatively low molecular weight (usually in the 20 000–40 000 range) and in possession of a preponderance of acidic over basic amino acid residues. Another noticeable feature is their marked stability to heat and other forms of denaturation treatment.

More recent studies on highly purified cod fish and ragweed pollen allergens, and active proteolytic cleavage fragments of these, have suggested that protein allergens can be of relatively lower molecular weight (for example as low as 3500). Further, the primary structural analysis of these allergenic constituents has failed to reveal any chemical characteristics of this type of biologically active molecule, although this work has initiated speculation about the nature of allergenic determinants. Thus the sequencing of the low-molecular-weight allergenic

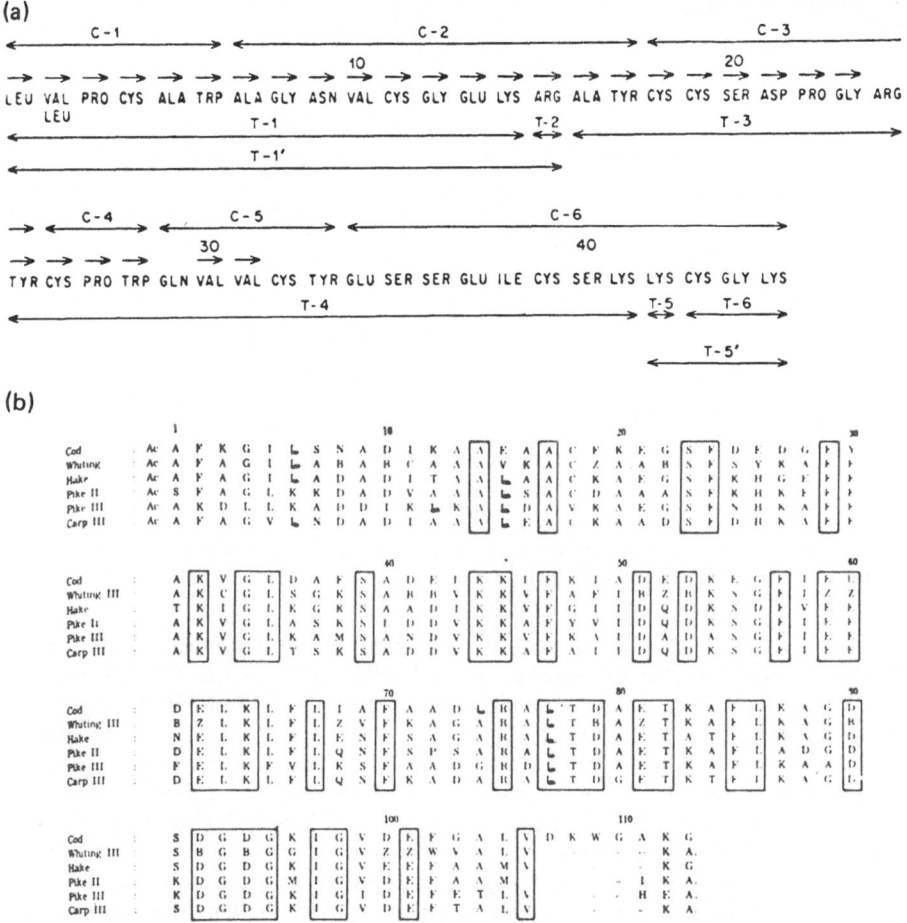

Figure 10.3 (a) The complete amino acid sequence of ragweed allergen Ra5 (reproduced by courtesy of Dr. L. E. Mole and associates, 1975). (b) The tentative complete amino acid sequence of cod fish allergen M, compared with the corresponding calcium-binding muscle albumins of other fish (reproduced by courtesy of Drs. S. Elsayed and H. Bennich, 1975). A, Ala; B, Asx; C, Cys; D, Asp; E, Glu; F, Phe; G, Gly; H, His; I, Ile; K, Leu; M, Met; N, Asn; P, Pro; Q, Gln; R, Arg; S, Ser; T, Thr; V, Val; W, Trp; Z, Glx.

constituent (Ra5) of ragweed pollen, which comprises 45 amino acid residues, has revealed no detectable carbohydrate, four disulphide bridges and a relatively high proportion (11 per cent) of aromatic amino acid residues, which could have an influence on its immunogenicity. Its only structural similarity to the recently sequenced cod fish allergen M, of 113 residues, appears to be an Arg-Ala doublet in positions 15–16 (as will be seen from a comparison of figures 10.3a and 10.3b). It has been suggested that the amino acid sequence illustrated in figure 10.4, which is seen in several positions in cod fish allergen M, might comprise an allergenic determinant (Aas, 1976). This proposal should be confirmed by the experiments now in progress in Scandinavia on the synthesis of peptides comprising fish allergen sequences.

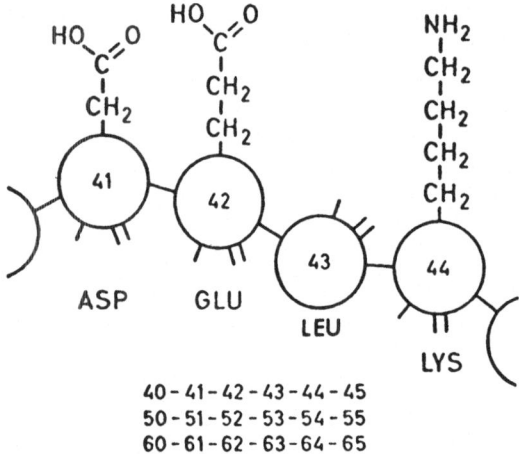

Figure 10.4 A possible allergenic determinant amino acid sequence, seen in cod fish allergen M (reproduced by courtesy of Dr. K. Aas, 1976).

What, however, is the relevance of such observations on the physical form and structural basis of activity of native protein allergens to the question of the potential allergenicity of high-molecular-weight therapeutic compounds? With regard to their mode of presentation to the atopic individual, it is important to recognise that, as is often the case even with fish allergens, they could be absorbed by inhalation, either in purified form or, for example, in the form of a mould in the case of antibiotics. Another major consideration is the conjugation of drugs to carrier proteins within the patient, with the formation of an effective sensitogen comparable with the hapten–protein conjugates that have been widely used in animal-sensitisation studies. In this connection, it is worth drawing attention to studies in spontaneously ragweed-sensitive dogs (Schwarzman *et al.*, 1971), which showed that a single injection of dinitrophenylated (DNP) ragweed allergen induced the formation of anti-DNP IgE antibody in contrast to repeated exposure to DNP-canine serum albumin by nebulisation. These early observations are consistent with findings from more recent studies on the important role of carrier protein determinants specific for T cells which can be distinguished from antigen (hapten) specific for B cells (Takatsu and Ishizaka, 1977). Thus in cases of drug-induced immediate hypersensitivity responses involving the formation of drug–protein conjugates *in vivo*, the drug can be expected to confer additional allergenic specificities on a protein carrier capable of mobilising T cells to help in IgE antibody production. Although, in contrast, long-term immune therapy of allergic (hay fever) patients is thought to result in the generation of *suppressor* T cells (Ishizaka, 1976).

As will be discussed in the next section, it is likely that the extent of chemical substitution of a carrier protein by a particular drug, and more particularly the distribution of such haptenic groups, is important at the stage of triggering of anaphylactic antibody-sensitised mast cells by specific allergen.

THE MOLECULAR BASIS OF ALLERGEN-INDUCED TRIGGERING OF ANTIBODY-SENSITISED MAST CELLS

The availability of myeloma forms of human IgE, the immunoglobulin class to which immediate sensitising antibody molecules belong, have greatly facilitated attempts to elucidate, at the molecular level, the manner in which interaction of allergen and sensitising IgE antibody, at the mast cell (or basophil) surface, initiates the release of histamine and other mediators. As far as the role of the allergen is concerned, the crucial event would seem to be the bridging of adjacent cell-bound

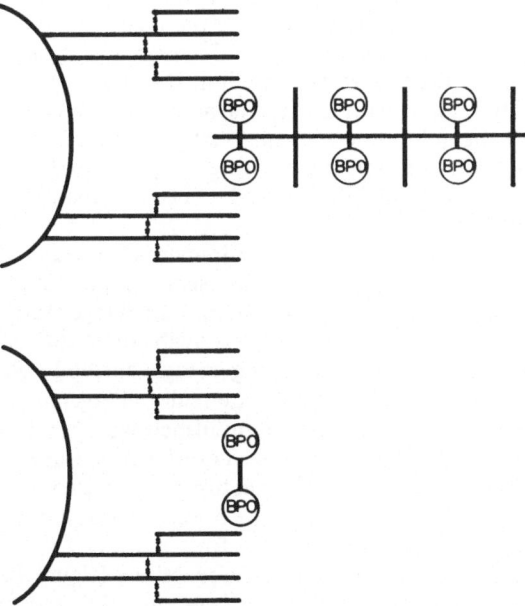

Figure 10.5 Schematic representation of the bridging of anaphylactic antibodies, bound to a target cell via sites in their Fc regions, by BPO–carrier conjugates (reproduced from Stanworth, 1973).

IgE antibody molecules. These, as our inhibition PK and PCA (passive cutaneous anaphylaxis) test studies with protolytic cleavage fragments of myeloma IgE showed (Stanworth *et al.*, 1968), are bound to mast cells via sites within their Fc regions, thereby leaving the Fab regions accessible to subsequent interaction with allergenic determinants (as shown in figure 10.4). This is concluded from various types of experimental approach, including studies of the influence of the size of hapten carrier (for example, penicilloyl–polylysine conjugates) on the ability to evoke PCA reactors in guinea pigs (Levine, 1965; De Weck and Schneider, 1968). Thus the crucial requirement for the induction of an immediate reaction in a pre-sensitised animal (or animal's tissue) was a valency (i.e. anaphylactic antibody-binding capacity) of at least two, rather than the overall size of the hapten carrier (figure 10.5). Taking this line of investigation further, studies on the induction of specific histamine release from the basophils of presensitised rabbits by bivalent hapten-carrier (polymethylene) conjugates have actually permitted the determination of the optimal spacing of the hapten (benzyl penicilloyl, BPO) groups for maximal release; compounds in which the two BPO groups were separated by 6-9 methylene groups proved to be the most active (Siraganian *et al.*, 1975). Moreover, as in the earlier studies, monovalent haptens were inactive. We have obtained similar results from the experimental sensitisation of guinea pigs with heat-aggregated human IgG. The induction of histamine release from the animals' tissue (ileum) *in vitro* could only be effected by challenge with aggregated IgG, but not with monomer which is nevertheless able to inhibit the activity of the aggregate (D. R. Stanworth and A. K. Smith; unpublished work).

De Weck (1972) has gone as far as exploring the possibility of exploiting inhibition of sensitivity by monovalent antigen and hapten as a means of preventing anaphylactic reactions to drugs such as penicillin. But this is a practice that would seem to be potentially fraught with clinical hazards, if one accepts the validity of occasional reports of the induction of anaphylactic reaction in experimentally sensitised animals by injection of *monovalent* antigen, quite apart from the observations that certain drugs like penicillin can under certain circumstances associate into multivalent forms *in vitro*.

Hence, in addition to the sensitogenic requirements for drug-induced immediate hypersensitivity reactions (considered in earlier sections), it would seem that there is a need of polyvalency at the subsequent allergen challenge stage. I have suggested (Stanworth, 1973) that native protein allergens might meet this requirement by the association of structural subunits carrying a single antibody binding site and there is some evidence that β-lactoglobulin, the major allergenic constituent of cow's milk, and horse (D. R. Stanworth, unpublished work) and cat (Stokes and Turner, 1975) dandruff allergens meet these requirements. But reports (Aas, 1976) of the induction of immediate sensitivity reactions by injection of relatively low-molecular-weight fragments of cod fish allergen might suggest otherwise. Nevertheless, it is noteworthy that such a requirement for a minimal two subunit allergen structure is ideally met in reverse anaphylactic reactions (figure 10.6), where presensitisation of animals' skin sites (or mast cells *in vitro*) by transfer of non-antibody IgE (or IgG) is followed by challenge with anti-antibody, which itself is effectively a dimeric form of a heavy–light chain subunit each with a single antibody binding site.

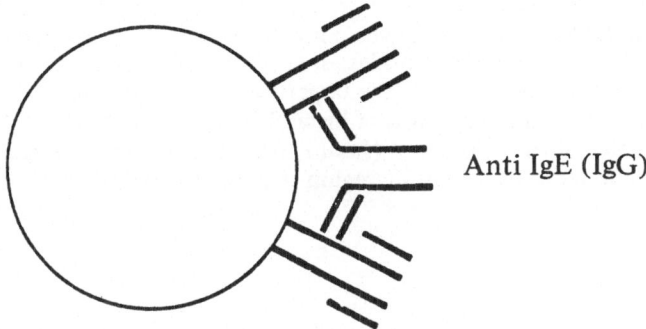

Anti IgE (IgG)

Figure 10.6   Diagram illustrating how cell-bound antibody is bridged by anti-antibody, rather than specific allergen, in reverse anaphylactic reactions.

It is noteworthy that, like the regular allergen challenge of antibody-sensitised mast cells, cross-linking of bound immunoglobulin molecules by anti-immunoglobulin initiates the active secretion of histamine and other mediators in a Ca^{2+} ion and energy-dependent manner. Indeed, there is reason to suppose (Stanworth, 1973)

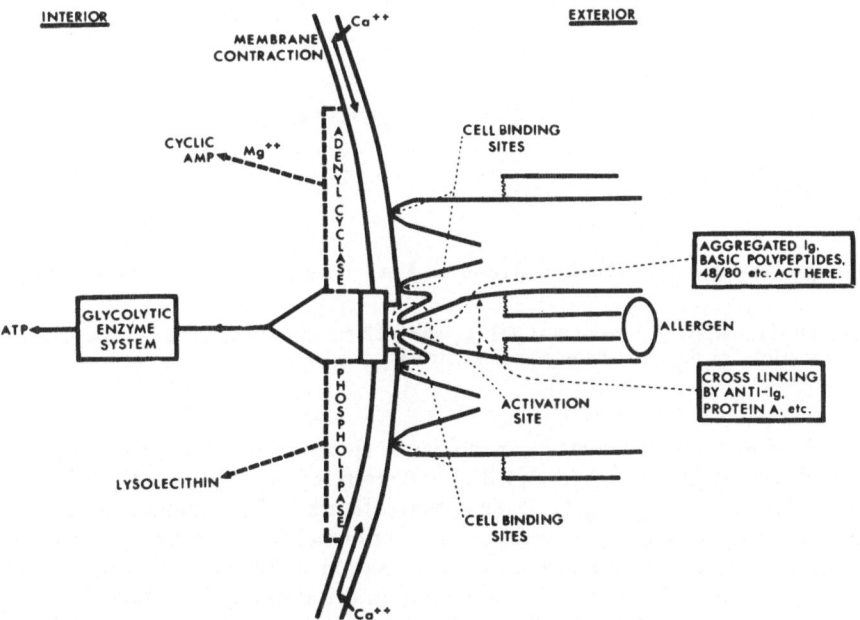

Figure 10.7   Summary diagram of various direct and indirect methods of triggering mast cells into histamine release, suggesting a common activation site on the plasma membrane (reproduced from Stanworth, 1973).

that this, and other forms of artificial triggering involving for instance the action of preformed anaphylactic antibody–allergen complexes or basic compounds like compound 48/80 and certain polypeptides on normal mast cells, leads to activation of the same site on the surface of the target mast cell (figure 10.7). Moreover, our studies on the structural basis of histamine-releasing activity of ACTH (corticotropin) and melittin derivatives (Jasani *et al.*, 1973), and more recently synthetic peptides representative of IgE Fc region sequences (Stanworth *et al.*, 1978),

MELITTIN

```
    1                            7
NH₂–Gly–Ile–Gly–Ala–Val–Leu–Lys–

8                                    19
Val–Leu–Thr–Gly–Leu–Pro–Ala–Leu–Ile–Ser–Trp–

20                          26
Ile↓Lys–Arg–Lys–Arg┤Gln–Gln–CONH₂
```

ACTH

```
1                                                                        16
NH₂–Ser–Tyr–Ser–Met–Glu–His–Phe–Arg–Trp–Gly–Lys–Pro–Val–Gly–Lys–Lys–

17               24
Arg–Arg┤Pro–Val–Lys–Val–Tyr–Pro–

25                                                           39
Asp–Gly–Ala–Glu–Asp–Glu–Leu–Ala–Glu–Ala–Phe–Pro–Leu–Glu–Phe–COOH
```

Figure 10.8 Primary structures of β-ACTH₁₋₃₉ and melittin showing clusters of basic amino acids responsible for their histamine-releasing activity.

have enabled us to predict that the anaphylactic antibody effector site comprises a cluster of basic amino acid residues with contiguous hydrophobic residues with potential for penetrating target cell membranes (figure 10.8). It should also be emphasised that this postulated mechanism of immunological triggering of mast cells (figure 10.9) supposes that the first sensitisation step involves the 'addressing' of target mast cells (or basophils) by a site within the antibody Fc region. Subsequent bridging of the adjacent cell-bound antibody molecules by allergen leads to the mobilisation of distinctive Fc effector sites, which are responsible for the conveyance of the 'message' responsible for the ultimate release of histamine and other mediators of immediate-type allergic reactions.

As already mentioned, it seems to be possible therefore to 'short circuit' the standard release process, not only by artificially cross-linking the cell-bound antibody molecules, but also by means of compounds capable of acting directly on the activation site. Included in this category are certain drugs, which themselves fulfil the requisite standard requirements or alternatively are able to initiate the formation of anaphylatoxic fragments C3a and C5a, which are themselves basic polypeptides (table 10.2) capable of triggering histamine release from mast cells. This question of drug-induced, non-immunologically-mediated and non-IgE-mediated release will be considered in the final section.

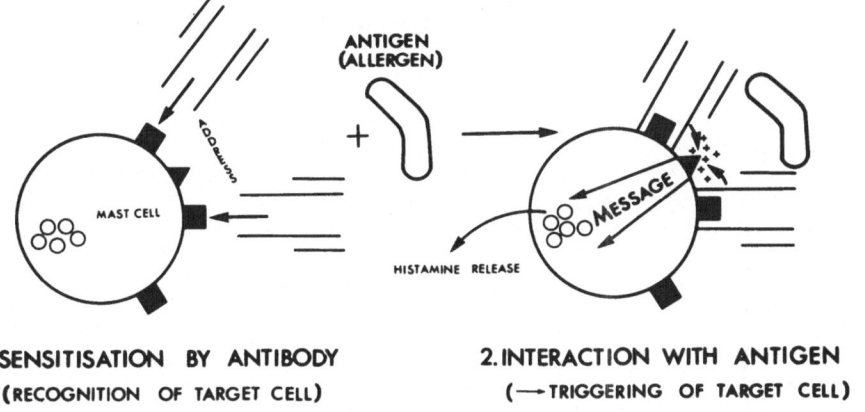

1. SENSITISATION BY ANTIBODY
(RECOGNITION OF TARGET CELL)

2. INTERACTION WITH ANTIGEN
(→ TRIGGERING OF TARGET CELL)

Figure 10.9 Postulated molecular basis of immunological triggering of mast cells.

Table 10.2 Properties of the human anaphylatoxins (Müller-Eberhard, 1976)

	C3a	C5a
Electrophoretic mobility	+ 2.1	−1.7
Diffusion coefficient	−	12.1
Frictional ratio	−	1.05
Molecular weight:		
Gel filtration	8700	17500
Gel electrophoresis	7200	16500
Amino acid analysis	8900	9000
Carbohydrate content	none	30%
Total molecular weight	8900	12000
Amino acid residues	77	73
COOH-terminus	Arginine	Arginine
Activity:		
Ileum contraction	13 nM	0.4 nM
Leukotaxis	Inactive	7 nM
Wheal and flare	2 pmol	1 fmol

DRUG-INDUCED IMMEDIATE HYPERSENSITIVITY REACTIONS NOT MEDIATED BY IgE ANTIBODY

Out of the wide variety of drug-induced allergic reactions that are suspected to fall into this category, two examples will be considered which illustrate what appear to be major ways of short-circuiting the initiation of mediator release by anaphylactic IgE antibody–allergen interaction (by the classical mechanism discussed in the previous section). In my own experience, and that of others, it has never proved possible to demonstrate specific IgE antibodies directed against the drug in the sera of such patients.

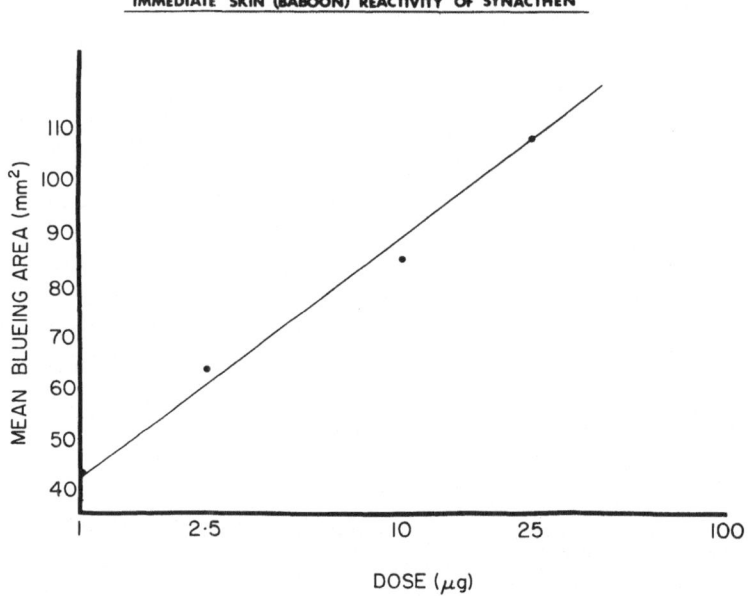

Figure 10.10 Dose–response curve obtained by prick-testing solutions of Synacthen in the skin of a normal baboon.

The first example is the clinically serious (and occasionally fatal) anaphylactic-type reaction shown rarely by patients injected with Synacthen depot. In collaborative studies with the Ciba Company, we examined sera from around 20 such cases for the presence of IgE antibodies by passive-transfer tests in baboons; none showed a positive PCA response after challenge with various Synacthen preparations at 4 or 24 h. Possibly our failure could be attributed to the testing of sera taken from the patients after the incident, but it is noteworthy that physiologically significant doses of synthetic hormone preparation (ACTH β^{1-24} peptide) can initiate histamine release from non-sensitised mast cells. This has been demonstrated *in vivo* by tests in guinea pig and rat skin (Jaques, 1965) and in primates (figure 10.10). It is possible to demonstrate that around 1 μM Synacthen is capable of inducing the release of 50 per cent of the available histamine from purified rat peritoneal mast-cell preparations (figure 10.11).

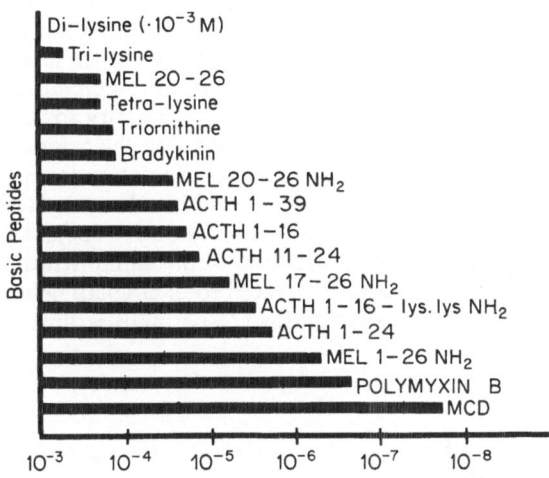

H.R. Activity, Molar Concentration At 50% Release

Figure 10.11   Relative histamine-releasing (HR) activities expressed as the molar concentration giving 50 per cent histamine release: MCD refers to mast cell degranulation substance from bee venom (reproduced from Jasani *et al.*, 1973).

As mentioned above, our structure–activity studies on the rat mast-cell system *in vitro* (Jasani *et al*, 1973) have indicated that the crucial structural feature responsible for such normal rat mast-cell triggering is the cluster of basic amino acid residues in positions 15–18 of the ACTH sequence (figure 10.8). Thus, as would be expected on this basis, the native ACTH hormone (β^{1-39} polypeptide) has an appreciably lower histamine-releasing capacity, because the 25–39 region contains acidic rather than basic amino acid residues which (as our studies showed) dampen the histamine-releasing activity of the basic residues.

As our work has also shown that such therapeutic compounds are, like the anaphylactic antibody–allergen reaction, capable of effecting an active secretion of histamine from mast cells (rather than having a cytolytic effect on them), it is possible that such a 'short circuiting' process is responsible for the pseudoanaphylactic reactions demonstrated by those patients who react adversely to Synacthen depot. If this is the case, it is necessary to explain why the vast majority of patients treated with this drug never encounter this type of problem.

The second example of the non-immunological release of mediators of immediate hypersensitivity reactions to which I want to refer concerns adverse reactions to colloid volume substitutes, and in particular dextran preparations. The incidence of adverse anaphylactoid reactions induced by such substance is fortunately very rare. For instance, a recent multi-centre prospective trial (Ring and Messner, 1977) has indicated that the incidence of severe reactions (shock, cardiac and/or respiratory arrest) to infusion of dextran was as low as 0.008 per cent and that most of these appear to be to dextran 60/75 rather than dextran 40, which is less highly cross-linked. This has handicapped the systematic study of the immunological basis of such reactions so that I have personally had an opportunity to study only one local case of apparent allergic reactivity to dextran. As with the cases of adverse reactivity to Synacthen mentioned above, I was unable to obtain from passive-transfer tests in baboons any evidence of production of either short-term sensitising antibody or specific IgE antibody against dextran, although a specimen of serum taken a few days after one patient's allergic reaction to the administration of Rheomacrodex during surgery did show a slightly elevated total circulating level of IgE (470 ng/ml compared with a normal range of 25–375 ng/ml of serum).

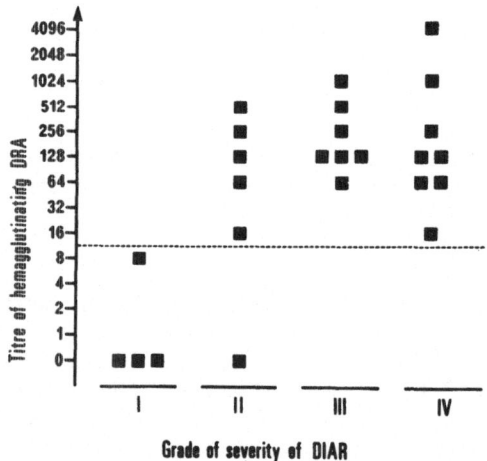

Figure 10.12 Relation between titres of haemagglutinating dextran-reactive antibody (DRA) in the sera of dextran-reactive patients (*n* = 25) and severity of dextran-induced anaphylactoid reactions (DIAR). Titres were estimated before the reaction (reproduced by courtesy of Dr. Harriet Hedin, 1977). Grades of severity: I, skin symptoms and/or mild fever reaction; II, measureable, but not life-threatening (cardiovascular reaction (tachycardia, hypotension), gastrointestinal disturbance (nausea), respiratory disturbance); III, shock, life-threatening spasm of smooth muscle (bronchi, uterus, etc.); IV, cardiac and/or respiratory arrest.

It should be pointed out, however, that a recent comprehensive study (Hedin, 1977) of a large number (123) of cases of dextran-induced anaphylactoid reactions in humans conducted in Sweden has likewise failed to obtain any evidence of the involvement of IgE-mediated reactions, either from testing for specific IgE antibody in the patients' sera by passive transfer to monkey skin or by the *in vitro* radio-allergosorbent test (RAST) employing dextran-coupled absorbent. Significantly, too, measurement of serum levels of factor B failed to provide any indication of activation of the alternative pathway of complement; thus seemingly ruling out the possibility that histamine release from mast cells in such patients was being accomplished by short-circuiting of the regular anaphylactic antibody–allergen interaction by the formation of the basic C3a and C5a anaphylatoxic fragments (referred to in the previous section). On the other hand, Richter and his associates have observed a positive correlation between the haemagglutination titres of dextran-reactive antibody and increasing severity of dextran-induced anaphylactoid reactions (figure 10.12), which has prompted the suggestion that specific immune complexes initiate mediator release through activation of the classical complement pathway. In this event, it is possible that the primary immunological triggering is on polymorphonuclear leucocytes with the release of mediators such as slow-

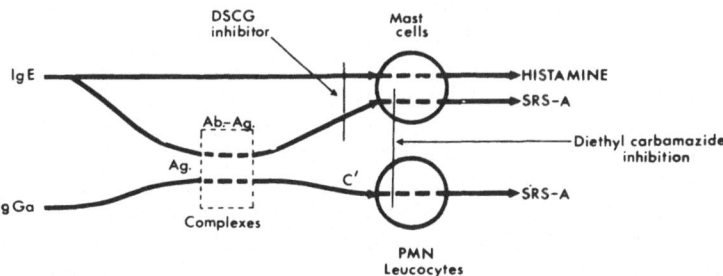

Figure 10.13 Diagrammatic representation of supposed manner in which rat IgE and IgG anaphylactic antibodies initiate the release of mediators of immediate-type hypersensitivity reactions, based on the findings of Orange *et al.* (1970) (reproduced from Stanworth, 1973).

reacting substance of anaphylaxis (SRS-A), in the manner attributed to complement-dependent release from target neutrophils initiated by rat IgG antibody–antigen complexes (Orange *et al.*, 1970) (figure 10.13). In this connection, it is also worth mentioning that a relatively low-molecular-weight (1200–2400) arginine-rich cation peptide with potent mast-cell rupturing activity has been isolated from the lysosomes of rabbit polymorphonuclear leucocytes (Seegers and Janoff, 1966). This might offer a means of switching to the regular pathway of release of mediators responsible for the clinical manifestations of immediate-type hypersensitivity reactions, without the need for mounting an IgE antibody-mediated response.

It could be significant that, unlike protein and mucopolysaccharide immunogens which elicit in humans IgG antibodies representative of all four IgG subclasses, pure polysaccharides such as dextran invoke an IgG antibody response solely in the IgG2 subclass. It is immunoglobulin of this human IgG subclass that has proved to be incapable of binding to heterologous (guinea pig) mast cells (Yount *et al.*, 1968). This could mean that release of histamine, by combination of antibody of this subclass with specific antigen, would probably have to rely on an alternative trigger process from the classical one involving presensitisation of the mast cell by cytophilic antibody (by the mechanism discussed in the previous section).

SUMMARY

In the limited space available an attempt has been made to outline the main factors controlling IgE-mediated immediate hypersensitivity responses in mammals before discussing the physical and structural features characteristic of well-defined inhalant and ingestant sensitogens, and their possible relevance to the type of high-molecular-weight therapeutic compound likely to elicit a similar clinically significant allergic response.

Attention has also been drawn to the apparent allergenic structural requirements necessary for the initiation of mediators after subsequent challenge of IgE antibody-sensitised mast cells and basophils (*in vivo* or *in vitro*). This has led to a brief description of the supposed molecular basis of the classical immunological trigger process and a consideration of feasible ways of short-circuiting this. Of the latter, two examples have been considered which could be of clinical significance in cases of adverse drug reactivity where IgE-mediated hypersensitivity is not demonstrable. First, the direct triggering of non-sensitised mast cells by basic polypeptides like ACTH and secondly, dextran-induced anaphylactoid reactions that appear to be mediated via activation of the classical complement pathway, by IgG antibody-polysaccharide antigen complexes. It is suggested, however, that the latter could result in a secondary switch-over to mast-cell triggering, by the release from target neutrophils of a basic polypeptide. In future studies, it will be important to investigate the possible involvement of immune complexes comprising the so-called short-term sensitising anaphylactic antibodies of the IgG class, which appear to be implicated in some incidents of drug-induced immediate hypersensitivity reactions not mediated by IgE antibodies, and are probably representative of the IgG4 subclass.

REFERENCES

Aas, K. (1976). Common characteristics of major allergens. In *Molecular and Biological Aspects of the Acute Allergic Reaction*, (eds. S. S. O. Johansson, K. Strandberg and B. Uvnäs), Nobel Foundation Symp. No. 33, Plenum Press, p. 3

De Weck, A. L. and Schneider, C. H. (1968). Immune and non-immune responses to monovalent low-molecular-weight penicilloyl-polylysines and penicilloyl-bacitracin in rabbits and guinea pigs. *Immunology*, 14, 1457

De Weck, A. L. (1972). Immunochemical mechanisms in drug allergy. In *Mechanisms in Drug Allergy* (eds. C. H. Dash and H. E. H. Jones), Churchill Livingstone, p. 2

Elsayed, S. and Bennich, H. (1975). *Primary structure* of allergen M from cod. *Scand. J. Immunol.*, 4, 203

Hamburger R. N., Orgel, H. A. and Bazaral, M. (1973). Genetics of human serum IgE levels.

In *Mechanisms in Allergy; Reagin-mediated hypersensitivity*, (eds. L. Goodfriend, A. H. Sehan and R. P. Orange), Marcel Dekker, New York, p. 131

Hedin, H. (1977). Dextran-induced anaphylactoid reactions in man. Immunological *in vitro* and *in vivo* studies. *Acta Univ. upsal.*, 432

Ishizaka, K. (1976). Induction and suppression of IgE antibody response. In *Molecular and Biological Aspects of the Acute Allergic Reaction*, (eds. S. G. O. Johansson, K. Strandberg and B. Uvnäs), Nobel Foundation Symp. No. 33, Plenum Press, p. 59

Jaques, R. (1965). Non-specific effects of synthetic corticotrophin peptides. *Int. Archs Allergy. appl. Immun.*, 28, 221

Jarrett, E. E. E., Haig, D. M., McDougall, W. and McNulty, E. (1976). Rat IgE production. II Primary and booster reaginic antibody responses following intradermal or oral immunization. *Immunology*, 30, 671

Jasani, B., Stanworth, D. R., Mackler, B. and Kreil, G. (1973). Studies on the mast cell triggering action of certain artificial histamine liberators. *Int. Archs Allergy appl. Immun.*, 45, 74

Knox, R. B., Heslop-Harrison, J. and Reed, C. (1970). Localization of antigen associated with the pollen grain wall by immunofluorescence. *Nature*, 225, 1066

Levine, B. B. (1965). The nature of antigen-antibody complexes which initiate anaphylactic reactions. II. The effect of molecular size on the abilities of homologous multivalent benzyl penicilloyl haptens to evoke PCA and Arthus reactions in guinea pigs. *J. Immun.*, 94. 121

Marsh, D. G. (1976). Allergy: a model for studying the genetics of human immune responses. In *Molecular and Biological Aspects of the Acute Allergic Reaction.*, (eds. S. G. O. Johansson, K. Strandberg and B. Uvnäs), Nobel Foundation Symp. No. 33, Plenum Press, p. 3

Müller-Eberhard, H. J. (1976). The anaphylatoxins: formation, structure function and control. In *Molecular and Biological Aspects of the Acute Allergic Reaction*, (eds S. G. O. Johansson, K. Strandberg and B. Uvnäs), Nobel Foundation Symp. No. 33, Plenum Press, p. 3

Orange, R. P., Stechschulte, D. J. and Austen, K. F. (1970). Immunochemical and biologic properties of rat IgE. II. Capacity to mediate the immunologic release of histamine and slow-reacting substance of anaphylaxis (SRS-A). *J. Immun.*, 105, 1087

Orr, T. C., Riley, P. and Doe, J. E. (1969). Potentiated reagin response to egg-albumin and ovalbumin in *N. brasiliensis* injected rats. *Life Sci.*, 8, part II, 1073

Pauwels, R., Bazin, H., Platteau, B. and van der Straeten, M. (1978a). The influence of genetic factors and antigen dose on IgE production in rats. *Immunology*, (in press)

Pauwels, R., Bazin, H., Platteau, B. and van der Straeten, M. (1978b). The effect of age on IgE-production in rats. *J. exp. Med.* (in press)

Ring, J. and Messmer, K. (1977). Incidence and severity of anaphylactoid reactions to colloid volume substitutes. *Lancet*, i, 466

Schwartzman, R. M., Rockey, J. H. and Halliewell, R. E. (1971). Immune reaginic antibody. Characterisation of the spontaneous anti-ragweed and induced anti-DNP reaginic antibodies of the atopic dog. *Clin. exp. Immun.*, 9, 549

Seegers, W. and Janoff, A. (1966). Mediators of inflammation in leukocyte lysosomes. VI. Partial purification and characterisation of a mast cell rupturing component. *J. exp. Med.*, 124, 833

Siriganian, R. P., Hook, W. A. and Levine, B. B. (1975). Specific *in vitro* histamine release from basophils by bivalent haptens: evidence for activation by simple bridging of membrane-bound antibody. *Immunochemistry*, 12, 149

Stanworth, D. R. (1957). The isolation and identification of horse dandruff allergen. *Biochem. J.*, 65, 582

Stanworth, D. R. (1973). Immediate hypersensitivity. The molecular basis of allergic responses mediated by humoral antibodies. *Frontiers of Biology*, Vol. 28, North Holland, Amsterdam.

Stanworth, D. R., Humphrey, J. H., Bennich, H. and Johansson, S. G. O. (1968). Inhibition of Prausnitz–Küstner reaction by proteolytic cleavage fragments of a human myeloma protein of immunoglobulin class E. *Lancet*, ii, 17

Stanworth, D. R., Kings, M., Roy, P. D., Moran, J. M. and Moran, D. M. (1978). Synthetic peptides comprising sequences of the human IgE heavy chain capable of releasing histamine. Submitted for publication

Stokes, C. R., Taylor, B. and Turner, M. W. (1974). Assocation of house dust and grass pollen allergies with specific IgA antibody deficiency. *Lancet*, ii, 485

Stokes, C. R. and Turner, M. W. (1975). Isolation and characterization of cat allergens. *Clin. Allergy*, 5, 241

Tada, T. (1975). Regulation of reaginic antibody formation in animals. *Prog. Allergy*, 19, 122

Takatsu, K. and Ishizaka, K. (1977). Reaginic antibody formation in the mouse. IX. Enhancement of suppressor and helper cell activities of primed spleen cells. *J. Immun.*, 118, 151

Taylor, B., Norman, A. P., Orgel, H. A., Stokes, C. R., Turner, M. W. and Soothill, J. F. (1973). Transient IgA deficiency and pathogenesis of infantile atopy. *Lancet*, ii, 111

Thomas, W. R., Watkins, M. C. and Asherson, G. L. (1978). Reaginic antibody to contact sensitising agents. Occurrence of cells which suppress IgG and not reagin responses. *Immunology*, (in press)

Yount, W. J., Dormer, M. M., Kunkel, H. G. and Kabat, E. A. (1968). Studies on human antibodies. VI. Selective variations in subgroup composition and genetic markers. *J. exp. Med.*, 127, 633

11
Tolerance in delayed hypersensitivity

Ladislav Polak
(Pharma Research Department, F. Hoffmann-La Roche & Co., Ltd,
Basle, Switzerland)

Specific immunological unresponsiveness, called tolerance, has been described in almost all immunological systems (Katz and Benacerraf, 1974; Howard and Mitchison, 1975; Nossal, 1974). It is of interest that the demonstration of tolerance in delayed hypersensitivity was one of the earliest to be reported (Sulzberger, 1929; Chase, 1946). Burnet's formulation of the clonal selection theory (Burnet and Fenner, 1949) and Medawar's (1958) concept of clonal deletion initiated a flood of experimental research that resulted in the general acceptance of a unifying theory of tolerance as an annihilation of the immunocompetent specific cells which was thought to be valid for all immunological systems.

This unifying theory of tolerance is, however, difficult to accept since immune responses, in general, are not affected by one single mechanism, since different immune reactions realised by different mechanisms can hardly be controlled by one and the same mechanism. Recently it was shown that besides the deletion of the competent lymphocytes (negative tolerance), an activation of specific suppressor elements such as enhancing antibodies (Voisin, 1971), suppressor cells (Droege, 1973) or antigen-antibody complexes (Hellström and Hellström, 1974) was able to suppress the existing, or prevent the induction of, an immune hypersensitivity state (positive tolerance). Moreover, Turk et al. (1972) have shown that such an activation of suppressor elements also occurs under conditions of conventional immunisation and does not require special conditions such as dose and route of antigen application or immunological incompetence of the animals.

In view of the complexity of the problem of specific unresponsiveness, I have chosen for the present study tolerance to DNCB (dinitrochlorobenzene) contact sensitivity in guinea pigs to illustrate one of the mechanisms responsible for the phenomenon of tolerance, namely suppressor cells.

In this system tolerance is induced by an i.v. (intravenous) application of dinitrobenzenesulphonic acid (sodium salt; $DNBSO_3$) (Turk and Stone, 1963; Frey et al., 1964). Animals treated in such a way failed to respond to a sensitising attempt performed 14 days later. The assumption that this tolerance is based

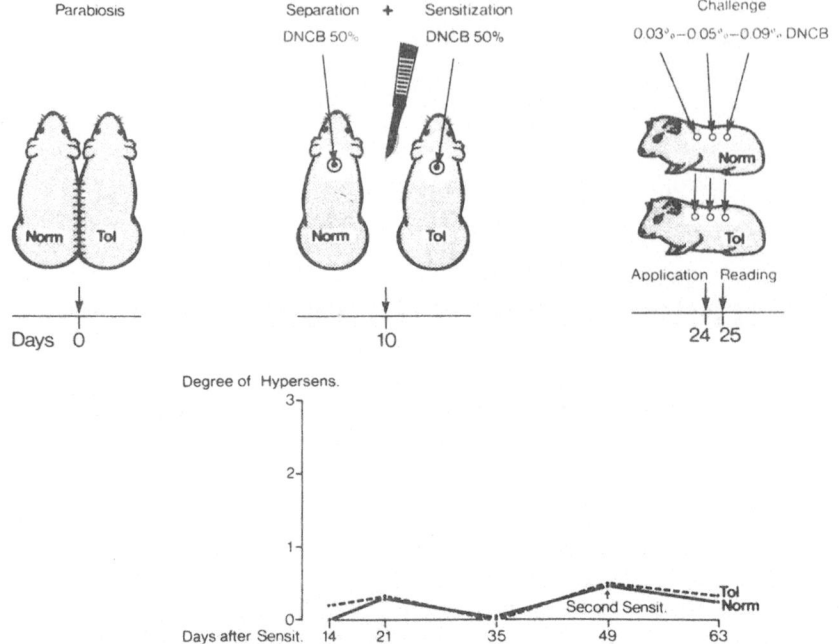

Figure 11.1 Transfer of tolerance by parabiosis
Tolerant (tol.) and normal (norm.) syngeneic guinea pigs were united by a skin-to-skin anastomosis for 10 days and sensitised immediately after separation. Animals were challenged 14, 21 and 35 days later. A second attempt at sensitisation was performed 49 days later and a second challenge 14 days after the second sensitising attempt.

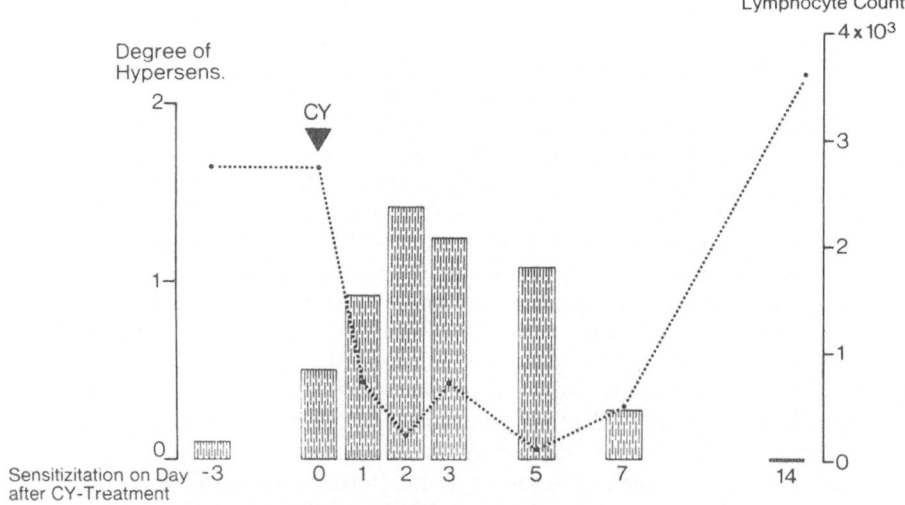

Figure 11.2 Reversal of tolerance by CY treatment
Tolerant guinea pigs were injected with 250 mg of CY/kg i.p. and sensitised at the same time or 1, 2, 3, 5, 7 or 14 days after or 3 days before the CY treatment and challenged 14 days later. Columns represent the degree of hypersensitivity and the dotted line the number of lymphocytes in mm³ in the peripheral blood.

on suppressor cells rests on two main facts. (1) Transfer of tolerance from tolerant to normal partners. (2) Reversal of tolerance by cyclophosphamide (CY) treatment known to eliminate suppressor cells.

Transfer of tolerance to DNCB contact sensitivity in guinea pigs was achieved with lymph node or spleen cells. This unresponsiveness was, however, only partial (Polak, 1976). A complete and stable tolerance was transferred in our system only by parabiosis (Polak, 1975). Pairs of syngeneic guinea pigs, one normal and one tolerant, were united by a skin-to-skin anastomosis for 10 days and sensitised at the time of separation (figure 11.1). Both partners became completely tolerant. According to the clonal deletion theory the results should have been the opposite.

Turk *et al.* (1972) have shown that CY given shortly before immunisation enhanced the resulting degree of contact sensitivity by elimination of the precursors of suppressor cells. The same treatment reversed the state of specific unresponsiveness in animals made previously tolerant by an i.v. injection of DNBSO$_3$ (figure 11.2). Since suppressor cells were already activated in these animals one has to accept that, in this case, active suppressor cells were eliminated by CY treatment (Polak and Turk, 1974; Polak and Geleick, 1975). It was therefore of interest to investigate whether in this system precursors of suppressor cells can also be eliminated by CY treatment.

Normal guinea pigs were treated with CY and 3 days later injected i.v. with the tolerogenic DNBSO$_3$. Under these conditions, however, the animals remained tolerant independent of whether the sensitising attempt was performed immediately

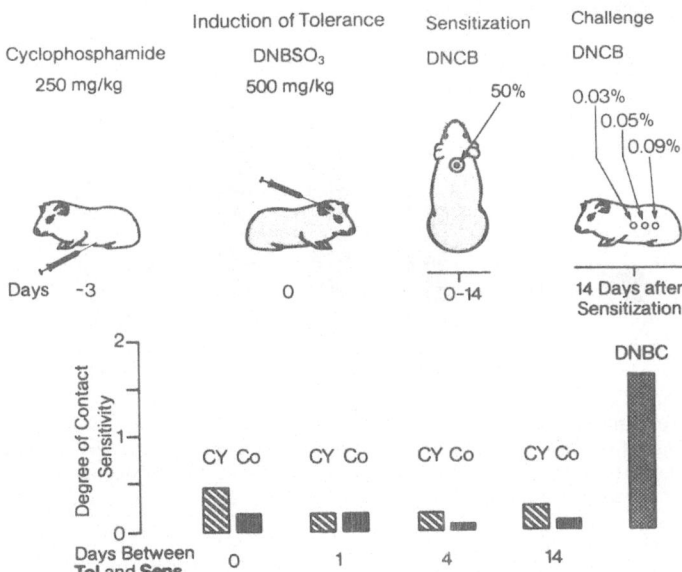

Figure 11.3 Attempt to prevent induction of tolerance by pretreatment with CY
Normal guinea pigs were injected i.p. with 250 mg of CY/kg and 3 days later i.v. with 500 mg of DNBSO$_3$/kg. Sensitising attempt with DNCB e.c. was performed either at the day of the i.v. injection of DNBSO$_3$ or 1, 4 or 14 days later. Non-CY-pretreated animals served as controls (Co). All animals were challenged 14 days after the sensitising attempt and the skin reaction was evaluated 24 h later.

after the induction of tolerance or several days later (figure 11.3). This result agrees
with the finding of Miller *et al.* (1977) in mice and indicates a certain difference between suppressor cells activated by the antigen during a conventional sensitisation
and suppressor cells activated by the tolerogen during induction of tolerance.

Little is known about the nature and mode of action of suppressor cells in guinea
pig contact sensitivity. In contact sensitivity in mice, it has been shown that several
types of suppressor cells exist. They are either of the T or of the B type and some
of them are CY sensitive and others CY resistant (Asherson *et al.*, 1977). However,
contact sensitivity in mice is different from contact sensitivity in guinea pigs (and in
man) in several aspects and therefore all analogies between the mechanism of contact
sensitivity in these two species should only be made with great reservation.

That the main activity of suppressor cells in guinea pig contact sensitivity is on
the afferent part of the immune response is evident from the following experiments. (1) The proliferation of the paracortical area of the draining lymph nodes
which is a common feature in the process of sensitisation does not occur in tolerant
guinea pigs (Turk, 1965). (2) Lymphoid cells from hypersensitive syngeneic donors
are not inhibited in their function when transferred to tolerant recipients either by
an i.v. transfusion or by parabiosis (figures 11.4 and 11.5) (Polak *et al.*, 1974; Polak,
1975). On the contrary, tolerance is reversed when tolerant guinea pigs are parabiosed

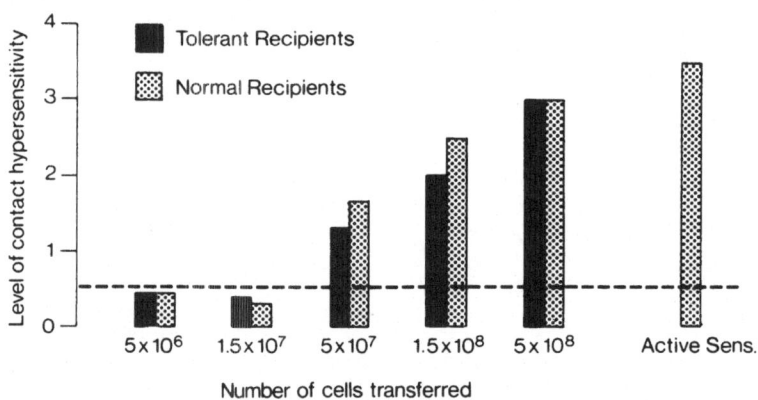

Figure 11.4   Termination of tolerance by transfer of cells from hypersensitive donors
Various numbers of peritoneal exudate cells from strongly DNCB contact-sensitive guinea pigs
were injected i.v. into normal or tolerant syngeneic recipients. The recipients were skin-challenged
14 days after the transfer.

with sensitised partners. (3) Moreover, CY applied to sensitised guinea pigs 3 days
before a skin challenge neither suppressed nor enhanced the intensity of the resulting
skin reaction (Polak and Rinck, 1977). Since CY eliminates suppressor cells without
affecting the activity of effector cells this result somehow excludes the effect of
suppressor cells on the efferent branch of this immune response.

The predominantly afferent effect of suppressor cells in contact sensitivity has also been demonstrated by Claman's group in contact sensitivity in mice (Phanuphak *et al*., 1974; Moorehead, 1976). However, under certain conditions suppressor cells may also affect the activity of effector cells in guinea pigs (Parker *et al*., 1976) and in mice (Asherson and Zembala, 1974). Whether suppressor cells affecting the afferent or the efferent part of the immune response in guinea pigs belong to the same type is not yet decided. In mice it has been shown that they are different.

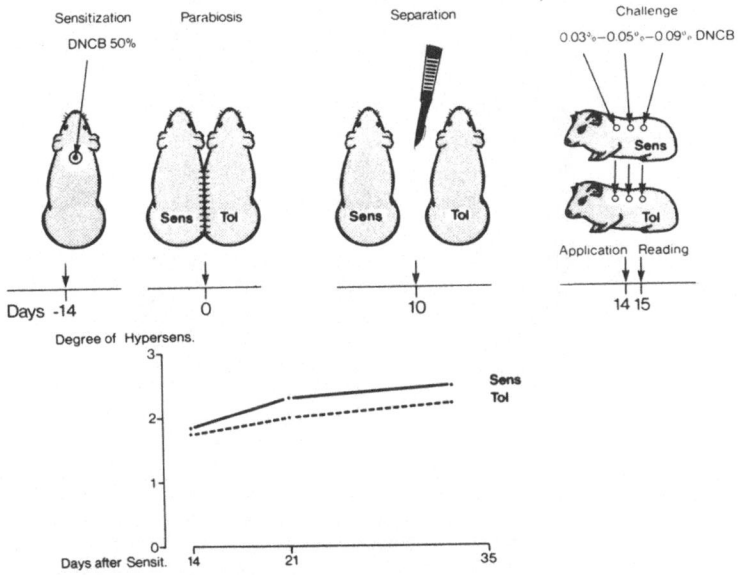

Figure 11.5   Transfer of DNCB contact sensitivity from hypersensitive to tolerant partners by parabiosis
Contact sensitive and tolerant syngeneic guinea pigs were united by a skin-to-skin anastomosis for 10 days and skin-challenged 14 days after separation.

An interesting feature of suppressor cells in tolerant guinea pigs is their persistence. Whereas in mice tolerance, as well as contact sensitivity, are relatively short-lasting phenomena, in guinea pigs a spontaneous disappearance of sensitivity and of tolerance are seen only as an exception. Guinea pigs injected i.v. with $DNBSO_3$ are resistant to contact sensitisation performed 6 or 12 months later. Moreover, active suppressor cells eliminated by CY treatment, 6 or 12 months after the induction of tolerance are still able to regenerate in about 14 days (figure 11.6). At that time the tolerogenic $DNBSO_3$ is almost completely eliminated from the organism. This would indicate that the renewal of suppressor activity is not tolerogen-dependent. To confirm this hypothesis, the following experiments were performed. It was established that in the blood the last traceable amount of $DNBSO_3$ was detected not later than 3 months after the induction of tolerance (table 11.1). Tolerance, however, could be transferred by parabiosis even 6 months after its induction (figure 11.7). In such a

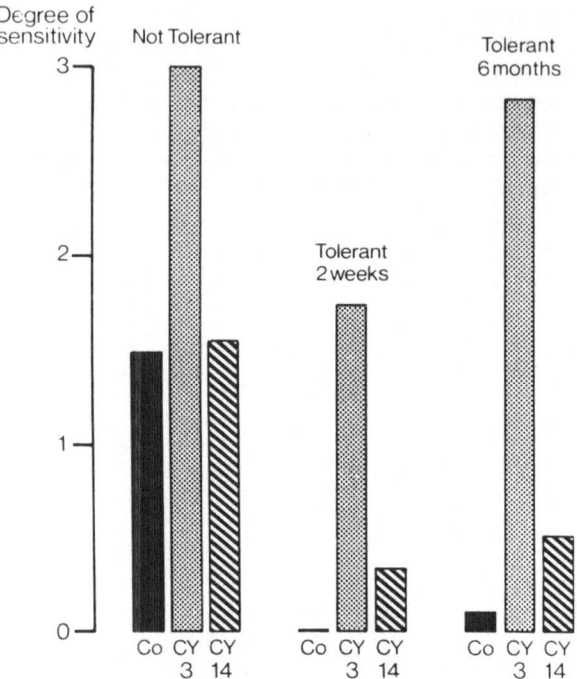

Figure 11.6 Reversal of tolerance and regeneration of suppressor cells after CY treatment
Normal guinea ɾigs or guinea pigs made tolerant by two i.v. injections of DNBSO₃ 2 weeks or
6 months before were injected i.p. with 250 mg of CY/kg. All animals were sensitised e.c. with
DNCB 3 (CY 3) or 14 (CY 14) days later, challenged 14 days after the sensitising procedure and
the skin reaction was evaluated after 24 h. Non-CY-treated animals served as controls (Co).

Table 11.1 Elimination of DNBSO$_3$ from the blood after
two i.v. injections of 500 mg/kg

No. of animals	Months after i.v. injection	DNBSO$_3$ (ng/50 μl of blood)
8	1	117 ± 11
8	2	71 ± 7
8	3	2.9 ± 0.14
8	4	0
8	6	0

A group of eight guinea pigs was injected with 500 mg of radioactive DNBSO₃ per kg
(specific radioactivity 50 μCi/mg) twice with a 14 days' interval. A sample (50 μl) of
blood was taken from the ear vein 1, 2, 3, 4 and 6 months after the last i.v. injection
and the content of DNBSO₃ was estimated. The lowest detectable amount of DNBSO₃
was 1.5 ng/50μl of blood. Values are means ± s.d. for eight animals.

way, animals were obtained that were made tolerant without actually seeing the tolerogen. As one would expect, it was possible to reverse this tolerance by CY treatment, as it was in the tolerance actively induced by an i.v. injection of $DNBSO_3$ (figure 11.8). Under these conditions suppressor cells were able to regenerate in about 2 to 3 weeks after CY treatment without any further contact with the antigen or tolerogen.

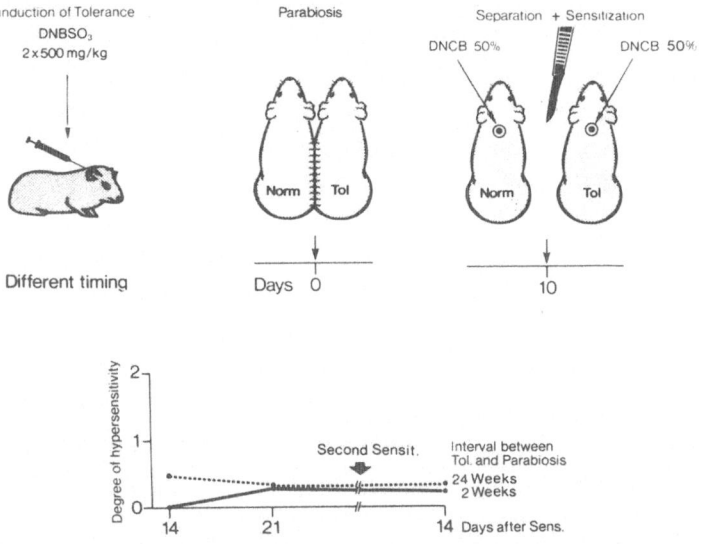

Figure 11.7 Transfer of tolerance by parabiosis 2 or 24 weeks after induction of tolerance Guinea pigs rendered tolerant to DNCB by two i.v. injections of $DNBSO_3$ 2 or 24 weeks before were united by a skin-to-skin anastomosis with normal syngeneic partners. The parabiosed pairs were separated 10 days later, sensitised e.c. with DNCB at the day of separation and challenged 14 and 21 days after the sensitising attempt. A second sensitising attempt with DNCB was performed 2 weeks later followed by a challenge after 14 days. Skin reactions were read 24 h after the challenges.

There are at least three ways of explaining this regeneration of suppressor cell activity under conditions of an evident absence of tolerogen. (1) For the activation of precursors of suppressor cells a relatively high dose of tolerogen is necessary. By its application, in analogy to the process of sensitisation, two populations of suppressor cells are formed. Active suppressors which prevent sensitisation and memory cells of suppression which are able to produce, on request, new active suppressor cells without any further antigenic or tolerogenic stimulus. These memory cells, however, have no suppressor effect. In contrast to active suppressors, which are CY sensitive, memory cells of suppression, as well as their precursors, are CY resistant. These memory cells are then transferred together with active suppressors by parabiosis and are able to produce new active suppressor cells when the transferred generation is eliminated by CY in recipients.

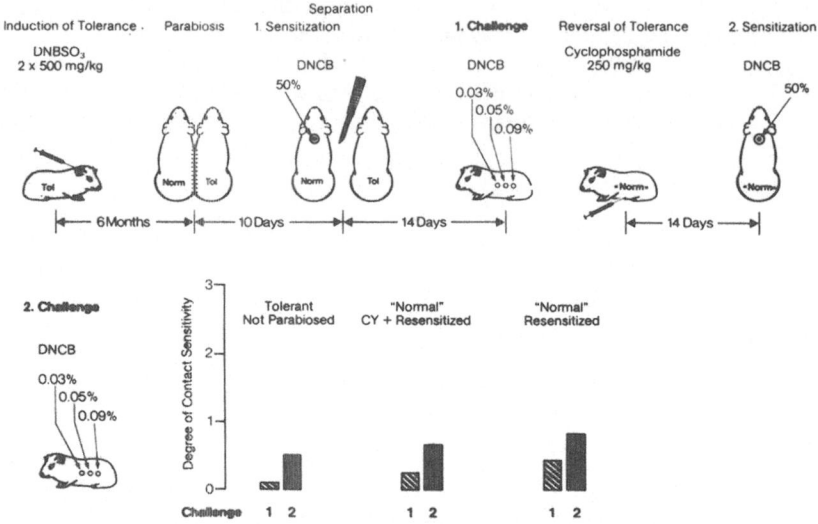

Figure 11.8   Regeneration of suppressor cells after CY treatment in guinea pigs made tolerant
by parabiosis with partners tolerised 6 months before
Guinea pigs tolerant to DNCB contact sensitivity were parabiosed with normal partners 6
months after the induction of tolerance. The parabiosed pairs were separated 10 days later,
sensitised e.c. with DNCB at the day of separation, challenged e.c. with DNCB (1. challenge)
and divided into two groups. One group was injected i.p. with 250 mg of CY/kg, the other one
remained untreated. Both groups were sensitised e.c. with DNCB 14 days later and challenged
14 days after sensitisation (2. challenge). No difference between conventionally tolerised,
tolerised by parabiosis and tolerised by parabiosis and CY-treated groups could be observed.

(2) It might, however, be possible that the CY treatment does not eliminate all
active suppressor cells and that the suppressor activity is restored by multiplication
and division of those not fully destroyed suppressor cells. This hypothesis does not
require the existence of a special population of memory cells of suppression. However, it presumes the existence of both a CY-resistant and CY-sensitive subpopulation of active suppressor cells.

(3) There is, however, a third possibility based on the recent discovery of the
role of macrophages in contact sensitivity. Activation of precursors of suppressor
cells may possibly require stimulator cells, which are formed by the processing of
the tolerogen by blood monocytes. These stimulator cells may contain undetect-
able amounts of tolerogen and secure a continuous stimulation of specific precursors
of suppressor cells. A precondition would be that these stimulator cells of suppression would be CY-resistant and would be transferred by parabiosis to normal
recipients making them tolerant.

Further evidence that tolerance in contact sensitivity is mediated by cellular
mechanism was revealed by experiments attempting to induce tolerance in offspring
by tolerisation of their mothers. Offspring of guinea pigs tolerised before pregnancy
were sensitised as normal. Since non-cellular elements of the blood, for example antibodies but not leucocytes, are capable of passing the placental barrier, this result

a)

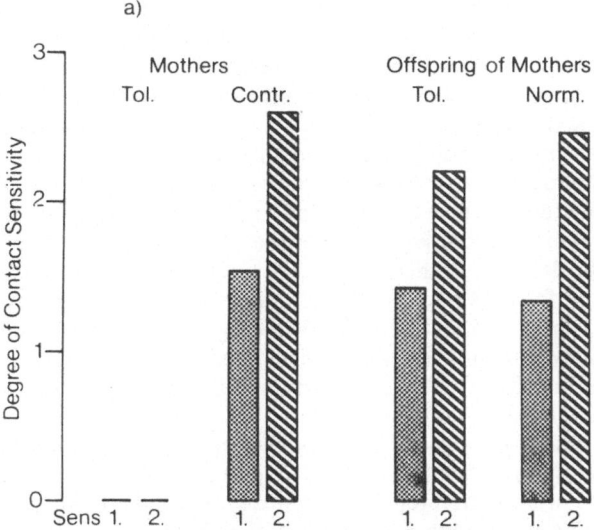

Figure 11.9a Transfer of tolerance during pregnancy: (a) Mothers tolerised before pregnancy
Female guinea pigs were rendered tolerant by two i.v. injections of DNBSO$_3$ and 14 days later
made pregnant. Both mothers and offspring were sensitised e.c. with DNCB 1 month after
birth, challenged 14 days later, resensitised after 1 week and challenged again 14 days later.
No difference between offspring of tolerant (Tol.) and control (Contr.) mothers could be
observed.

b)

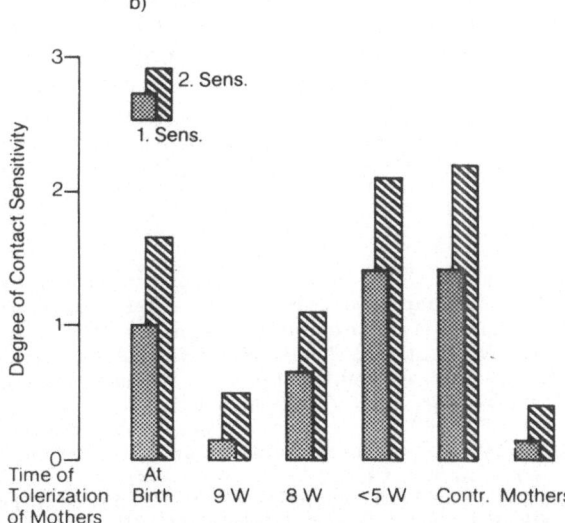

Figure 11.9b Transfer of tolerance during pregnancy: (b) Mothers tolerised during pregnancy
Guinea pigs at different stages of pregnancy were injected i.v. with 500 mg of DNBSO$_3$/kg and
both mothers and offspring sensitised with DNCB 1 month after birth, challenged 14 days later,
resensitised after 1 week and challenged again 14 days later.

indicated that transfer of tolerance cannot be accomplished when cells cannot pass the barrier (figure 11.9a). On the other hand, offspring of mothers tolerised during week 9 of pregnancy, just before birth, were completely tolerant (figure 11.9b). In this case, the unresponsiveness was not transferred from mothers to their offspring but rather actively induced in foetuses by the tolerogen that passed the placental barrier. This induction of tolerance requires a certain state of immunological maturity of the foetuses. Offspring of guinea pigs tolerised in week 8 of pregnancy were only partially tolerant and the offspring of mothers tolerised in the earlier period of pregnancy were not tolerant at all, despite the fact that a certain level of the tolerogen could be detected in their blood. This indicates that for the induction of unresponsiveness in foetuses two factors are important: the immunological maturity and the level of tolerogen in the foetuses. Offspring of mothers tolerised earlier than week 8 of pregnancy were not tolerant because the level of tolerogen at the time of their immunological maturity, i.e. later than week 8 of pregnancy, decreased below the level required for induction of tolerance.

In conclusion our knowledge about suppressor cells in contact sensitivity in guinea pigs may be summarised by the following hypothesis. In normal guinea pigs, specific precursors of both effector and suppressor cells are present which themselves do not exhibit any immunological functions. Both these subpopulations can be activated by a contact with the specific antigen. Depending on the dose of the antigen, the route of its application and the immunological state of the animals the activation of either effector or suppressor cells is favoured, resulting on one hand in a state of hyperimmunisation and on the other hand in tolerance.

In tolerant animals the activity of suppressor cells leads to a prevention of the generation of effector cells. Active effector cells are, however, to a large extent resistant to the inhibitory effects of suppressor cells. Stimulation of precursors of suppressor cells requires the tolerogen to be present at a certain high level. If this condition is fulfilled besides active suppressor cells, memory cells of suppression are generated. These cells are capable of generating active suppressor cells which continuously keep animals tolerant for an unlimited period of time. They are also able to restore the tolerant state when active suppressor cells have been eliminated, for instance by CY treatment. Memory cells of suppression are CY-resistant.

REFERENCES

Asherson, G. L. and Zembala, M. (1974). Suppression of contact sensitivity by T cells in the mouse. 1.Demonstration that suppressor cells act on the effector stage of contact sensitivity; and their induction following *in vitro* exposure to antigen. *Proc. R. Soc. B.*, **197**, 320

Asherson, G. L., Mayhew, B., Pereira, M., Thomas, W. R., Wood, P. and Zembala, M. (1977). Distinct suppressor cells which act at different stages of the immune response to contact sensitizing agents in the mouse. *Scand. J. Immun.*, **6**, 677

Burnet, F. M. and Fenner, F. (1949). *The production of antibodies.* McMillan, Melbourne

Chase, M. W. (1946). Inhibition of experimental drug allergy by prior feeding of the sensitizing agent. *Proc. Soc. exp. Biol. N.Y.*, **61**, 257

Droege, W. (1973) Five questions on the suppressive effect of thymus-derived cells (Part I and Part II). *Current titles in Immunol. Transpl. & Allergy*, 1/4, 95 (Part I) 1/5, 131 (Part II)

Frey, J. R., de Weck, A. L. and Geleick, H. (1964). Immunological unresponsiveness in allergic contact dermatitis to dinitrochlorobenzene in guinea pigs. *J. invest. Derm.*. **42**, 41

Hellström, K. E. and Hellström, I. (1974). Lymphocyte-mediated cytotoxicity and blocking serum activity to tumor antigens. *Adv. Immun.*, **18**, 201

Howard, J. G. and Mitchison, N. A. (1975). Immunological tolerance. *Progr. Allergy*, 18. 43

Katz, D. H. and Benacerraf, B. (eds) (1974). *Immunological tolerance. Mechanisms and potential therapeutic applications*. Academic Press, Inc., New York, San Francisco and London

Medawar, P. B. (1958). The Croonian Lecture. The homograft reaction. *Proc. R. Soc. B.*, 149, 145

Miller, S. D., Sy, M. S. and Claman, H.N. (1977). The induction of hapten-specific T cell tolerance using hapten-modified lymphoid membranes. II. Relative roles of suppressor T cells and clone inhibition in the tolerant state. *Eur. J. Immun.*, 7, 165

Moorhead, J. W. (1976). Tolerance and contact sensitivity to DNFB in mice. VI. Inhibition of afferent sensitivity by suppressor T cells in adoptive tolerance. *J. Immun.*, 117, 802

Nossal, G. J. V. (1974). Principles of immunological tolerance and immunocyte receptor blockade. *Adv. Cancer Res.*, 20, 93

Parker, D., Turk, J. L. and Scheper, R. J. (1976). Central and peripheral action of suppressor cells in contact sensitivity in the guinea pig. *Immunology*, 30, 593

Phanuphak, P., Moorhead, J. W. and Claman, H. N. (1974). Tolerance and contact sensitivity to DNFB in mice. III. Transfer of tolerance with 'suppressor T cells'. *J. Immun.*, 113. 1230

Polak, L. (1975). The transfer of tolerance to DNCB contact sensitivity in guinea pigs by parabiosis. *J. Immun.*, 114, 988

Polak, L. (1976). Studies on the role of suppressor cells in specific unresponsiveness to DNCB. *Immunology*, 31, 425

Polak, L. and Geleick, H. (1975). Differing mechanisms of tolerance and desensitization to DNCB in guinea pigs. *Eur. J. Immun.* 5, 94

Polak, L. and Rinck, C. (1977). Effect of the elimination of suppressor cells on the development of DNCB contact sensitivity in guinea pigs. *Immunology*, 33, 305

Polak, L. and Turk, J.L. (1974). Reversal of immunological tolerance by cyclophosphamide through the inhibition of suppressor cell activity. *Nature*, 249, 654

Polak, L., Geleick, H. and Frey, J. R. (1974). The cellular mechanism of tolerance and desensitization in contact hypersensitivity to DNCB in guinea pigs. In *Contact Hypersensitivity in Experimental Animals* (eds. J. L. Turk and D. Parker), *Monogr. Allergy*, vol. 8, p. 168, Karger Basel.

Sulzberger, M. D. (1929) Hypersensitiveness to neoarsphenamine in guinea pigs. *Archs Derm. Syph. (Chic.)*, 20, 669

Turk, J. L. (1965). An experimental model for the investigation of the cellular bases of desensitization in contact sensitivity. *Int. Archs Allergy*, 28, 105

Turk, J. L. and Stone, S. H. (1963). Implications of the cellular changes in lymph nodes during the development and inhibition of delayed type hypersensitivity. In *Cell-Bound Antibodies*, (eds. Amos and Koprowski). Wistar Inst. Press., Philadelphia, p. 51

Turk, J. L., Parker, D. and Poulter, L. W. (1972). Functional aspects of the selective depletion of lymphoid tissue by cyclophosphamide. *Immunology*, 23, 493

Voisin, G. Y. (1971). Immunological Facilitation, a broadening of a concept of the enhancement phenomenon. *Progr. Allergy*, 15, 328

12

Adverse reactions to practolol

G. E. Davies* (Imperial Chemical Industries Ltd, Pharmaceuticals Division,
Alderley Park, Maccledfield, Cheshire, U.K.)

Practolol was introudced in 1970 as a cardio-selective β-adrenoceptor antagonist.
In 1973 there were two reports of a systemic lupus erythematosus-like syndrome
in a few patients receiving the drug (Assem and Banks, 1973; Raftery and Denman,
1973). During 1974 a hitherto undescribed adverse reaction complex was discerned
(Nicholls, 1976). The main features of this rare syndrome are skin rashes (Felix *et
al.*, 1974), ocular involvement (Wright, 1975) and a sclerosing peritonitis (Brown

Symptoms

Skin rashes:	Psoriasiform eruptions
Ocular involvement:	Hyperaemic conjunctivae
	Reduced tear flow
	Conjunctival scarring
	Fornix obliteration
	Corneal opacification
Impairment of hearing	
Fibrosing polysercsitis of:	Peritoneum
	Pleura
	Pericardium

Effects occur both in isolation and in combination

Effects are unrelated to: Sex (male = female)
Age (60 – 65 years)
Dose (mean 300 mg/day:
1–24 months' treatment)

Disease state

Figure 12.1 Practolol-induced oculomucocutaneous syndrome.

*Present address: Imperial Chemical Industries Ltd., Central Toxicology Laboratory, Alderley
Park, Macclesfield, Cheshire.

et al., 1974) (figure 12.1). This syndrome of adverse reactions is so far unique to practolol and although a variety of minor symptoms and signs have been attributed to other β-blockers there is no reason to associate them to the very specific features of the practolol-induced oculomucocutaneous syndrome — as is shown very forcibly by the fact that many patients suffering from the practolol adverse reaction have been treated with other β-blockers without untoward effect (Nicholls, 1976).

This present paper has a single, well-defined objective in that I intend to review the reported effects of practolol on the immune system of man to see if such effects can offer an explanation of the cause of the untoward practolol syndrome.

ANTINUCLEAR FACTOR (ANF)

The first reported occurrence of ANF in association with the administration of practolol was by Assem and Banks (1973). They described a single patient with skin lesions which fluctuated in quality, being at times psoriasiform and at other lichenoid. Tests for ANF were positive on three occasions and LE (lupus erythematosus) cells were present. Raftery and Denman (1973) examined three patients with symptoms of drug-induced SLE. All three were positive for ANF and LE cells. It is also worth noting at this point that all three had raised ESR (erythrocyte sedimentation rate) values and there was an altered response of their lymphocytes to mitogens (table 12.1)—a remark that will be put into context when I come to discuss the paper by Pugh and his colleagues. Many subsequent authors have reported a high incidence of ANF in association with practolol administration. The syndrome of drug-induced LE associated with administration of practolol has all the features of similar reactions produced by a number of other drugs (procainamide, hydrallazine etc.), but is not related to the practolol oculomucocutaneous syndrome and I will not refer to it again.

Table 12.1 Response to mitogens of lymphocytes from patients treated with practolol (Raftery and Denman, 1973). PHA, phytohaemagglutinin; Con. A, concanavalin A; PWM, pokeweed mitogen.

	MITOGENS		
	PHA	Con A	PWM
Case 1	Normal only to highest concentration	Normal	Normal
Case 2	Depressed	Normal to highest concentration	Depressed
Case 3	Depressed	Depressed	Depressed

OTHER AUTO-ANTIBODIES

Amos *et al.* (1975) demonstrated, by indirect immunofluorescence, deposition of immunoglobulin in the intercellular spaces of squamous allogeneic or xenogeneic tissue treated with sera from patients with specific conjunctival eye signs associated with the administration of practolol. Staining was confined to the intercellular region and was present in 27/29 sera. The authors commented on the possible significance of the fact that the two negative sera came from patients who were still taking practolol at the time of sampling.

No convincing intercellular staining was found in sera from patients who had some kind of skin rash due to practolol, from two patients with a possible LE syndrome thought to be induced by practolol or from those with mucous membrane pemphigoid and concomitant eye damage who had never taken practolol. Sera from all three groups contained ANF, but its titre did not seem to correlate with the level of intercellular antibody (table 12.2). Conjunctival biopsy specimens from

Table 12.2　Antibody titres in sera from three groups of patients (Amos *et al.*, 1975).

	NUMBERS OF SERA WITH TITRE OF:					
Antibody	1/10	1/80	1/60	1/320	1/640	1/1280
Intracellular	3	3	3	7	3	8
Anti-nuclear	7	18	2		2	

three patients with eye damage were shown, by direct immunofluorescence, to have IgG in the intercellular region. The intercellular antibodies were differentiated from similar antibodies found in the sera of patients with pemphigus by the inability of the practolol-associated antibodies to bind to isolated epidermal cells. The authors were unable to come to any conclusion about the association of intercellular antibody and tissue damage; they suggested that the antibody might behave as a cytophilic antibody and attach itself to Fc receptors in target tissue — they also suggested that it might have specificity for antigens such as drug determinants.

Intercellular deposition of immunoglobulin was also found by Rahi *et al.* (1976) not only in the intercellular spaces of acanthotic epithelium, corneal epithelium and lens epithelium of patients with eye damage but also in the intercellular spaces of the squamous epithelium of buccal mucosa, tongue, oesophagus and skin, where there was no associated tissue damage. They were unable to find C3 in ocular tissue and concluded that the deposited antibodies were not cytotoxic and that the formation of auto-antibodies in patients with practolol-induced eye disease is more likely to be secondary to epithelial damage than its cause.

Table 12.3　Deposition of IgM, IgC and C3 in dermo-epidermal junction (Dahl *et al.*, 1975).

Positive in lesional skin only	7
Positive in lesional and non-lesional skin	5
No deposits	7
19 patients	

Dahl *et al.* (1975) demonstrated granular deposits of IgM, IgG and C3 in the dermo–epidermal junction (DEJ) of lesional skin in 12/19 patients with psoriasiform and lichenoid skin lesions. Incidentally eight patients had circulating ANF and all of them had DEJ deposits in lesional skin—five of the eight had deposits also in non-lesional skin. However, seven patients had neither circulating ANF nor DEJ deposits (table 12.3) yet they did not differ clinically from the others; four of these seven reacted positively when challenged with practolol. Behan *et al.* (1976) carried out an extensive series of immunological tests in five groups of patients: (i) 15 in whom either skin or skin and eye lesions developed during practolol therapy; (ii) three with sclerosing peritonitis; (iii) nine who had been on practolol for 2 years but had shown no adverse reaction; (iv) five who had been on practolol for 3–6 months and (v) 35 healthy controls. They found intercellular antibody in 2/15 patients in group (i); 2/3 in group (ii) and 3/9 in group (iii) (table 12.4). Other autoantibodies appeared to be raised in patients given practolol but here again there was no obvious relationship between their presence and tissue damage (table 12.4).

Table 12.4   Presence of intercellular antibody in five groups of patients (Behan *et al.*, 1976).

Intercellular antibody	
Patient	Proportion positive
Eye or eye and skin lesions	2/15
Sclerosing peritonitis	2/3
Long-term practolol: no side effects	3/9
Healthy controls	0/35

Auto-antibodies were also studied by Garner and Rahi (1976) and by Jachuck *et al.* (1977). A synthesis of the findings of these three groups of workers is shown in table 12.5. The only finding to emerge clearly is that there is an increased incidence of antinuclear antibody (ANA) in patients given practolol but there is no clear evidence of agreed association between the incidence of this antibody and tissue damage nor is there evidence of such a relationship for the other auto-antibodies (tables 12.4 and 12.5).

DEPRESSION OF LYMPHOCYTE FUNCTION

Behan *et al.* (1976) also studied lymphocyte function in the five groups. Full data are presented only for what the authors refer to as 'protein synthesis' which was estimated by the uptake of [^{3}H] leucine by peripheral lymphocytes stimulated with phytohaemagglutinin (PHA) over a 22 h period (table 12.6). Stimulation ratios for 35 healthy controls lay between 2.0 and 3.3; 11/15 patients with lesions had ratios below 2.0 as did the three patients with sclerosing peritonitis. But 5/6 patients who had been on practolol for 2 years without untoward effect also had ratios below 2.0. Again we can see an association between alteration of immune

Table 12.5 Presence of auto-antibodies in various patients

Auto-antibody	Behan et al. (1976)			Garner and Rahi (1976)		Jachuck et al. (1977)	
	Practolol with lesions	Practolol without lesions	Control	Practolol with lesions	Control	Practolol without lesions	Control
Nuclear	50	44	3	50	15	19	4
Smooth muscle	11	11	0	25	16	7	3
Rh. F	39	22	0	0	9	–	–
Parietal cell	10	0	0	0	3	9	6

Table 12.6   Protein synthesis by lymphocytes (Behan *et al.*, 1976).

Patients	Proportion with decreased synthesis
Lesion	11/15
Sclerosing peritonitis	3/3
Practolol − no lesions	5/6
Healthy controls	0/35

function and the administration of practolol, but not with side effects. More conventional lymphocyte-transformation tests were carried out by measuring uptake of [³H] thymidine in response to PHA or streptokinase–streptodornase (SKSD) during 3 or 6 days respectively. No results were given, but the responses are said to be decreased in the patients with eye and skin manifestations, in the three with sclerosing peritonitis and in three of the patients on long-term practolol who did not have untoward reactions. In contrast to these findings, Amos and Brigden (1976) found responses to PHA to be normal in the lymphocytes of 16 patients with severe eye damage, all of whom had not taken practolol for some months.

Pugh *et al.* (1976) defined depressed lymphocyte responses as subnormal responses to one or more mitogens. They were able to correlate this depression only with a raised ESR and not with either practolol administration or the presence of ANA (table 12.7). Following this study, 20 consecutive patients were tested; four developed untoward effects but only one showed any evidence of depression of lymphocyte function and even here the relationship between treatment with practool and the patients disease was said to be uncertain.

Behan *et al.* (1976) also carried out skin tests to the common antigens *Candida albicans* and SKSD: 12 of 15 of the patients with side effects did not respond to *C. albicans*, 12 did not respond to SKSD and 9 did not respond to either antigen. Unfortunately the authors did not carry out skin tests in the group of nine on long-term practolol, without side effects, so it is not possible to assess the significance of their findings in terms of untoward effects.

Table 12.7   Lymphocyte response to mitogens (Pugh *et al.*, 1976).

Patients	% with depressed lymphocyte response			
	ANF negative		ANF positive	
	ESR < 20 mm/h	ESR > 20 mm/h	ESR < 20 mm/h	ESR > 20 mm/h
Not on practolol	16 (3/18)	53 (7/13)	0 (0.3)	0 (0/2)
On practolol	16 (6/36)	64 (11/17)	23 (3/13)	45 (5/11)

Total on practolol: 32% depressed
Total not on practolol: 26% depressed

RESULTS OF CHALLENGE TESTS

One of the explanations suggested for the untoward effects resulting from practolol treatment is that they represent an allergic reaction to practolol, or to some metabolite. The diagnosis of drug allergy is exceedingly difficult to carry out by laboratory test and often the only sure procedure is to challenge the patient with the suspected drug. Naturally, such challenge tests have been carried out with practolol, but there again the results are equivocal if we attempt to interpret them in terms of drug allergy.

Assem and Banks (1973) gave practolol i.d. (intradermally) to a patient with a skin rash and found that it produced a 10 mm lesion after 48 h. Felix *et al.* (1974) produced a positive result to a patch test in 1/14 patients with skin lesions but it is not clear from their paper what was used for challenge — pure practolol 50 per cent and 10 per cent in yellow soft paraffin or the 'injectable form made up in propylene glycol at 50% and 10%'; 3/13 showed a reaction to 0.05 μg of practolol injected i.d. in 0.05 ml, but again no detail is provided. The same authors challenged with oral practolol given daily until untoward effects were reported; nine patients reported after 36 h, 1 after 4 days and 1 after 5 days. Each patient first reported itching followed by the appearance of an erythematous macular eruption 4 h after taking one 100 mg tablet. Felix *et al.* (1974) concluded, however, 'we have probably excluded immediate and delayed-type allergies'. Mikkelsen (1974) found a reaction to oral challenge after 1 day: patch test with 5 per cent practolol was negative. The same author with co-workers (Mikkelsen *et al.*, 1975) reported recurrence of skin changes 0.5 to 3 days after daily oral challenge. I.d. tests with practolol 0.5–5 per cent in 10 patients gave an atypical positive response. In a report of a patient with exfoliative dermatitis who experienced intense itching within 5 days of the re-start of practolol treatment, Kauppinen *et al.* (1976) remarked that the interval between challenge and eruption was very long for a drug eruption and they also commented that the histological changes were unlike those of any other drug eruption.

IMMUNE MECHANISMS DIRECTED AGAINST THE DRUG

Only one claim has been made of a positive lymphocyte transformation to practolol (Assem and Banks, 1973). Negative results with practolol, des-acetyl practolol and des-isopropyl practolol are reported by Behan *et al.* (1976) and to practolol and practolol–albumin conjugates by Amos and Brigden (1976).

Some very interesting work has been carried out by Amos and his collaborators (Amos *et al.*, 1977, 1978) on antibodies apparently specific for a metabolite of practolol. Both these papers describe the use of a microsomal mixed-function oxidase complex *in vitro* (figure 12.2) to generate metabolites and link them to a protein present at the time of their formation. In the earlier paper microsomal fractions from rat liver were used and the carrier protein was a rabbit non-agglutinating antibody to human 0 erythrocytes. The reaction mixture, after incubation, was centrifuged and the supernatant, containing the putative antigen, used in an agglutination assay (figure 12.3). Four of six sera from patients with severe adverse effects due to practolol agglutinated the treated cells in the presence of anti-μ. There was no corresponding agglutination with sera from patients given practolol who were without side effects or from a control group, matched for age and medical disability, who had not received practolol (table 12.8). Marked inhibition of the response was obtained

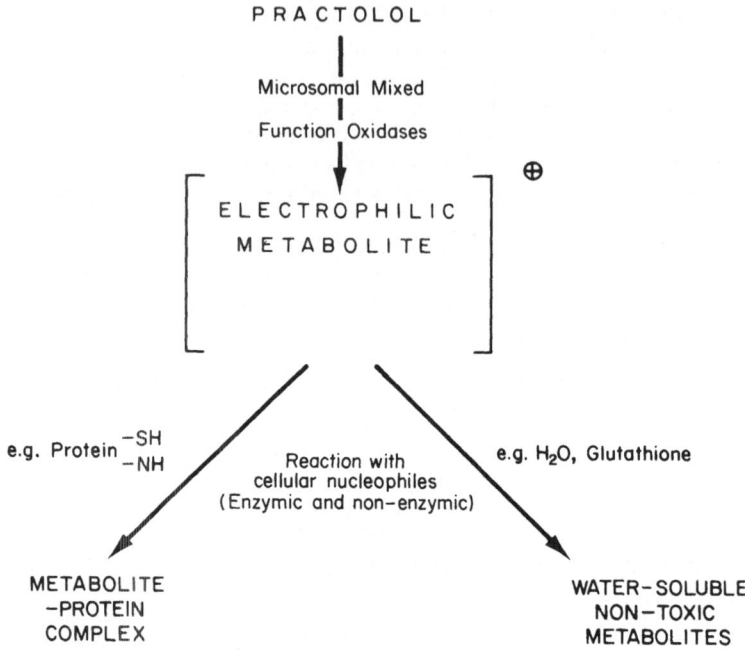

Figure 12.2 Formation of practolol-derived antigen.

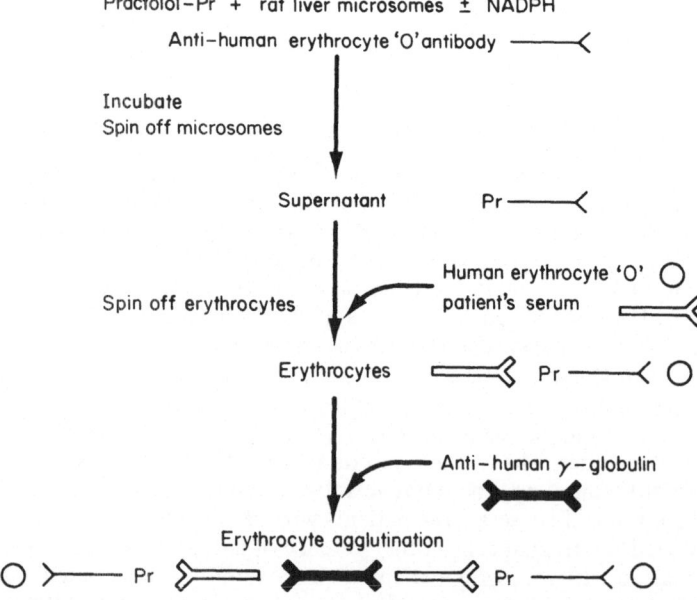

Figure 12.3 Demonstration of antibodies to practolol metabolite in serum of patients with severe reaction.

Table 12.8 Anti-practolol antibody and auto-antibodies (Amos *et al.*, 1977).

Patient no.	Haemagglutination titre (anti-μ)	Auto-antibody	
		ANA	IC
1	128	80	Negative
2	356	Negative	Negative
3	712	20	Negative
4	2	80	1280
5	8	640	1280
6	128	160	Negative

when antisera were preincubated with the microsomal antigen reagent and there was partial inhibition by practolol, its des-acetyl and des-isopropyl derivatives and diol derivatives. The intriguing observation was made that the sera from the two patients with side effects, although not containing antibody, nevertheless gave significant titres of the intercellular antibody (it is not stated whether or not the patients had recently received practolol since its presence in the sera could be an alternative explanation for the apparent absence of antibody). The second paper confirms and extends these observations. A slightly different system was used: hamster microsomes were used since they are metabolically more active than those of the rat (Orton and Lowery, 1977) and ^{125}I-labelled human serum albumin was used as the carrier protein and antibody was estimated by Farr's ammonium sulphate method (table 12.9). All of 28 sera from patients with side effects precipitated more than 10 per cent of the added antigen at a dilution of 1:10 as did 10 or 15 patients who had been treated with practolol but had no adverse effects (again it is not stated whether or not these patients were still receiving the drug). The level of antibody could be increased by challenge of the patient with oral practolol. The very high potency of some of the antisera is particularly impressive – one serum precipitated nearly 50 per cent of the added antigen at a dilution of 1:100.

Table 12.9 Presence of antibody in sera from various patients (Amos *et al.*, 1978).

Patients	Proportion of 1/10 sera precipitating > 10% antigen
Adverse effect (practolol)	28/28
No adverse effect (practolol)	9/15
Other β-blocker – no adverse effect	0/10
Controls (no β blocker)	0/21

Unfortunately no quantitative results for the amount of antigen added or the degree of binding are given. The nature of the antigen is unknown, but from studies by Orton and his colleagues the 3-hydroxy derivative is a likely candidate but this substance is a very minor metabolite of practolol, 74–90 per cent of which is excreted unchanged (Case *et al.*, 1978) (figure 12.4).

It is virtually impossible to derive any meaningful conclusion from these various studies on the immunology of the practolol syndrome. Very few of the findings have received independent confirmation. Many difficulties of interpretation stem from the many variables inherent in the problem, nature of side effect, age and medical disability, period on (and off) the drug and so on. Nor is interpretation

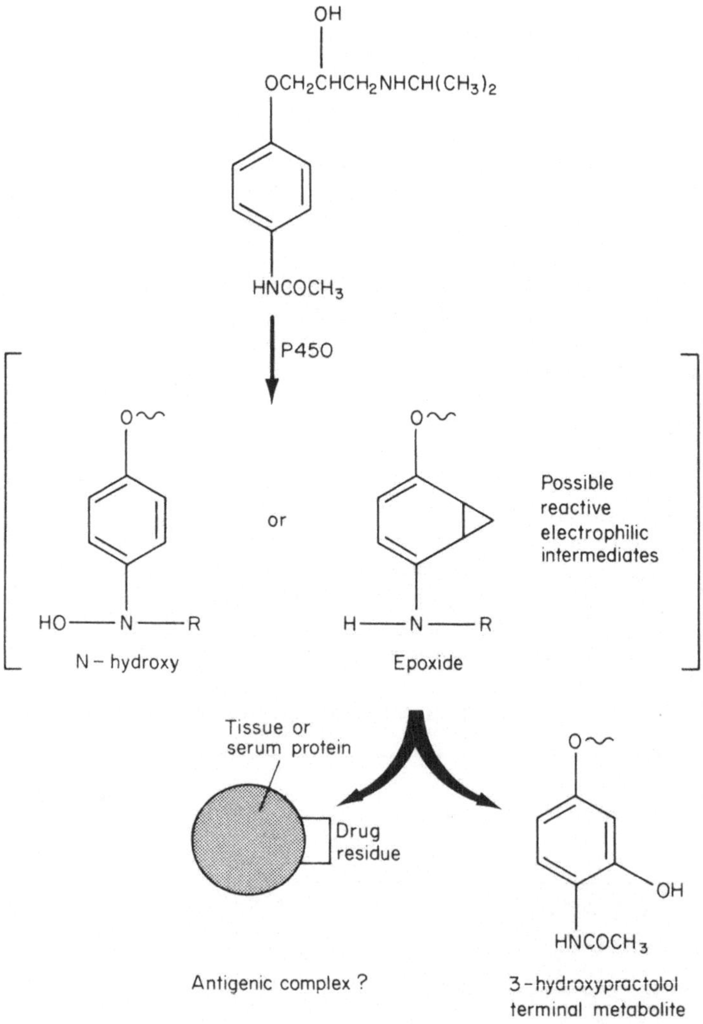

Figure 12.4 Reaction mechanism of practolol.

helped by differences in technique, or inadequate description of technique or failure to provide important information or the use of inappropriate controls or their complete absence.

The most important aspect is the association, if any, between the immunological phenomena and tissue damage produced by practolol administration. Most of the reported changes are also seen in patients who have taken practolol without untoward effect. This, of course, could have two explanations; either the change is not related to damage or damage has not yet become overt. It also seems possible that some of the changes are a consequence of the damage rather than its cause.

A naive and simplistic view might account for most of the reported phenomena. From first principles it is not surprising that antibodies are produced to drugs or their metabolites: the situation with penicillin is well known and antibodies to procaine amide have been demonstrated in a high proportion of people taking the drug (Russell and Ziff, 1968). But no evidence has been produced that they are the cause of tissue damage (with the possible exception of reaginic antibodies to penicillin) and the pathology of the practolol syndrome is not that of an allergic reaction. Secondly, it is not entirely unexpected that auto-antibodies appear in response to marked tissue damage of the kind seen.

REFERENCES

Amos, H. E. and Brigden, W. D. (1976). Immunological changes and practolol. *Lancet*, ii, 1298

Amos, H. E., Brigden, W. D. and McKerron, R. A. (1975). Untoward effects associated with practolol: demonstration of antibody binding to epithelial tissue. *Br. med. J.*, I, 598

Amos, H. E., Lake, B. G. and Atkinson, H. A. C. (1977). Allergic drug reactions; an *in vitro* model using a mixed function oxidase complex to demonstrate antibodies with specificity for a practolol metabolite.

Amos, H. E., Lake, B. G. and Artis, J. (1978). Possible role of antibody specific for a practolol metabolite in the pathogenesis of oculomucocutaneous syndrome. *Br. med. J.*, I, 402

Assem, E. S. K. and Banks, R. A. (1973). Practolol induced drug eruption. *Proc. R. Soc. Med.*, 66, 179

Behan, P. O., Behan, W. M. H., Zacharias, F. J. and Nicholls, J. T. (1976). Immunological abnormalities in patients who had the oculomucocutaneous syndrome associated with practolol therapy. *Lancet*, ii, 984

Brown, P., Baddeley, H., Read, A. E., Davies, J. D. and McGarry, J. (1974). Sclerosing peritonitis, an unusual reaction to a beta-adrenergic blocking drug (practolol). *Br. med. J.*, I, 598

Case, D. E., Lindup, W. E., Lowery, C., Orton, T. C., Reeve, P. R. and Whittacker, S. L. (1978). Metabolism studies with practolol. Communication to British Pharmacological Society.

Dahl, M. G. C., Felix, R. H., Ive, F. A. and Wilkins, D. S. (1975). Immunologic aspects of practolol-induced lupus erythematosus. *J. invest. Derm.*, 64, 299

Felix, R. H., Ive, F. A. and Dhal, M. G. C. (1974). Cutaneous and ocular reactions to practolol. *Br. med. J.*, 2, 321

Garner, A. and Rahi, A. H. S. (1976). Practolol and ocular toxicity. *Br. J. Ophthal.*, 60, 684

Jachuck, S. J., Stephenson, J., Bird, T., Jackson, F. S. and Clark, F. (1977). Practolol-induced autoantibodies and their relation to oculocutaneous complications. *Postgrad. med. J.*, 53, 75

Kauppinen, K., Niemi, K. M. and Salo, O. P. (1976). Cutaneous reactions to practolol. *Ann. clin. Res.*, 8, 232

Mikkelsen, H. I. (1974). Psoriasiforme hudforandringer under praktol (Eraldin) behandling. *Ugeskr. Laeg.*, 136, 2358

Mikkelsen, H. I., Jensen, H. E., Wadskov, S. and Sondergaard J. (1975). Hud-og ojenforandringer ved langtidshehandling med prakotol (Eraldin). *Ugeskr. Laeg.* 137, 2188

Nicholls, J. T. (1976). Adverse effects of practolol. *Ann. clin. Res.*, 8, 229

Orton, T. C. and Lowery, C. (1977). Irreversible protein binding of [^{14}C]-practolol metabolites to hamster liver microsomes. *Br. J. Pharmac.*, 60, 319P

Pugh, S., Pelton, B., Raftery, E. B. and Denman, A. M. (1976). Abnormal lymphocyte function is secondary to drug-induced autoimmunity. *Ann. rheum. Dis.*, 35, 344

Raftery, E. B. and Denman, A. M. (1973). Systemic lupus erythematous syndrome induced by practolol. *Br. med. J.*, 2, 452

Rahi, A. H. S., Chapman, C. M., Garner, A. and Wright, P. (1976). Pathology of practolol-induced ocular toxicity. *Br. J. Ophthal.*, 60, 312

Russell, A. S. and Ziff, M. (1968). Natural antibodies to procaine amide. *Clin. exp. Immun.*, 3, 901

Wright, P. (1975). Untoward effects associated with practolol administration: Oculomucocutaneous syndrome. *Br. med. J.*, I, 595

13

Approaches to prevention and treatment of drug allergy

Alain L. de Weck (Institute for Clinical Immunology,
University of Bern, Inselspital, Bern, Switzerland)

The problem of allergic reactions to drugs continues to plague patients, physicians and drug manufacturers. Most drug-monitoring studies record about 10 to 15 per cent untoward reactions of hospitalised patients to one or the other drug administered to them; among these 40 to 50 per cent are felt to be of allergic nature (Klein *et al.*, 1972), which leaves us with an overall incidence of about 5 per cent of allergic reactions to drugs in a population of hospitalised patients.

What can be done to remedy this unpleasant situation? Obviously, it is not possible in the frame of this presentation to discuss all aspects of drug allergy; I shall restrict this discussion to some general comments on prevention of drug allergy, with illustrations drawn from our experience. In so doing, we may consider approaches based on the drug itself, i.e. means to make a given drug less allergenic than usual, or on the already allergic patient, namely the prevention of clinical allergic reactions in such individuals.

MODIFICATIONS OF THE ALLERGENIC POTENTIAL FROM DRUGS

To induce an immune response of the immediate or cell-mediated type, most chemotherapeutic agents, as low-molecular-weight compounds, are supposed to bind covalently to autologous proteins and cell-membrane proteins, forming thereby immunogenic conjugates (de Weck, 1971). Whether the binding of the allergenic drug to an autologous carrier molecule always has to be of covalent nature might be doubted, various examples in basic immunology suggest that non-covalent binding to carriers, provided sufficiently strong, is also capable of inducing an antibody response (Green *et al.*, 1966). Accordingly, an allergenic drug should be considered first from two angles, (a) the presence of reactive groups enabling covalent binding to proteins and (b) the presence of structures favouring attachment to cell membranes, especially to macrophages. These considerations are valid not only for the drug itself, but also for its derivatives and its metabolites. Further, they apply

211

to all chemical contaminants of a drug preparation; these may be either biological or chemical side products resulting from the process used in preparation of the drug or additives and preservatives consciously added to the drug. Some examples of allergenic by-products in drug preparations are given in table 13.1. Obviously, a

Table 13.1 Some examples of allergenic by-products
in drug preparations

---

(1) *Reactive derivatives and degradation products*

Benzylpenicillenic acid, benzylpenicilloic acid
in aged penicillin solutions. Penicillin (especially
ampicillin) polymers.

(2) *Reactive metabolites*

Phenetidin and its oxydation products in phenacetin
allergy. Quinones in allergy to compounds of the
'para' group (paraphenylenediamine).

(3) *Reactive chemical impurities as by-products of synthesis*

Acetylsalicylsalicylic acid and acetylsalicylic
anhydride in aspirin.

(4) *Immunogenic biological impurities*

Mycelial proteins in penicillins extracted from broth;
Escherichia coli penicillin amidase in 6-aminopenicillamic
acid used for synthesis of semi-synthetic pencillins

(5) *Additives with immunogenic potential or serving as
inert carriers*

Tartrazine, azodyes, parabens.
Carboxymethylcellulose, starch.

---

thorough immunochemical analysis of all factors and compounds involved in the occurrence of sensitisation to a given drug may suggest preventive measures. For example the elimination of high-molecular-weight impurities of biological origin in penicillin allergy (Batchelor *et al.*, 1967), the prevention of degradation to allergenic derivatives, such as penicillenic or penicilloic acids (de Weck and Eisen, 1960; Levine, 1966) or of the formation of allergenic polymers (de Weck *et al.*, 1968; Dewdney, 1977) by appropriate storage conditions, the minimisation of the forma-tion of allergenic side-products of synthesis such as aspirin anhydride and acetylsali-cylic acid in aspirin allergy (Bundgaard and de Weck, 1975) and the avoidance of potentially allergenic additives such as a number of dyestuffs (for example carboxy-methylcellulose in penicillin preparations). This approach, however, has its limita-tions. In a number of instances, with penicillins or cephalosporins for example, chemically reactive groups responsible for the allergenic potential are also required for the desired pharmacological activity. This is why despite 20 years of intensive research and the synthesis of literally thousands of penicillin and cephalosporin derivatives, it has not been possible, to my knowledge, to produce a totally non-immunogenic penicillin while fully maintaining antibiotic activity. However, there are obviously differences between the degree by which structural modifications of the basic penicillin structure will affect antibiotic activity on the one hand and allergenic potential on the other hand.

When allergy to a drug is not due to the drug itself, but to a metabolite (for example phenetidin in phenacetin allergy), it could appear at first glance that not much can be done about it. However, the fact that metabolic pathways of a drug may vary from one individual to another and also that they can sometimes be influenced by the concomittant administration of another drug or by nutritional and environmental factors should be kept in mind by people concerned with the prevention of drug allergies. Genetic and environmental factors may well be responsible, at least in part, for regional or racial differences in the frequency of allergic reactions to some drugs.

Obviously, allergenic impurities and additives should be removed from drug preparations. How far the increased consciousness about high-molecular-weight impurities in penicillin preparations is responsible for the apparent decline in the incidence of severe allergic reactions to penicillin during the past 5 years (table 13.2) is not entirely clear. Other factors, such as the increased awareness of physicians and patients about penicillin allergy have probably also played a role. Studies form

Table 13.2   Clinical cases of penicillin allergy within two different periods

Main symptoms	1962–1966 (311 cases)	1971–1976 (231 cases)
Urticaria	102 (33)	90 (39)
Anaphylactic shock	59 (19)	8 (3)
Anaphylactoid symptoms		7 (3)
Serum-like disease	43 (14)	6 (3)
Angioneurotic oedema	28 (9)	31 (14)
Generalised exanthema	25 (8)	65 (28)
Contact dermatitis	15 (5)	3 (1)
Blood dyscrasias	13 (4)	4 (2)
Generalised pruritus	6 (2)	7 (3)
Local reactions	7 (2)	4 (2)
Asthma	4 (1)	0 (–)
Miscellaneous	9 (3)	6 (3)

Relative percentages are given in parentheses.

Kristofferson *et al.* (1977), however, suggest that significant amounts of immunogenic high-molecular-weight impurities are still present in most commercial penicillin preparations. Although high-molecular-weight impurities may undoubtedly contribute to penicillin immunogenicity and should therefore be eliminated as far as technically possible, it is my conviction, based on several lines of evidence, that even the purest penicillin obtainable would still be responsible for a significant number of allergic reactions. In fact penicillins remain the most common cause of allergic reactions to a drug.

A problem frequently facing drug manufacturers is the assessment of potential allergenicity of a new drug. In general, considerations of pharmacological efficiency, absorption and pharmacokinetics, as well as toxicological findings, have priority in the assessment of new drugs, and more accurate prediction of the allergenic potential on the basis of animal experiments is still faced with difficulty. However, increasing attention is being paid to this problem and endeavouring to ensure low allergenicity slowly begins to play a role in drug development. Of course, this problem has long been recognised for those drugs primarily used for topical application and potentially inducing contact dermatitis (Magnusson and Kligman, 1970).

PREVENTION OF ALLERGIC REACTIONS BY ACCURATE DIAGNOSIS OF DRUG ALLERGY IN THE ALLERGIC PATIENT

Aside from measures taken by the drug manufacturer, which should lead to the availability of pharmacologically active drugs devoid as much as possible of allergenic potential, the physician may also significantly contribute to the prevention of such reactions. Besides limiting the prescription of known allergenic drugs such as penicillin and other antibiotics to serious clinical indications, objective and reliable methods for the diagnosis of drug allergy would also be a great contribution to prevention.

At present, the diagnostic tests available for drug allergics are still relatively unsatisfactory, except for penicillin allergy. The main reasons for the difficulty encountered daily in establishing an objective diagnosis of drug allergy in a given patient are the following. (a) The immunological mechanisms of allergic reactions to drugs are varied, therefore an accurate diagnosis will require several types of tests; (b) in numerous instances, the immunochemical mechanisms leading to sensitisation to a given drug are not precisely known, accordingly, the reagents required for peforming appropriate immunological tests are not available; (c) immunological tests indicate whether the patient has made an immunological response to the drug, but they do not have absolute predictive value about the re-occurrence of an overt clinical allergic reaction on re-administration of the drug.

A list of tests potentially useful in the diagnosis of drug allergy is given in table 13.3. I would like to discuss briefly here only two types of tests: those designed to detect specific IgE antibodies (RAST test) and those based on the presence in the blood of specifically sensitised lymphocytes.

The RAST test has for the time being been applied only to the diagnosis of penicillin allergies (Wide and Juhlin, 1971; Kraft *et al.*, 1977; de Weck, 1978) where it is undeniably quite useful. Correlation between skin tests detecting anaphylactic hypersensitivity to the major and minor determinants of penicillin allergy (table 13.4) is undeniably present, especially if only highly sensitive patients are considered. On the other hand, the RAST test, like many other similar tests based on the detection of circulating anti-drug antibodies, has a severe drawback: in more than 50 per cent of the cases, the antibody level decreases within 1 year after the last clinical

Table 13.3   Diagnostic tests in drug allergy

---

(1)   *Skin tests.*   (a)   Immediate-type: scratch or prick,
                                     if possible with
                                     drug–polylysine conjugates

                     (b)   Delayed-type: epicutaneous, with drugs
                                     or allergenic drug derivatives

(2)   *Detection of antibodies*
       (a)   Haemagglutination, detects mostly IgM and IgG
       (b)   RAST test, for IgE
       (c)   Inhibition of drug-coated bacteriophages,
             detects mostly IgM and IgG
       (d)   Ig binding of radiolabelled drug
       (e)   Passive degranulation of basophils

(3)   *Cellular tests*
       (a)   Lymphocyte-transformation test (blasts
             count or [^{3}H] thymidine uptake)
       (b)   Macrophage migration inhibition (MIF) test
       (c)   Leucocyte migration inhibition (LIF) test
       (d)   Specific rosette tests

---

allergic reaction to a point where the test becomes negative (Kraft *et al.*, 1977; de Weck, 1978). It is not yet known why, without apparent further contact with the drug, the antibody levels may remain high for years in some patients but decrease massively within a few months in others.

Tests based on the reactivity of peripheral blood lymphocytes hold, in my opinion, a much greater promise in the diagnosis of drug allergy for the following reasons. (a) Sensitive lymphocytes appear to remain detectable for years in the peripheral blood of allergic patients; (b) lymphocytes are apparently capable of metabolising a large number of drugs, which explains why positive reactions may be obtained even when the drug itself, and not one of its allergenic metabolites, is used for the test; (c) such tests will detect delayed-type allergic hypersensitivity, which is more frequently involved in allergic reactions to drugs than antibodies.

However, most tests based on lymphocyte cultures *in vitro* are still relatively cumbersome and expensive. For clinical and practical purposes, we feel that epicutaneous tests should receive more attention and credit in the diagnosis of drug allergy. Their value has probably been underestimated (Felix and Comaish, 1974) and could still be improved by using the appropriate allergenic derivatives (for example phenetidin in phenacetin allergy; Ruegger *et al.*, 1973) and appropriate vehicles facilitating penetration of the skin. In penicillin allergy also, epicutaneous tests are frequently positive not only in those cases where IgE antibodies are responsible for the clinical manifestations but mostly in those clinical reactions (for example morbilliform exanthema) where a cell-mediated mechanism is primarily involved (table 13.5). The frequent ocurrence of positive reactions after epicutaneous application of the allergen in individuals or experimental animals, which have been senitised by intramuscular injection or ingestion of the

Drugs and Immune Responsiveness

Table 13.4   Comparison of skin tests and RAST test in patients with
history of penicillin allergy

		High reactors	Low reactors	Negative
	Skin test BPO-PLL:			
	+++	3	0	1
	++	13	0	0
RAST	+	22	2	1
	−	39	44	47
	Skin test BPN:			
	+++	1	2	1
	++	8	2	3
RAST	+	9	4	12
	−	38	23	68
	Skin test BPNCO:			
	+++	1	1	2
	++	5	4	4
RAST	+	5	2	17
	−	21	24	85

For details of skin-testing procedures and evaluation, see de Weck *et al.* (1975). BPN,
Benzylpenicillin; BPO-PLL, benzylpenicillinoyl-polylysine; BPNCO, benzylpenicilloic acid.

drug, suggests that primary sensitisation through the skin and formation of drug
conjugates to skin proteins are not essential for the development of allergic contact reactions to drugs (deWeck, 1977).

SPECIFIC INHIBITION OF ANTIBODY-MEDIATED REACTIONS TO DRUGS

All antibody-mediated allergic reactions encompass the binding of antibodies to
antigen through the combining sites of antibodies. It is well-known since Landsteiner that an excess of monovalent free antigenic determinants (or haptens)
specifically inhibit antigen–antibody reactions *in vitro*. Since it has been shown
that anaphylactic reactions to haptenic determinants in experimental animals
in vivo may also be inhibited by monovalent haptens (Farah *et al.*, 1960; Ovary
and Karush, 1960), the application of this principle to the clinical prevention of
allergic reactions to penicillin was a logical development. After a number of pre-
liminary experiments (de Weck and Schneider, 1972; de Weck and Girard, 1972),
an extensive clinical trial was performed, demonstrating that a monovalent benzyl
penicilloyl hapten (BPO-FLYS or Ro 6-0787) is capable of preventing the great

Table 13.5   Results of epicutaneous tests with BPN in patients with history of penicillin allergy

Main clinical symptoms			Patch test with BPN	
			+ve	−ve
Urticaria	Immediate	+ve	12	7
(38 cases)	skin tests	−ve	11	8
Patch test +ve: 23/38 (60%)				
Exanthema	Immediate	+ve	15	1
(56 cases)	skin tests	−ve	34	6
Patch test +ve: 49/56 (87%)				

Patch test with BPN, 200 000 units/ml was for 24 h.
Scratch and intradermal skin tests were with BPO-PLL, BPN and BPNCO. For details, see de Weck *et al*. (1975).

majority of allergic reactions to penicillin in man (de Weck *et al*., 1975). However, during the course of that trial, an unexpected finding impaired widespread use of the monovalent hapten: in 5 to 10 per cent of the allergic patients, especially in those with a high degree of sensitivity, the hapten elicited the allergic reaction instead of inhibiting it as it did in 90 per cent of the patients. Although the paradoxical elicitation of anaphylactic reactions by apparently monovalent haptens has been encountered before in a few experimental systems (Amkraut *et al*., 1963; Frick *et al*., 1968; de Weck *et al*., 1973), the mechanism of such reactions has not been elucidated. Reactions to the monovalent BPO hapten in man were apparently due to the development of some minor determinant, but the precise immunochemical identity of the minor determinants of penicillin allergy has not yet been worked out. In recent years, our laboratory has developed an experimental model of sensitisation to penicillins in guinea pigs, which will permit a serious immunochemical investigation of the minor determinants (de Weck *et al*., 1976). Sensitisation of guinea pigs by BPO–protein conjugates and/or BPN in such a way as to raise high levels of reaginic (IgE-like) antibodies yielded animals reacting anaphylactically not only to the injection of preformed multivalent penicilloyl conjugates but also to BPN itself and to penicillin derivatives, such as BPNCO and penicilloyl amides. Accordingly, we now have a true model of penicillin allergy in which the percentage of reactions to the major and various minor determinants appears quite similar between man and guinea pig (table 13.6). Immunisation of a large number of outbred guinea pigs with the same BPO–protein conjugates under identical conditions yields animals showing strikingly dissimilar patterns of sensitisation (table 13.7). This points to the probable role of genetic factors, to which the minor determinants presented in low dose to the organism should be particularly sensitive.

In any case, it now appears likely that the problem of minor determinants in penicillin allergy will soon find its immunochemical conclusion. Accordingly, the development of combined penicillin preparations, in which not only the major BPO

Table 13.6   Comparative frequency of reactions to penicillin derivatives in humans allergic to penicillin and in guinea pigs immunised with penicillin–protein conjugates.

Penicillin derivative	Immediate-type skin reactivity in humans		PCA with serum of outbred guinea pigs immunised with BPO-BGG	
BPO-PLL	152/249	(61)	156/157	(99)
BPN	108/246	(44)	43/157	(27)
BPNCO	76/248	(30)	47/116	(40)
BPO-FLYS	35/248	(14)	15/157	(9)
N-Formyl benzylpenicilloylformyl-lysine	57/203	(28)	1/22	(4)
BPO-PLL	49/96	(51)	1/58	(1)

Outbred guinea pigs were repeatedly immunised with 1μg of benzylpenicilloyl–bovine gamma-globulin (BPO-BGG) in aluminium hydroxide (A1(OH)$_3$). Percentage values are given in parentheses. BPO-FLYS, Benzylpenicilloylformyl-lysine; PCA, passive cutaneous anaphylaxis.

contingent but also the minor determinants would be prevented from interacting with their corresponding antibodies by addition of suitable monovalent haptens, may become reality. It should be pointed out, however, that this mode of specific

Table 13.7   Patterns of PCA reactivity to various BPN derivatives in outbred guinea pigs immunised with BPO-BGG

Number of animals	BPO-PLL	PCA elicited by: BPN	BPNCO	BPO-FLYS
26	+	−	−	−
6	+	+	−	−
31	+	+	+	−
3	+	+	+	+
3	+	+	−	+
1	+	−	−	+
1	+	−	+	−

For abbreviations and conditions of immunisation, see tables 13.5 and 13.6.

inhibition only applies to antibody-mediated allergic reactions. Clinical and experimental experience has shown that the monovalent BPO hapten does not inhibit lymphocyte-induced reactions to penicillin (de Weck, 1975).

INDUCTION OF LONG-LASTING TOLERANCE TO DRUGS

Most attempts to achieve long-lasting desensitisation to drugs in allergic patients by repeated and progressive administration of the drug have been unsuccessful and are also quite dangerous. In special cases, however, a 'rush' desensitisation in which a massive therapeutic dose is reached by progressive administration of the drug may be justified (Reisman *et al.*, 1962; Zolov *et al.*, 1967). This procedure is not without danger, has to be performed under emergency conditions and has no long-term protective effects. In penicillin allergy, it may in most cases be advantageously replaced by the procedure of hapten inhibition described above (de Weck *et al.*, 1975).

On the basis of experiments designed to achieve immunological tolerance to a number of chemically defined haptens, several new approaches potentially useful for the induction of prolonged desensitisation to drugs have emerged in recent years. Characteristics for these approaches are: (a) the fact that they induce a long-lasting state of specific unresponsiveness to the hapten in animals that had already developed a full-fledged immune response; they are therefore relevant to the clinical situation where patients are usually encountered only after they have become allergic; (b) the specific impairment of B cells and of antibody production (B-cell tolerance) but cellular immunity appears not to be affected. This form of long-lasting unresponsiveness is brought about by the injection in a sensitive animal of the hapten coupled to a so called 'tolerogenic carrier'. Tolerogenic carriers that have been described up to now are: (a) a D-amino acid copolymer, D-glutamyl-D-lysine (Katz *et al.*, 1972); (b) polysaccharides such as pneumococcal polysaccharide (Mitchell *et al.*, 1972), levans (Howard and Mitchison, 1975) and dextrans (Coutinho *et al.*, 1974); (c) homologous gamma-globulins (Lee and Sehon, 1975; Paley *et al.*, 1975). Although this phenomenon was originally described for haptens without drug activity, such as dinitrophenyl (DNP), its validity for the BPO determinant has been confirmed (Lee and Sehon, 1976). In recent years, we have studied systematically the molecular properties required of amino acid polymers and of dextrans as tolerogenic carriers in the penicillin system. The main conclusions of these studies (Otz *et al.*, 1978; Schneider *et al.*, 1978) are as follows: (a) a large number of amino acid polymers and copolymers may serve as tolerogenic carriers, even with a molecular weight as low as 3000; (b) a D-configuration is not essential, provided a high degree of hapten substitution is achieved; efficiency is probably correlated with low biodegradability.

The main practical obstacle to the clinical trial of such compounds in penicillin-allergic patients is their high efficiency in eliciting anaphylactic reactions, since they are multivalent. However, various possibilities may be visualised to overcome this difficulty (for example protracted administration, antianaphylactic medication, etc.).

Another potential approach to the problem of drug allergy would be the administration of drugs in such a way as to induce preferentially an immunological tolerance, possibly by the preferential induction of suppressor cells. Oral administration of haptens is well known to favour the induction of immunological tolerance (Chase, 1946). The common experience that allergic reactions to drugs, although possible, are much less frequent after p.o. administration than after injection or application to the skin may be related, at least in part, to that phenomenon.

In conclusion, although from the point of view of diagnosis and therapy, allergies to drugs are still more difficult to manage than the common allergies to protein or polysaccharide antigens, the application of immunological principles to drug allergy appears to open new possibilities for its prevention and management.

ACKNOWLEDGEMENT

This work has been supported in part by the Swiss National Research Foundation (Grant no. 3.468.75).

REFERENCES

Amkraut, A. A., Rosenberg, L. T. and Raffel, S. (1963). Elicitation of PCA by univalent and divalent haptens. *J. Immun.*, 91, 644

Batchelor, F. R., Dewdney, J. M., Feinberg, J. G. and Weston, R. D. (1967). A penicilloylated protein impurity as a source of allergy to benzylpenicillin and 6-aminopenicillanic acid. *Lancet*, i, 1175

Bundgaard, H. and de Weck, A. L. (1975). The role of amino-reactive impurities in acetylsalicylic acid allergy. *Int. Archs Allergy appl. Immun.*, 49, 119

Chase, M. W. (1946). Inhibition of experimental drug allergy by prior feeding of the sensitizing agent. *Proc. Soc. exp. Biol. Med.*, 61, 257

Coutinho, A., Möller, G. and Richter, W. (1974). Molecular basis of B cell activation. I. Mitogenicity of native and substituted dextrans. *Scand. J. Immun.*, 3, 321

De Weck, A. L. (1971). Drug reactions. In *Immunological diseases*, (ed., M. Samter), Little Brown and Co.,Boston, p. 415

De Weck, A. L. (1975). Molecular mechanisms of T and B lymphocyte triggering. *Int. Archs Allergy appl. Immun.*, 49, 247

De Weck, A. L. (1977). Immune responses to environmental antigens which act on the skin (with special reference to the role of lymphokines in contact dermatitis). *Fedn Proc.*, 36, 1742

De Weck, A. L. (1978). Application du RAST dans l'allergie à la pénicilline. *Med. Hyg.*, 36, 118

De Weck, A. L. and Eisen, H. N. (1960). Some immunochemical properties of penicillenic acid, an antigenic determinant derived from penicillin. *J. exp. Med.*, 112, 1227

De Weck, A. L. and Girard, J. P. (1972). Specific inhibition of allergic reactions to penicillin in man by a monovalent hapten: II. Clinical studies. *Int. Archs Allergy appl. Immun.*, 42, 798

De Weck, A. L. and Schneider, C. H. (1972). Specific inhibitionof allergic reactions to penicillin in man by a monvalent hapten: II. Clinical studies. *Int. Archs Allergy*, 42, 789

De Weck, A. L., Schneider, C. H. and Gutersohn, J. (1968). The role of penicilloylated protein impurities, penicillin polymers and dimers in penicillin allergy. *Int. Archs Allergy appl. Immun.*, 33, 535

De Weck, A. L., Schneider, C. H., Toffler, O. and Lazary, S. (1973). Inhibition of allergic reactions by monovalent haptens. In *Mechanisms of reaginic allergy*, (ed., A. Sehon) Dekker, New York, p. 323

De Weck, A. L., Jeunet, F., Schulz, K. H., Louis, P., Girard, J. P., Grilliat, J. P., Moneret-Vautrin, D., Storck, H., Wüthrich, B., Spengler, H., Juhlin, L., Scheiffarth, F., Warnatz, H., Wortmann, F. and Vigary, S. (1975). Clinical trial of Ro 6-0787: a monovalent specific hapten inhibitor of penicillin allergy. *Z. Immunitätsforsch.*, 150, 138

De Weck,, A. L., Toffler, O., Koleckarova, M. and Spengler, M. (1976). Theoretical basis and experimental studies on the prevention of allergic reactions to penicillins by a monovalent benzylpenicilloyl hapten. *Chemotherapy*, 4, 345

Dewdney, J. (1977). Immunology of the antibiotics. In *The Antigens, IV*, (ed., M. Sela), Academic Press, New York, p.74

Farah, F. S., Kern, M. and Eisen, H. N. (1960). Specific inhibition of wheal-and-erythema responses with univalent haptens and univalent antibody fragments. *J. exp. Med.*, 112, 1211

Felix, R. H. and Comaish, J. S. (1974). The value of patch and other skin tests in drug eruptions. *Lancet*, i, 1017

Frick, O. L., Nye, W. and Raffel, S. (1968). Anaphylactic reactions to univalent haptens. *Immunology*, 14, 563

Green, I., Paul, W. E. and Benacerraf, B. (1966). The behavior of hapten–poly-L-lysine conjugates as complete antigens in genetic responders and as haptens in nonresponder guinea pigs. *J. exp. Med.*, 123, 859

Howard, J. G. and Mitchison, N. A. (1975). Immunological tolerance. *Progr. Allergy*, 18, 43

Katz, D. H., Hamaoka, T. and Benacerraf, B. (1972). Immunological tolerance in bone marrow-derived lymphocytes. I. Evidence for an intracellular mechanism of inactivation of hapten-specific precursors of antibody-forming cells. *J. exp. Med.*, 136, 1404

Klein, U., Gikalov, I., Keller, M. and Hoigné, R. (1972). Drug monitoring in der medizinischen Abteilung eines Regionalspitals. *Schweiz. Med. Wschr.*, 102, 1083

Kraft, D., Roth, A., Mischer, P., Pichler, H. and Ebner, H. (1977). Specific and total serum IgE measurements in the diagnosis of penicillin allergy. A long-term follow-up study. *Clin. Allergy*, 7, 21

Kristofferson, A., Ahlstedt, S., Pettersson, E. and Svärd, P. O. (1977). Antigens in penicillin allergy. I. A radioimmunoassay for detection of penicilloylated protein contaminants in penicillin preparations. *Int. Archs Allergy appl. Immun.*, 55, 13

Lee, W. Y. and Sehon, A. H. (1975). Suppression of reaginic antibody formation. II. The use of adoptive transfer system for the study of immunological unresponsiveness. *J. Immun.*, 114, 837

Lee, W. Y. and Sehon, A. H. (1976). Suppression of reaginic antibody formation. IV. Suppression of reaginic antibodies to penicillin in the mouse. *J. Immun.*, 117, 927

Levine, B. B. (1966). Immunochemical mechanisms of drug allergy. *A. Rev. Med.*, 17, 23

Magnusson, B. and Kligman, A. M. (1970). *Allergic contact dermatitis in the guinea pig*, C. C. Thomas, Springfield, Illinois, U.S.A.

Mitchell, G. F., Humphrey, J H. and Williamson, A. R. (1972). B cell tolerance induced by polymeric antigens. I. Comparison of the dose and epitope density requirements for inactivation of primed and unprimed B cells *in vivo*. *Eur. J. Immun.*, 5, 361

Otz, U., Schneider, C. H., de Weck, A. L., Gruden, E. and Gill, T. G. (1978). Induction of immunological tolerance to the penicilloyl antigenic determinant. I. Evaluation of BPO-amino acid polymers and copolymers in mice. *Eur. J. Immun.*, (in press)

Ovary, Z. and Karush, F. (1960). Studies on the immunologic mechanism of anaphylaxis: I. Antibody–hapten interactions studied by passive cutaneous anaphylaxis in the guinea pig. *J. Immun.*, 84, 409

Paley, R. S. Leskowitz, S. and Borel, Y. (1975). Effect on tolerance induction of the mode of attachment of the hapten to the carrier. *J. Immun.*, 115, 1409

Reismann, R. E., Rose, N. R., Witebsky, E. and Arbesman, C. (1962). Penicillin allergy and desensitization. *J. Allergy clin. Immun.*, 33, 178

Rüegger, R., Spengler, H., de Weck, A. L. and Dubach, U. C. (1973). Immunologische Aspekte der Sensibilisierung auf Phenacetin. *Dtsch. Med. Wochenschr.*, 98, 762

Schneider, C. H., Otz, U. and Gruden, E. (1978). Induction of immunological tolerance to the penicilloyl antigenic determinant. II. Evaluation of stable and unstable penicilloyl-dextrans. *Eur. J. Immun.*, (in press)

Wide, L. and Juhlin, L. (1971). Detection of penicillin allergy of the immediate-type by radioimmunoassay of reagins (IgE) to penicilloyl conjugates. *Clin. Allergy*, 1, 171

Zolov, D., Redmond, A. P. and Levine, B. B. (1967). Immunological studies of desensitization in penicillin allergy. *J. Allergy clin. Immun.*, 39, 107

14
Principles, technical difficulties and developments of radioimmunoassay procedures

Leif Wide (Department of Clinical Chemistry, University Hospital
Uppsala, Sweden)

The introduction of a group of assay methods called 'binding assays' or 'ligand assays or ligand-binding assays' has had a great impact on biomedical science. In general, these assay methods combine high specificity, high sensitivity with a high practicability when compared with previously used 'chemical' or 'biological' methods. It is characteristic for these assays that the substance to be measured is bound to a binding reagent and that the reaction is governed by the law of mass action:

$$P + Q \rightleftharpoons PQ$$

The term ligand (P) is used in this survey for every compound that will bind to the appropriate binding site on the binding reagent (Q). The second characteristic for most binding assays is the presence of a label which is used as a marker. The binding assays may be classified into two groups (a) those using a labelled ligand and (b) those using a labelled binding reagent.

The principles of eight different binding assays are shown schematically in figure 14.1. All methods using a labelled ligand are competitive binding assays. In its simplest form (figure 14.1(Aa)) the labelled ligand is added simultaneously with the unlabelled ligand, which is the compound to be assayed, and the two different ligands compete for a limited number of sites on the binding reagent. The reaction may or may not go to equilibrium. The labelled and unlabelled ligand have as a rule different binding constants in the reaction. After the reaction has been interrupted the bound and/or free fraction of labelled ligand is determined. The effect of increasing amounts of unlabelled ligand is a decrease in amounts of labelled ligand bound. The reaction for the unknown ligand is compared with that of a standard solution with known concentration.

If the labelled ligand is given a 'handicap' by later addition to the incubation mixture, sequential incubation (figure 14.1(Ab)), and the reaction is then interrupted before it has reached equilibrium an increased sensitivity of the assay method may be obtained. This method is often used when assaying by radioimmunoassay larger

PRINCIPLES OF BINDING ASSAYS

(A) Labelled ligand

(1) *Competitive binding assays*

(a) Simultaneous incubation

$$Q + P \rightleftharpoons QP$$
$$+ P^* \rightleftharpoons QP^*$$

(b) Sequential incubation

$$Q + P \rightleftharpoons QP$$
$$+ P^* \rightleftharpoons QP^*$$

(c) Solid phase ligand–coupled binding reagent

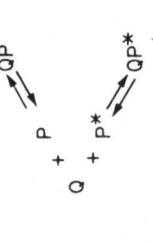

(B) Labelled binding reagent

(1) *Non-competitive binding assays* 'Sandwich' binding assays

(a) Two separation step assay

$$\boxed{Q_1} + P \rightleftharpoons \boxed{Q_1}P$$
$$+ Q_2^* \rightleftharpoons \boxed{Q_1}PQ_2^*$$

(b) Three separation step assay

$$\boxed{Q_1} + P \rightleftharpoons \boxed{Q_1}P$$
$$+ Q_2 \rightleftharpoons \boxed{Q_1}PQ_2$$
$$+ R^* \rightleftharpoons \boxed{Q_1}PQ_2R^*$$

(c) One separation step assay, sequential incubation

$$P + Q_1^* \rightleftharpoons PQ_1^*$$
$$+ Q_2 \rightleftharpoons \boxed{Q_2}PQ_1^*$$
$$(\boxed{Q_2}P)$$

(B) Labelled binding reagent

(2) *Competitive binding assays*

(a) One separation step assay, sequential incubation

$$P + Q^* \rightleftharpoons PQ^*$$
$$\boxed{P} Q^*$$
$$+ \boxed{P} \rightleftharpoons$$
$$(\boxed{P} Q^*P)$$

(b) Two separation step assay, sequential incubation

$$P + Q \rightleftharpoons PQ$$
$$\boxed{P} + \rightleftharpoons \boxed{P} PQ$$
$$+ R^* \rightleftharpoons \boxed{P} QR^*$$

P   = Ligand
Q   = Binding reagent
*   = Label
R   = Binding reagent for Q, different from P
$\boxed{P}$ = Solid phase coupled ligand
$\boxed{Q}$ = Solid phase coupled binding reagent

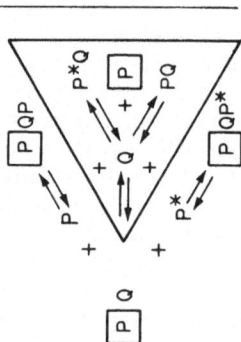

Figure 14.1 Principles of binding assays.

Table 14.1 Binding assays 1956 – 1978.

Year	Description	Reference
1956	'Erythroimmunoassay' for insulin. Homogeneous labelled ligand competitive-binding assay.	Arquilla and Stavitsky, 1956 *a,b*
1959–60	Radioimmunoassay for insulin. Radioligand, competitive binding. Non-immunological radioligand binding assay for thyroxin.	Yalow and Berson, 1959, 1960 Ekins, 1960
1962	The chloramine T method for labelling with ^{131}I.	Hunter and Greenwood, 1962 Greenwood *et al.*, 1963
1966	Radioimmunoassay for a hapten.	Oliver *et al.*, 1966
1966	Solid-phase radioimmunoassays.	Catt *et al.*, 1966 Wide and Porath, 1966
1967–69	Sandwich radioimmunoassays. Labelled binding reagent (antibodies) non-competitive binding assay.	Wide *et al.*, 1967*b* Wide, 1969
1968	Immunoradiometric assay. Labelled binding reagent (antibodies) competitive binding assay.	Miles and Hales, 1968
1971–72	Enzymoimmunoassays. Competitive and sandwich binding assays.	Engvall and Perlmann, 1971, 1972 van Weemen and Schuurs, 1971
1972–73	'Homogeneous' electron-spinimmunoassays and enzymoimmunoassays	Leute *et al.*, 1972 Schneider *et al.*, 1973
1973	Method for conjugation-labelling of proteins.	Bolton and Hunter, 1973

proteins with a low dissociation rate constant in the binding reaction.

Some milestones in the history of the binding assays are given in table 14.1. The first binding assays described were based on this principle of labelled ligand competitive assay and were used for the assay of insulin. One method was developed by Arquilla and Stavitsky in 1953–56 (Stavitsky and Arquilla, 1953; Arquilla and Stavitsky, 1956*a,b*). Insulin was labelled with erythrocytes and the labelled and unlabelled insulin competed for the binding sites on a limited number of antibodies to insulin. The antibody-bound labelled insulin was then detected by addition of complement which caused a release of haemoglobin from the antibody– insulin-erythrocyte complex. They showed clearly the relationship between dose and response in this type of assay and how a decrease in amount of antibodies increased the sensitivity of the assay. Their method, which is of great historical interest as being the first in a long series of binding assays, had a sensitivity of about 100 ng of insulin per test tube which was too low for clinical use.

This assay technique for insulin was considerably improved by Yalow and Berson (1959, 1960) who replaced the erythrocyte by a radioactive label, ^{131}I, which increased the sensitivity of the assay. They separated antibody-bound and free labelled ligand by chromato-electrophoresis before measuring the radioactivity of the two fractions. The first radioimmunoassay had been developed. At the same time Ekins (1960) introduced the use of a ligand labelled with a radioactive isotope in a non-immunological competitive binding assay. It was an assay for thyroxin where the binding reagent was thyroxin-binding globulin (TBG). A stage in the development of binding assays had now been reached where two different markers were used for labelling and two different groups of binding proteins used as binding reagents. Ekins (1963) emphasised the general principle of this group of binding assays by suggesting the name saturation analysis, a name that has not been generally accepted.

Table 14.2   Examples of labels and binding reagents used in binding assays

Label	Binding reagents
Radioactive isotopes	Antibodies
Enzymes	Antigens
Fluorescent markers	Plasma-binding proteins
Phages	Receptors
Free radicals	Enzymes
Enzyme inhibitors	
Erythrocytes	
Metals	

A series of examples of labels and binding reagents that have been used are given in table 14.2. The different binding assays have been named according to the nature of the label and the binding reagent and names such as radioimmunoassay, enzymo-immunoassay, radioreceptorassay, etc. are now commonly used. Such names are in general used for all binding assays with a particular type of label and binding reagent independent of whether it is a labelled ligand or a labelled binding reagent or if it is a competitive or a non-competitive binding assay. In the early 1960's, it was technically difficult and sometimes also hazardous to label minute amounts of proteins to high specific radioactivity with a radioactive isotope like [131]I. Therefore it was a major advance when Hunter and Greenwood (1962) described the so-called chloramine T method for labelling with [131]I. As a result most clinical laboratories were able to label a small amount, about 1 µg, of proteins with ^{131}I or ^{125}I to high specific radioactivities using acceptable amounts of radioactive material. A number of different techniques for labelling, in particular for ^{125}I, have been developed since then. Of these the lactoperoxidase technique (Thorell and Johansson, 1971) and the methods for conjugation-labelling of proteins (Bolton and Hunter, 1973) seem to be the most important.

Oliver *et al.* (1966) widened the field of application of this assay principle considerably by the use of haptens, small compounds that are intrinsically non-immunogenic. Highly specific antisera to haptens like steroids, thyroid hormones, and a number of different drugs could be obtained by coupling them in a suitable way to a carrier protein to render them immunogenic. The principles of the radioimmunoassays used for the assay of these haptens were the same as those used for the assay of protein antigens. Labelling of haptens with ^{125}I could be made after conjugation of, for example, tyrosine methyl ester to the hapten.

Three different groups of techniques have been used to distinguish between unbound and bound labelled ligand (see table 14.3). In the first group the reaction is performed in the liquid phase and a separation of bound and unbound labelled ligand is then made according to three different principles. (a) Precipitation of the bound labelled ligand, (b) adsorption of the free labelled ligand, and (c) different mobility of bound and free labelled ligand. The double antibody, the charcoal, the polyethylene glycol (PEG) and the ammonium sulphate techniques seem to be the most com-

Table 14.3 Techniques to distinguish between unbound and bound labelled ligand

---

(1) Separation by use of:

    (a) precipitation of bound labelled ligand: double antibody, solid-phase double antibody, PEG, ammonium sulphate, etc.

    (b) adsorption of free labelled ligand: charcoal, silica, talc, paper chromatography, ion-exchange, etc.

    (c) differential migration of free and bound labelled ligand: electrophoresis, gel filtration

(2) Solid-phase coupled binding reagent for ligand.

        Particles
        Discs
        Inside of test tube
        Gels in column

(3) Change in message from label when labelled ligand is bound. Homogeneous assays.

        Haemolysis
        Electron-spin label
        Enzymes

---

monly used at present. The second group comprises methods using solid-phase coupled binding reagent for the ligand. In the third group, the so called 'homogeneous' binding assays, the technique to distinguish between unbound and bound labelled ligand is based on a change in message from the label when the labelled ligand is bound. It is thus not necessary to remove the bound fraction from the unbound. The erythroimmunoassay of Arquilla and Stavitsky (1956 *a,b*), the electron-spinimmunoassay (Leute *et al.*, 1972) and some of the enzymoimmunoassays (Schneider *et al.*, 1973) belong to this group of binding assays.

The solid-phase radioimmunoassays (Catt *et al.*, 1966; Wide and Porath, 1966) were introduced to simplify the separation of unbound from bound labelled ligand. The binding reagent is coupled to a solid phase, which may have the form of small Sephadex or cellulose particles (Wide *et al.*, 1967a; Wide, 1969). The matrix may also be of a plastic or paper disc, or the inside surface of a test tube (Catt and Tregear, 1967). Separation is achieved by removing the liquid phase and usually includes several washings of the solid phase. The separation can be extremely efficient with a low misclassification error in such an assay. By coupling the binding reagent to a solid-phase conjugated ligand (indirect coupling) an increased specificity may be obtained. For example, the antibodies to a particular antigen are selectively 'extracted' from an antiserum by incubating the serum with the antigen, highly purified and covalently coupled to a solid phase (Wide *et al.*, 1973). The second binding site of the antibodies is then used in the competitive binding assay. An effect of the complicated reaction shown within the triangle in the figure 14.1(Ac) is an enhanced 'response' in the assay for increased amounts of unlabelled ligand when compared with assays using antibodies coupled directly to the solid phase.

A non-competitive radioimmunoassay using a labelled binding reagent (antibodies) instead of a labelled ligand was introduced by Wide *et al.* (1967b). This was the first in a series of 'sandwich' radioimmunoassays (Wide, 1969, 1971). The general principle is shown in figure 14.1 (B1a). It is a direct assay in which the effect of increasing amounts of ligand is an increase in amounts of labelled binding reagent bound. The method was first applied to the assay of reagins to specific allergens. This was developed because it was not possible to obtain the high degree of specificity, a double specificity, that was needed to measure specific reagins by the conventional radioimmunoassay. In the sandwich radioimmunoassay for specific reagins (the radioallergosorbent test, RAST) the reagins (P in figure 14.1 (B1a)) are first bound to a solid-phase coupled allergen (Q) and the bound reagins are then detected by their ability to bind ^{125}I-labelled immunosorbent-purified antibodies to IgE (Q$^*_2$). The same principle has been used for the assay of larger antigens and bivalent antibodies (Wide, 1969, 1971; Addison and Hales, 1971). The method is in principle applicable for all substances that have at least two binding sites. The 'sandwich' binding assays are so called reagent-excess methods whereas the competitive binding assays are limited-reagent assays (Ekins, 1976). Both the solid-phase coupled binding reagent and the labelled binding reagent are added in excess to each test tube and the exact amount is less critical in the sandwich assay than in the competitive binding assay. Therefore discs of plastic or paper or the inside surface of a test tube are suitable as matrices in the sandwich assay. A low dissociation rate, particularly in the first reaction, is a prerequisite for obtaining a high sensitivity in a 'sandwich' binding assay.

A variant of the sandwich assays is a three-separation-step method using three different binding reagents (Belanger *et al.*, 1973; Beck and Hales, 1975). For example, in an assay for a larger antigen this is first bound to a solid-phase coupled antibody (Q_1 in figure 14.1 (B1b)) from one species. An antibody (Q_2) from another animal species and directed to the same antigen is bound in the second stage. In the third stage of the assay a labelled antibody (R^*) directed to the immunoglobulin in the second stage is added. An advantage with this variant is that the same type of labelled antibodies can be used for the assay of several different antigens. Another variant of the sandwich binding assays is illustrated in figure 14.1 (B1c). This is a one-separation-step assay with sequential incubation in which the washing procedures have been reduced to one. A disadvantage is a lower sensitivity and larger 'hook effect' (Rodbard *et al.*, 1978) when the ligand is present in large amounts.

Two variants of competitive binding assays using a labelled binding reagent have been described. One was developed by Miles and Hales (1968) and was called the immunoradiometric assay. The labelled binding reagent was antibodies to insulin labelled with a radioactive isotope (^{125}I). This method is a one-separation-step assay with sequential incubation (figure 14.1 (B2a)). The labelled binding reagent should preferably be univalent to avoid a decrease in sensitivity due to the reaction shown in parenthesis in figure 14.1. A very similar technique was developed by our group for the assay of allergens (Wide *et al.*, 1971; Aronsson and Wide, 1974). The original study on RAST showed that the reaction could be inhibited by preincubating the reagins in serum with the allergen in solution (Wide *et al.*, 1967b). The general principle of this assay is shown in figure 14.1 (B2b). In the assay for allergen activity P is allergen, Q is reaginic antibody and R^* is the labelled antibody to IgE. The amount of binding reagent bound to the solid-phase coupled ligand is inversely correlated to the amount of ligand in the test solution. The similarity between immunoradiometric assay and the RAST allergen assay, one-separation-step and two-separation-step methods respectively, is evident from figure 14.1.

The main technical developments of radioimmunoassays during the last years concern automation, instruments for measurement of radioactivity and programs and computers for calculation of results and quality-control data. In 1975 it was estimated that in clinical laboratories throughout the world 100 million radioimmunoassays were done and by 1980 this would have increased to 250 millions. It seems likely that most laboratories will use semi-automatic systems in the near future and that the fully automated systems will be used only in centres where a very large number of tests are performed, in particular for screening purposes. However, this will of course depend on factors such as reliability, flexibility, speed and cost of the automatic systems.

Most of the new technical improvements for automation come from the commercial organisations. Union Carbide has a system called Centria in which the samples and reagents are added to cavities separated by ridges on a centrifuge disc. By the use of centrifugal force the reagents are mixed with the sample and when the centrifugation rate is increased the mixtures are transferred to Sephadex-gel-filtration columns to separate bound and free labelled ligand. The columns can be re-used after washing. The Micromedic System Concept 4 is based on the use of antibody-coated test tubes. They can easily be washed without a centrifugation step. The Becton Dickinson ARIA II system uses solid-phase coupled antibodies in a chamber as a separation device. The antibody chamber is regenerated after each test and is then ready for the next sample. Both the unbound and the bound (released by regenerating the chamber) flow through a counter. The Technicon Automatic

RIA System utilises continuous flow, magnetic fields and antibodies coupled to a solid phase containing ferric oxide (Nye *et al.*, 1976). The separation is made by holding the particles in the magnetic field while the unbound labelled ligand is washed away. The magnets are then de-energised and the particles with the bound labelled ligand are diverted to the detector. Another method that seems to be well suited for automation has been developed by Dr. W. M. Hunter and Mr. J. D. Lock in Edinburgh. In their system a vibratory conveyor is used to transport the test tubes. Labelled ligand bound to solid-phase (Sepharose) coupled antibodies is separated from free ligand in solution by letting the gel particles sediment through a sucrose solution (Hunter, 1977), which avoids centrifugation steps.

A number of facts such as the nature, size and availability of the substance and the degree of specificity, will determine which of the many variations of binding assays is to be chosen for the assay of a particular substance. However, the real problem with radioimmunoassay is not a 'pure technical' one. The schematic formulae in figure 14.1 are very much oversimplified. The ligand (P) is usually a mixture of several substances. Also the binding reagent (Q) is heterogeneous, both with regard to binding sites on P and to avidity in the binding reaction. 'Standard P' differs from 'Unknown P' and labelled P from both of these. Antisera show a large biological variation and every blood sample taken on a different occasion from an immunised animal should be regarded as unique with respect to specificity, avidity, etc. of the antibodies. A change of the labelled ligand, for example by storage, may change the specificity of the assay and give a different result for the unknown. However, these complications will in no way detract from the continued and increased use of radioimmunoassays in biomedical science and their great usefulness in clinical medicine is well established.

REFERENCES

Addison, G. M. and Hales, C. N. (1971). *Horm. Metab. Res.*, 3, 59
Aronsson, T. and Wide, L. (1974). *Int. Archs Allergy appl. Immun.*, 47, 224
Arquilla, E. R. and Stavitsky, A. B. (1956a). *J. clin. Invest.*, 35, 458
Arquilla, E. R. and Stavitsky, A. B. (1956b). *J. clin. Invest.*, 35, 467
Beck, P. and Hales, C. N. (1975). *Biochem. J.*, 145, 607
Belanger, L., Sylvestre, C. and Dufour, D. (1973). *Clin. Chim. Acta*, 48, 15
Bolton, A. E. and Hunter, W. M. (1973). *Biochem. J.*, 133, 529
Catt, K. J. and Tregear, G. W. (1967). *Science* 158, 1570
Catt, K. J., Niall, H. D. and Tregear, G. W. (1966). *Biochem. J.*, 100, 31C
Ekins, R. P. (1960). *Clin. Chim. Acta.*, 5, 453
Ekins, R. P. (1963). In *Radioactive Isotope in Klinik und Forschung*, Band V, (eds. K. Fellinger and R. Höfer), Urban and Schwarzenberg, München, p. 211
Ekins, R. P. (1976). In *Hormone Assays and their Clinical Application*, (eds. J. A. Loraine and E. T. Bell), Churchill Livingston, Edinburgh, p. 1
Engvall, E. and Perlmann, P. (1971). *Immunochemistry*, 8, 871
Engvall, E. and Perlmann, P. (1972). *J. Immun.*, 109, 129
Greenwood, F., Hunter, W. M. and Glover, J. S. (1963). *Biochem. J.*, 133, 529
Hunter, W. M. (1977). *Acta Endocr. Suppl.*, 212, 260
Hunter, W. M. and Greenwood, F. C. (1962). *Nature*, 194, 495
Leute, R., Ullman, E. F., Goldstein, A. and Hersenberg, L. A. (1972). *Nature New Biol.*, 236, 93
Miles, L. E. and Hales, C. N. (1968). *Nature*, 219, 186
Nye, L., Forrest, C . G., Greenwood, H., Garner, J. S., Jay, R., Roberts, J. R. and Landon, J. (1976). *Clin. Chim. Acta*, 69, 387

Oliver, G. C., Brasfield, D., Parker, B. M. and Parker, C. W. (1966). *Lab. clin. Med.*, 68, 1002
Rodbard, D., Feldman, Y., Jaffe, M. L. and Miles, L. E. M. (1978). *Immunochemistry*, 15, 77
Schneider, R. S., Lindquist, P., Tong-in Wong, E., Rubenstein, K. E. and Ullman, E. F. (1973). *Clin. Chem.*, 19, 821
Stavitsky, A. B. and Arquilla, E. R. (1953). *Fed. Proc.*, 12, 461
Thorell, J. I. and Johansson, B. (1971). *Biochim. Biophys. Acta*, 251, 363
Van Weemen, B. K. and Schuurs, A. H. W. M. (1971). *FEBS Lett.*, 15, 232
Wide, L. (1969). *Acta Endocr. Suppl.*, 142, 207
Wide, L. (1971). In *Radioimmunoassay Methods*, (eds. K. E. Kirkham and W. M. Hunter), Churchill Livingston, Edinburgh, p. 405
Wide, L. and Porath, J. (1966). *Biochim. Biophys. Acta*, 130, 257
Wide, L., Axen, R. and Porath, J. (1967a) *Immunochemistry*, 4, 381
Wide, L., Bennich, H. and Johansson, S. G. O. (1967b), *Lancet*, ii, 1105
Wide, L., Aronsson, T., Fagerberg, E. and Zetterström, O. (1971). In *Allergology*, (eds. J. Charpin *et al.*), Excerpta Medica Int. Congr. Series, 251, 85
Wide, L., Nillius, S. J., Gemzell, C. and Roos, P. (1973). *Acta Endocr. Suppl.*, 174, 1
Yalow, R. S. and Berson, S. A. (1959). *Nature*, 184, 1648
Yalow, R. S. and Berson, S. A. (1960). *J. clin. Invest.*, 39, 1157

15
Enzymoimmunoassays and related analytical techniques for drugs

Elizabeth Shaw,* J. Landon and R. S. Kamel (Departments of Microbiology*
and Chemical Pathology, St. Bartholomew's Hospital, London E.C.1, U.K.)

INTRODUCTION

Radioimmunoassay (RIA) has a number of advantages as an analytical technique
including its sensitivity, specificity, practicality and, in particular, wide applica-
bility. Thus it is not surprising that, since the development of the first RIA for a
drug, digitoxin (Smith et al., 1969), such assays have been introduced for over
60 drugs (Landon and Moffat, 1976), and have proved of great value to the clinical
pharmacologist and clinician. Nonetheless, RIA has a number of disadvantages such
as the need for radioisotope-counting equipment, a slight health hazard and, in the
case of RIA based on gamma-emitting radioisotopes (such as ^{125}I), which have a
relatively short half-life, the frequent need to prepare batches of the isotopically
labelled drug, with consequent problems of quality control and distribution.

The disadvantages of using a radioisotope for labelling purposes has led to a
search for appropriate non-radioactive labels. The dominant reactant in all immunoassays for drugs is the antibody, since it is this which, in large part, determines both
the specificity and ultimate sensitivity that can be achieved — the latter depending
on the affinity with which the antibody binds the antigen. The labelled drug is used
only as a tracer and any label would be suitable provided its determination is relatively simple, sufficiently precise and sensitive for the purpose to which the assay
will be applied, there are no marked problems with interfering materials present in
the sample, means are available to link the label to the drug, and the antibody does
not distinguish significantly between the labelled and unlabelled drug (Landon,
1977).

Many different materials have already been used for labelling purposes, in addition to gamma- and beta- emitting isotopes. These include free radicles, enzymes,
the coenzymes NAD and ATP, enzyme inhibitors, viruses, proteins, fluorescent
and chemiluminescent molecules, metals, erythrocytes, latex and other particles.
The first example of an alternative label was for the detection of drugs of abuse
in urine, by using drugs labelled with a free radicle. However, virtually all subse-

quent work related to the non-radioisotopic immunoassay (NIIA) of drugs has centred on the use of enzymes (enzymoimmunoassay, EIA) or fluorescent molecules (fluoroimmunoassay, FIA) as the label. This paper will concern itself only with EIAs and FIAs.

CLASSIFICATION OF NIIA USING LABELLED ANTIGENS

NIIAs requiring separation of the antibody-bound and free fractions

In an RIA it is impossible to distinguish between the radioactivity in the bound and free fractions and therefore a separation step is essential. For example, in one RIA for methotrexate it is necessary to add microlitre amounts of the sample (or standard), ^{125}I-labelled methotrexate and an appropriate dilution of the antiserum, incubate the tubes sufficiently long for equilibrium to be attained, precipitate the bound fraction by the addition of a suitable concentration of sodium sulphate, pour off the supernatant containing the free fraction, count the precipitate (bound fraction) for radioactivity in a gamma-counter, and, finally, construct a standard curve — by plotting the percentage of the labelled methotrexate in the antibody-bound fraction against the amount of drug present — from which the amount of methotrexate in each unknown sample can be read off.

The separation NIIAs (sometimes referred to as heterogeneous assays) are analogous to RIAs as exemplified by an FIA for the antiepileptic drug, phenytoin. The only differences involve the use of a phenytoin analogue labelled with fluorescein isothiocyanate (FITC) instead of a radioactive isotope and end-point detection by means of a fluorimeter in place of a scintillation counter. With FITC-labelled drugs, the excitation wavelength of the fluorimeter is set at approximately 480 nm and the emission wavelength at about 520 nm. In this example (figure 15.1) the fluorescence intensity can be determined either in the supernatant (representing the free fraction, in which case the signal will be related directly to the amount of unlabelled drug present), or in the precipitate after this has been redissolved in sodium hydroxide (representing the antibody-bound fraction, when the signal will be inversely proportional to the amount of unlabelled phenytoin present). As expected, the results obtained for a series of samples determined by both FIA and RIA correlated closely, as did those determined by FIA and a gas-liquid chromatographic procedure (R. S. Kamel *et al.*, unpublished work).

EIA involving the use of a separation step, termed ELISA (enzyme-labelled immunosorbent assays), have also been developed and proved sufficiently sensitive for the assay of a variety of steroids and other hormones. Although suitable for the purpose, they have not been used extensively for the determination of drugs in biological fluids, although a kit for digoxin is now commercially available.

It is important to appreciate that there may be a major advantage in including a separation step in a NIIA and determining the amount of label present in the precipitated fraction. Thus, in addition to separating the antibody-bound and free fractions, such a step enables removal of any endogenous materials present in the sample that might interfere with the signal. For example, bilirubin fluoresces when excited at 480 nm and in an icteric serum sample causes a high background signal which necessitates use of a blank in any FIA based on an FITC-labelled antigen — unless removed during the separation stage. Similarly, in the case of an EIA, the sample may contain an enzyme with activity similar to that being employed as the label or, alternatively, contain an enzyme inhibitor.

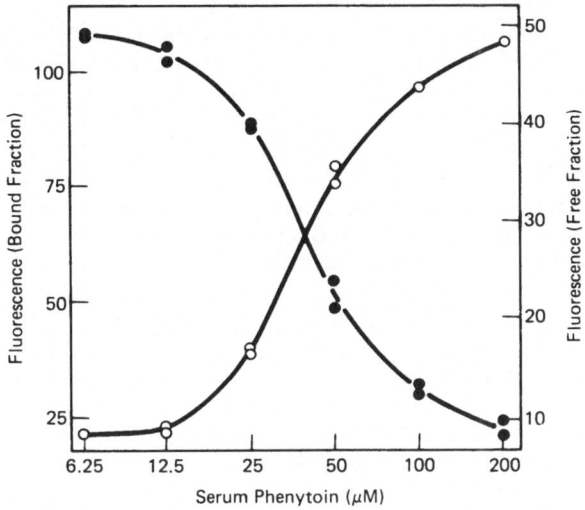

Figure 15.1   NIIA using FITC-labelled phenytoin analogue. ○, Free fraction; ●, bound fraction

NIIAs not requiring a separation step

The development of the first non-separation procedure (sometimes referred to as a homogeneous assay), an EIA for morphine by Rubenstein *et al.* (1972), is an important landmark in the history of immunoassay. Thus avoidance of a separation step simplifies an assay and removes a potential source of imprecision. It will be apparent that, in such NIIAs, there must be a significant difference between the signal given by the free and by the antibody-bound fraction and an appropriate classification can be based on which of the two retain activity (table 15.1).

Table 15.1   Immunoassays with non-isotopically labelled antigens

Involving separation of antibody-bound and free fractions (heterogeneous)	Non-separation immunoassays (homogeneous)	
	Signal from free fraction	Signal from bound fraction
	Quenching assays	Enhancement assays
		Indirect quenching assays
		Polarisation fluorescent assays

Polarisation fluorescent assays are applicable to fluoroimmunoassay only.

Non-separation NIIAs in which the signal is derived from the free fraction
Such assays, which can be regarded as 'direct quenching' procedures, are based on
the signal from the labelled antigen being decreased as a result of antibody binding,
with only the free fraction retaining full activity. Both EIAs and FIAs of this type
have been described. In the first it is assumed that the antibody sterically hinders
the reaction between the enzyme and its substrate, although other explanations
could be advanced, such as a change in the tertiary structure of the active site of
the enzyme being induced by antibody binding of the adjacent molecule. With regard
to FIAs, it is assumed that the presence of antibody interferes either with the excitation or emission of the fluorescent molecules.

Assays of the 'direct quenching' type are suitable for haptens, such as drugs, because their small size ensures that the antigenic determinant will lie in sufficiently
close proximity to the label so that antibody binding influences the signal. The
major contributors in this area have been Syva, who initially developed EIAs for a
variety of drugs of abuse in urine, aimed at detection rather than accurate quantitation. Subsequently they extended their range of assays to include several antiepileptic, cardioactive and other drugs (table 15.2), applied these assays to serum
and introduced various modifications to improve precision.

Table 15.2   Homogeneous enzymoimmunoassays for drugs

Drugs of abuse — urine	Anti-epileptic drugs — serum	Other drugs — serum
Opiates	Phenytoin	Digoxin
Methadone	Carbamazepine	Lidocaine
Propoxyphene	Phenobarbital	Theophylline
Amphetamine	Ethosuximide	
Cocaine	Primidone	
Barbiturates		
Benzodiazepine		

It should be noted that, in general, circulating drug concentrations are high compared with many other serum constituents. Thus, for example, most hormones and
vitamins circulate in the nmol/l or pmol/l range, whereas the majority of drugs lie
in the μmol/l range. This enables the Syva assays to require only a few μl of sample
and, since the time taken for an immunoassay to reach equilibrium is related to the
concentration of the reactants, for results to be available within minutes. An exception is digoxin, with serum concentrations in the low nmol/l range, for which an
incubation period of 30 min is required. Although probably slightly less precise
than RIAs (because, even at the extreme dilutions used, enzymes or enzyme inhibitors present in the serum may affect the result) and requiring a more time-con-
suming and less accurate end-point determination, the non-separation EIAs are
sufficiently precise for clinical and pharmacological purposes. The stability of the
reagents, avoidance of a separation step, ease of automation, suitability for laboratories that do not have radioactivity counting equipment and lack of any health
hazard will all ensure their continued and expanding use.

As a routine we use a 'direct quenching' FIA for gentamicin that has proved most suitable to monitor serum levels and ensure that they lie in the appropriate therapeutic range. This is of especial importance with the aminoglycoside antibiotics, since persistent circulating concentrations only slightly above the therapeutic range may result in nephrotoxicity or ototoxicity. The sample is diluted with FITC-labelled gentamicin and the decrease in fluorescence then determined after addition of an appropriate dilution of antiserum. Obviously, the more unlabelled gentamicin present in the sample or standard, the less FITC–gentamicin will be bound and the greater will be the fluorescence intensity (Shaw *et al.*, 1977). The FIA is much simpler and quicker than the usual microbiological assays and the results correlate closely. The results of the FIA and an RIA for gentamicin also correlate closely and the FIA has the additional advantage that it can be automated using existing standard Auto-Analyzer modules (Shaw *et al.*, 1976).

Non-separation NIIAs in which the signal is derived from the bound fraction
There are a number of non-separation NIIAs in which the labelled antigen in the antibody-bound fraction contributes the main component of the signal. One approach, termed 'indirect quenching' NIIAs, involves addition of a second antibody directed against the label (D. Nargessi, unpublished work). It was developed for the assay of large molecules, such as human albumin, but as it has not been used for haptens it will not be considered in this paper.

Enhancement NIIAs
Non-separation assays of the enhancement type are the exact reverse of direct-quenching assays in that antibody binding is associated with an increased signal. Such an assay has been described for thyroxine (T_4), using a T_4 derivative covalently linked to malate dehydrogenase such that the enzyme has little activity until the addition of anti-T_4 serum (Ullman *et al.*, 1975). An enhancement effect has also been noted when FITC-labelled T_4 is bound by a specific antibody — probably because the iodine atoms in the T_4 molecule quench the fluorescent signal until prevented from doing so by the presence of antibody (Smith, 1977). Although NIIAs of the enhancement type would seem feasible for drugs, we are unaware of their use in this context.

Polarisation fluorescence
The final type of non-separation assay to be discussed, termed polarisation fluorescence, is applicable only to FIAs. The technique requires the use of a polarisation fluorimeter, an instrument designed to excite the sample and to determine the emission from the sample in a specified plane. Polarisation fluorescence is based on the markedly enhanced signal that results when a hapten labelled with a fluorophor is bound by antibody, and has been applied to the assay of gentamicin in serum (Watson *et al.*, 1976). This approach has also been used to study the kinetics of the gentamicin FIAs and has shown that equilibrium is attained within 1 min. The assay is very simple to perform and would provide an excellent means of quantitating serum levels of many drugs. However, the widespread application of such assays must await the ready availability of the appropriate equipment which, at present, is expensive compared with standard fluorimeters.

CONCLUSION

NIIA for the detection and quantitation of a wide variety of drugs in biological fluids are being developed in several centres. Most success has been achieved with the introduction of non-separation EIAs of the 'direct quenching' type and these will probably continue to dominate this area for several years. Nonetheless, the relative imprecision and complexity of determining enzyme activity together with possible interference of the measurement by enzymes or enzyme inhibitors in the sample suggest that, in the future, improved NIIAs may be introduced based on other labels.

REFERENCES

Landon, J. (1977). *Nature*, **268**, 483
Landon, J. and Moffat, A. C. (1976). *The Analyst*, **101**, 1201, 225
Rubenstein, K. E., Schneider, R. S. and Ullman, E. F. (1972). *Biochem. Biophys. Res. Commun.*, **47**, 846
Shaw, E. J., Watson, R. A. A. and Smith, D. S. (1976). *Second International Symposium on Rapid Methods and Automation in Microbiology* (eds., H. H. Johnston and S. W. B. Newsom), Learned Information, (Oxford), p. 78
Shaw, E. J., Watson, R. A. A. and Landon, J. (1977). *J. clin. Path.*, **30**, 526
Smith, D. S. (1977). *FEBS Lett.*, **77**, 25
Smith, T. W., Buttler, V. P., Jr. and Haber, E. (1969). *New Engl. J. Med.*, **281**, 1212
Ullman, E. F., Blekemere, J., Leute, R. K., Eimsted, W. and Jaklitsch, A. (1975). *Clin. Chem.*, **21**, 1011
Watson, R. A. A., Landon, J., Shaw, E. J. and Smith, D. S. (1976). *Clin. Chim. Acta*, **73**, 51

16

New approaches to linkage of haptens for radioimmunoassay

J. E. T. Corrie (MRC Radioimmunoassay Team, 2 Forrest Road,
Edinburgh EH1 2QW, U.K.)

Although much of the basic understanding remains unclear, the practical metho-
dology of raising antibodies to small, intrinsically non-immunogenic molecules
(haptens) is now well established and is the subject of recent reviews (Kohen *et al.*,
1975; Kellie *et al.*, 1975 ; Parker, 1976). In particular, it is generally accepted that
the best results are obtained when the hapten is covalently linked to an immunogenic carrier protein and the nature and strategy of the linking process is the subject of this paper.

Desirable properties of the hapten—protein linkage include ease of introduction
and non-masking of immunoreactive sites in the hapten. The former is largely a
practical consideration for the preparation of the immunogen, and the latter may
vitally affect the utility of the eventual antiserum. The operation of these factors
may be considered in relation to some of the existing methods for hapten conjugation. Probably the most commonly used approach, at least in the raising of antisera for radioimmunoassay, is based on the method of Erlanger (Erlanger *et al.*,
1957, 1959) in which a carboxylic acid group, either pre-existing in the hapten or
chemically introduced, is used to form a peptide bond with the terminal amino
groups of lysine residues in the protein.

$$\text{Hapten—COOH} + \text{NH}_2\text{—Lys-protein} \longrightarrow \text{Hapten—CO-NH-Lys-protein}$$

Examples of inherent carboxyl groups used for this purpose, as shown in figure
16.1, are found in bile acids (Simmonds *et al.*, 1973), steroid glucuronides (Kellie
et al., 1972) and prostaglandins (PG) (Jaffe *et al.*, 1973). Figure 16.2 shows some of
the wide variety of means used to introduce carboxyl groups into molecules that
could not otherwise be conjugated by this method, carboxymethyloxime (CMO)
(Exley *et al.*, 1971), thioalkanoate (Rao and Moore, 1976), hemisuccinate (Steiner
et al., 1969), alkanamate (Robinson *et al.*, 1975) and carboxymethyl (Spector and
Parker, 1970).

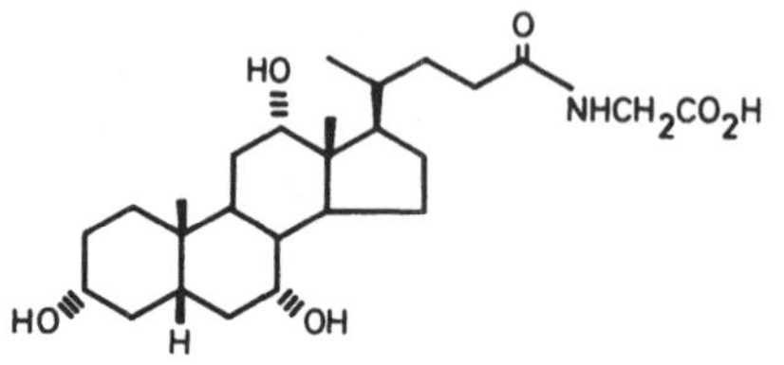

Glycocholic acid (1)

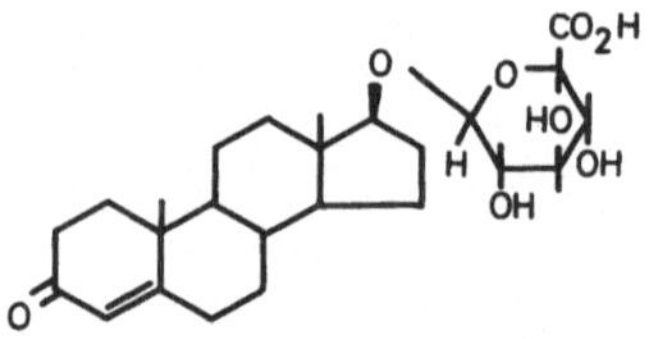

Testosterone - 17β-glucuronoside (2)

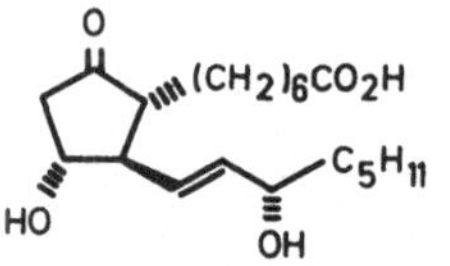

PGE₁ (3)

Figure 16.1   Haptens with an inherent carboxylic acid function.

In all these examples, activation of the carboxyl group for coupling to the protein can be readily achieved by standard methods, usually by an alkyl chloroformate in the Erlanger procedure or with a soluble carbodi-imide (Bauminger *et al.*, 1969), to afford conjugates in which the hapten remains chemically unaltered and with its unique point of attachment clearly defined. The latter consideration is very important, since many studies have shown that antibodies best recognise in the free hapten structural characteristics distal to the point of conjugation and are often insensitive to changes near that site. This may be either useful (see below) or deleterious, as for example when antibodies raised against a conjugate of 3-carboxymethylmorphine react more extensively with codeine than with morphine itself (Spector and Parker, 1970). Similar effects were observed when antisera to steroid hormones were first raised, since the tendency was to use one of the existing functional groups for conjugation, with the frequent result of serious reactivity for similar molecules. More recent preparations have used carefully chosen sites which allow for a fuller expression of structural characteristics (see for example Kohen *et al.*, 1975).

A case in which the poor recognition of changes near the conjugation site has been exploited is contained in a report (Grota and Brown, 1976) on metanephrine-binding antibodies which were raised by immunisation with a conjugate produced from incubation of bovine serum albumin and synephrine (compound 12) with formaldehyde. The structure of this conjugate, shown in figure 16.3, is sufficiently similar to that of metanephrine, a major adrenalin metabolite, to permit the development of a radioimmunoassay for metanephrine in urine (Lam *et al.*, 1977), but only because synephrine itself is absent from the material being analysed.

In the examples discussed, the chemistry of the conjugation reactions has led unambiguously to a uniquely defined point of attachment from each hapten to its carrier protein. However, cases exist in which the structure of the immunogen is less clearly specified, with serious consequences for the specificity of the derived antiserum. One such case reviewed by Parker (1976) concerns the conjugation of the octapeptide angiotensin II to protein. Angiotensin II, which differs from angiotensin I by two *C*-terminal amino acids, contains free *N*- and *C*-termini. Carbodi-imide-mediated conjugation therefore results not only in coupling of the *C*-

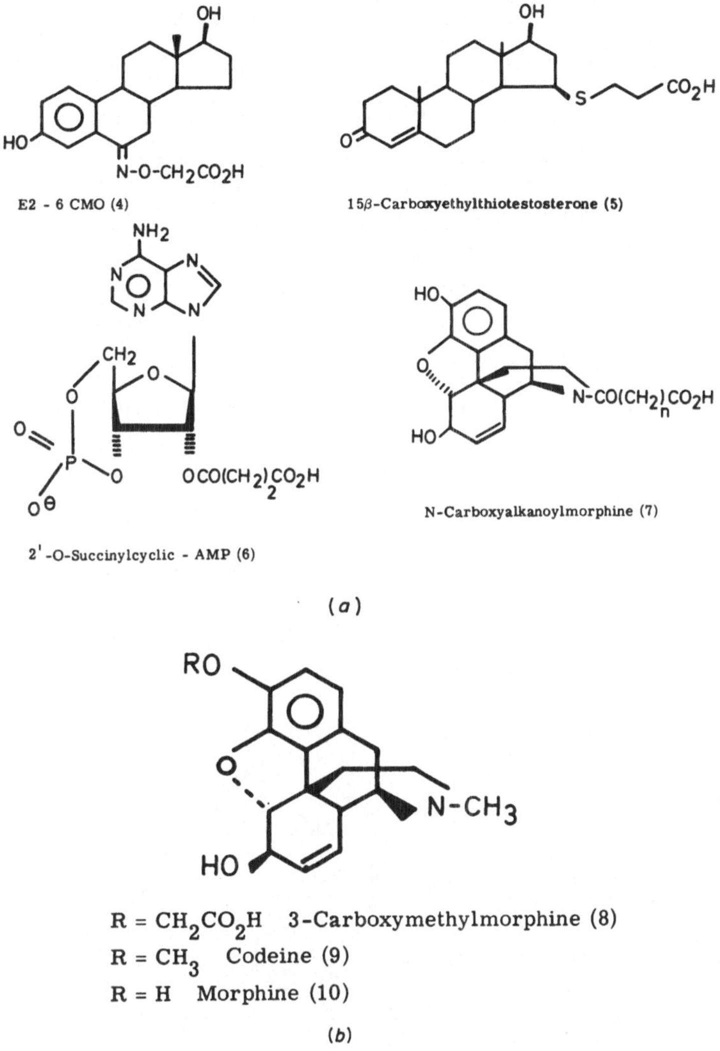

OH

HO

N-O-CH₂CO₂H

E2 - 6 CMO (4)

OH

S—CO₂H

15β-Carboxyethylthiotestosterone (5)

NH₂

N
N
N
N

CH₂

O

O

P
O
O⊖

OCO(CH₂)₂CO₂H

2'-O-Succinylcyclic - AMP (6)

HO

O

HO

N-CO(CH₂)ₙCO₂H

N-Carboxyalkanoylmorphine (7)

(*a*)

RO

O

N-CH₃

HO

R = CH₂CO₂H   3-Carboxymethylmorphine (8)
R = CH₃   Codeine (9)
R = H   Morphine (10)

(*b*)

Figure 16.2 Haptens with an introduced carboxylic acid function.

terminus to protein lysines but also in 'reversed' coupling, i.e. of the *N*-terminus to protein glutamate and aspartate (figure 16.4). The antiserum obtained from such conjugates reacts with approximately equal efficacy with angiotensins I and II. The problem can be circumvented by the use of a reagent specific for the *N*-terminus, namely toluene diisocyanate which reacts as shown in figure 16.4 to give only *N*-terminal-coupled angiotensin II.

Numerous other conjugation techniques are discussed in the review literature and need no further elaboration here. The examples and problems already men-

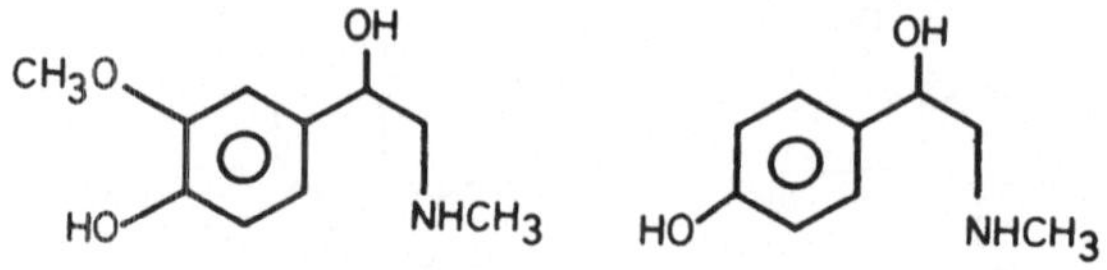

Metanephrine (11)

Synephrine (12)

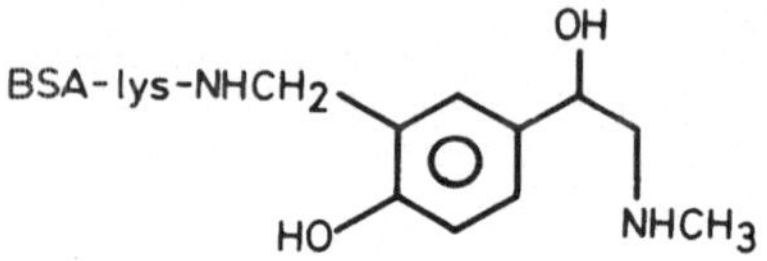

(13)

Synephrine - formaldehyde - BSA conjugate

Figure 16.3   Structures related to the production of the metanephrine-binding antibodies.

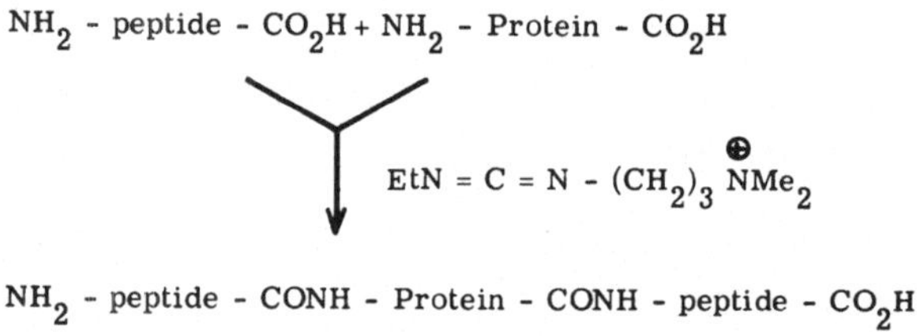

NH_2 - peptide - CO_2H + NH_2 - Protein - CO_2H

$EtN = C = N - (CH_2)_3 \overset{\oplus}{N}Me_2$

NH_2 - peptide - CONH - Protein - CONH - peptide - CO_2H

(*a*)

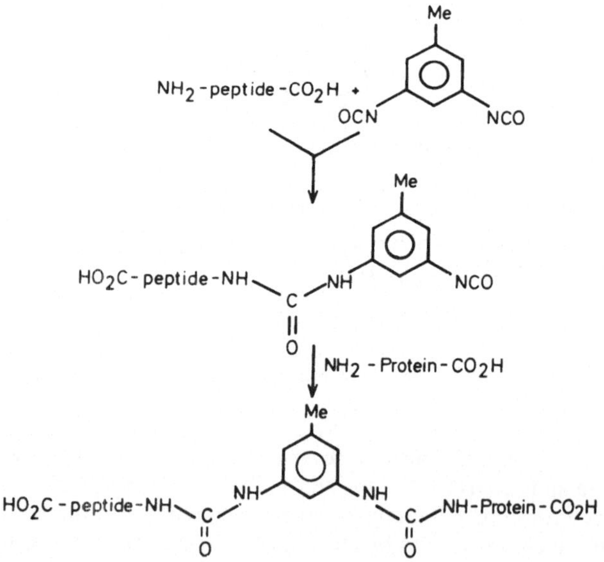

NH_2-peptide-CO_2H +

HO_2C- peptide -NH — C — NH — NCO

NH_2 - Protein-CO_2H

HO_2C - peptide-NH — C — NH — NH — C — NH-Protein-CO_2H

(*b*)

Figure 16.4   Random and controlled coupling of a peptide hapten.

tioned provide the background to our design of a novel conjugation method, which we believe will prove to be valuable in certain circumstances, notably those in which the hapten contains a primary or secondary amine function. Such a situation, which will serve purely as a paper exercise for discussion, would obtain if it were desired to raise an antiserum to desipramine (compound 14), a major metabolite of the tricyclic antidepressant imipramine (compound 15) (Osol and Pratt, 1973). Desipramine is further metabolised to *N*-hydroxydesipramine (16) (Beckett and Al-Sarraj, 1973) and there therefore exists a family of rather similar substances which differ only by a single substituent at precisely the site from which it would be easiest to construct a linkage (carboxymethyl or succinamate) for conjugation (figure 16.5).

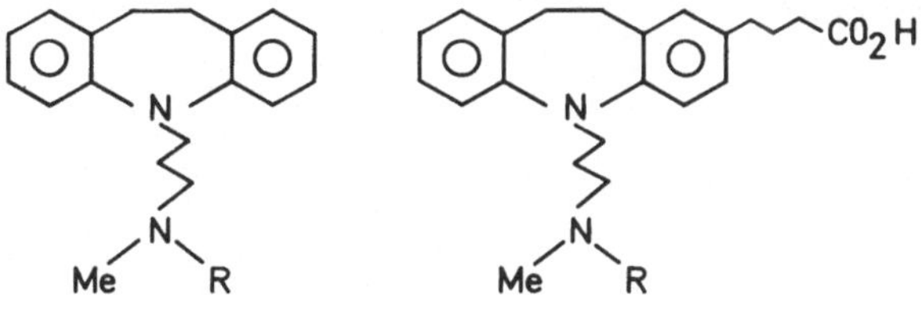

R = H   Desipramine (14)   R = H (17)
R = Me   Imipramine (15)   R = CO$_2$iBu (18)
R = OH   N-Hydroxydesipramine (16)

Figure 16.5 Tricyclic antidepressants and related compounds

It is clear that antisera raised to such a conjugate would be most unlikely to distinguish well between the three compounds. The answer generally applied to this problem would be to insert a carboxylic acid function elsewhere in the molecule to give a compound such as (17), but since compound (17) is an amino acid, attempts to activate the carboxylic acid group before protein coupling will result either in polymerisation of the hapten or in initial irreversible acylation of the nitrogen atom to yield compound (18). In the presence of excess of isobutyl chloroformate, the carboxyl group of compound (18) would be activated and could be coupled to protein, but the conjugate would still carry the unwanted substituent on the amino group and would be as unsatisfactory as a conjugate prepared by simple linkage through the amine function. Conjugation of compound (17) using a carbodi-imide would effect coupling through the carboxyl and amino groups, as previously shown for angiotensin, and would be similarly unsatisfactory.

Our solution to this dilemma derives from methods well known in protein chemistry for the modification of cysteine thiol groups (Means and Feeney, 1971). *N*-Ethylmaleimide reacts rapidly and very selectively with thiols below pH 7. It can also react with amines at higher pH, but at pH 7 the relative rates of reaction with thiols and amines differ by approximately three orders of magnitude. We reasoned that by incorporating maleimido groups into a carrier protein and a thiol group into the hapten (figure 16.6), it would be possible to achieve a clean, mild and selective conjugation procedure that would restore to the coupling of compounds such as desipramine the highly desirable property of a uniquely defined point of attachment. The execution of this scheme is shown in figure 16.7.

Bovine serum albumin (BSA) contains a single free thiol group and to avoid any problems of cross-linkage, this was first modified by exposure to *N*-ethylmaleimide. 'Reversed' maleimido groups were then incorporated by a standard Erlanger coup-

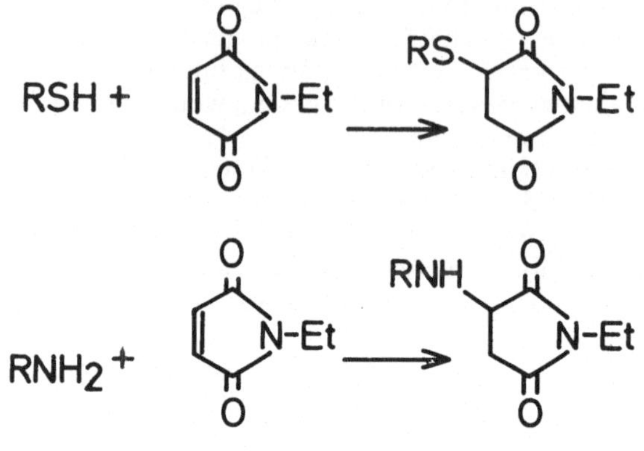

Figure 16.6 The reaction of thiols and amines with *N*-ethylmaleimide.

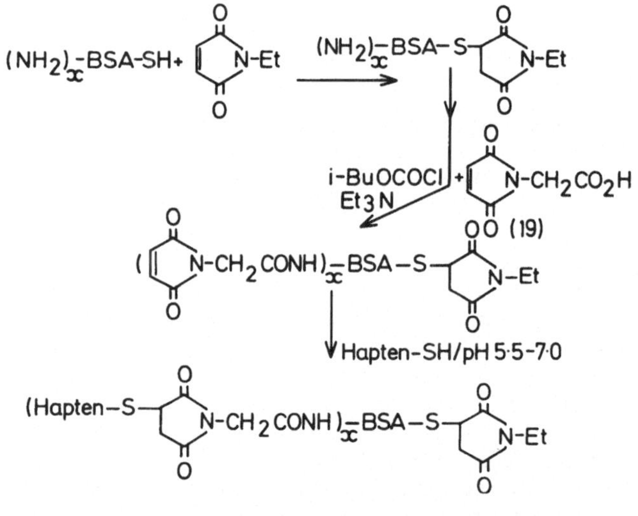

Figure 16.7 Scheme for the coupling to protein of a thiol-bearing hapten.

ling between maleoylglycine (19) (Rich *et al.*, 1975) and the modified BSA. After purification of the doubly modified protein by gel filtration, it was treated with radioactive cysteine, which we have used as a convenient model thiol, and residual free cysteine was separated by gel filtration. The effect of pH on the number of cysteine residues incorporated per molecule of protein is shown in table 16.1. Although the coupling reaction was usually allowed to proceed for 30 min, a four-fold decrease in reaction time left the incorporated cysteine/protein ratio virtually unaltered. Maleimido groups are susceptible to alkaline hydrolysis and it is likely that some are lost during the conjugation of maleoylglycine to the protein. However, those which survive this process appear to be relatively stable when the modified protein is stored at 4°C in pH 5.5. buffer. After 42 h under these conditions,

Table 16.1   Effect of pH on the number of cysteine residues incorporated per molecule of modified bovine serum albumin

pH	Cysteine : BSA
7.0	23.0
6.5	21.5
6.0	20.0
5.5	19.5

the loss of cysteine-binding capacity was less than 5 per cent. Alternatively the modified protein can be freeze-dried and stored for at least several weeks without change. It is therefore possible to treat the substituted protein as a 'stock' reagent which can be mixed with the hapten in an appropriate buffer solution when it is desired to prepare a hapten conjugate. Hence the actual conjugation procedure is extremely mild and this may be of some value when dealing with chemically sensitive haptens. The admitted drawback of the method lies in the construction of the thiol-bearing hapten. It is probable that this stage will always involve rather more chemical manipulation than has been required with previous procedures. Nevertheless, we believe that there are areas where such investment is worthwhile and we are continuing to work in this field.

In conclusion, we append two cautionary tales. First, it might be thought that another well-known protein/thiol reagent, iodoacetate (Means and Feeney, 1971) could be used in an analogous fashion. Our attempts to produce an iodoacetylated protein were uniformly unsuccessful, in that no cysteine-binding capacity could be observed. Presumably iodoacetate is too labile to survive the Erlanger conjugation. Secondly, our first attempts to incorporate a thiol into the maleoylated protein using 6-mercaptopurine, which has a readily observable chromophore that we hoped to use for quantitation purposes, were unsuccessful. Again, no hapten incorporation was observed, no doubt because of the reduced nucleophilicity of the sulphur when attached to the heterocyclic ring. Thus it is only electronically unperturbed thiols that are suitable for use in this procedure.

ACKNOWLEDGEMENT

We thank Miss J. S. Macpherson for skilled technical assistance.

REFERENCES

Bauminger, S., Lindner, H. R., Perel, E. and Arnon, R. J. (1969). *J. Endocr.*, **44**, 567
Beckett, A. H. and Al-Sarraj, S. (1973). *J. Pharm. Pharmac.*, **25**, 335
Erlanger, B. F., Borek, F., Beiser, S. M. and Lieberman, S. (1957). *J. biol. Chem.*, **228**, 713
Erlanger, B. F., Borek, F., Beiser, S. M. and Lieberman, S. (1959). *J. biol. Chem.*, **234**, 1090
Exley, D., Johnson, M. W. and Dean, P. D. G. (1971). *Steroids*, **18**, 605
Grota, L. J. and Brown, G. M. (1976). *Endocrinology*, **98**, 615
Jaffe, B. M., Behrman, H. R. and Parker, C. W. (1973). *J. clin. Invest.*, **52**, 398
Kellie, A. E., Samuel, V. K., Riley, W. J. and Robertson, D. M. (1972). *J. Steroid Biochem.*, **3**, 275

Kellie, A. E., Lichman, K. V. and Samarajeewa, P. (1975). In *Steroid Immunoassay*, (eds. E. H. D. Cameron, S. G. Hillier and K. Griffiths), Proceedings of the Fifth Tenovus Workshop, Cardiff, April 1974, Alpha Omega Publishing Ltd., Cardiff

Kohen, F., Bauminger, S. and Lindner, H. R. (1975). In *Steroid Immunoassay*, (eds. E. H. D. Cameron, S. G. Hillier and K. Griffitsh), Proceedings of the Fifth Tenovus Workshop, Cardiff, April 1974, Alpha Omega Publishing Ltd., Cardiff

Lam, R. W., Artal, R. and Fischer, D. A. (1977). *Clin. Chem.*, **23**, 1264

Means, G. E. and Feeney, R. E. (1971). *Chemical Modification of Proteins*, Holden-Day, San Francisco, p. 110

Osol, A. and Pratt, R. (1973). *The United States Dispensatory*, J. B. Lippincott Co., Philadelphia, p. 611

Parker, C. W. (1976). *Radioimmunoassay of Biologically Active Compounds*, Prentice-Hall, Englewood Cliffs

Rao, P. N. and Moore, P. H. (1976). *Steroids*, **28**, 101

Rich, D. H., Gesellchen, P. D., Tong, A., Cheung, A. and Buckner, C. K. (1975). *J. med. Chem.*, **18**, 1004

Robinson, J. D., Morris, B. A., Piall, E. M., Aherne, G. W. and Marks, V. (1975). In *Radioimmunoassay in Clinical Biochemistry*, (ed. C. A. Pasternak), Heyden, London, p. 113

Simmonds, W. J., Korman, M. G., Go, V. L. W. and Hofmann, A. K. (1973). *Gastroenterology*, **65**, 705

Spector, S. and Parker, C. W. (1970) *Science*, **168**, 1347

Steiner, A. L., Kipnis, D. M., Utiger, R. and Parker, C. W. (1969). *Proc. natn. Acad. Sci. U.S.A.*, **64**, 367

Index